Cancer and Cardiovascular Disease

Syed Wamique Yusuf • Jose Banchs
Editors

Cancer and Cardiovascular Disease

A Concise Clinical Atlas

Springer

Editors
Syed Wamique Yusuf
Department of Cardiology
University of Texas MD Anderson Cancer Center
Houston, Texas
USA

Jose Banchs
Department of Cardiology
University of Texas MD Anderson Cancer Center
Houston, Texas
USA

ISBN 978-3-030-09669-4 ISBN 978-3-319-62088-6 (eBook)
https://doi.org/10.1007/978-3-319-62088-6

Printed on acid-free paper

This Springer imprint is published by the registered company Springer International Publishing AG, part of Springer Nature.
The registered company address is: Gewerbestrasse 11, 6330 Cham, Switzerland

Foreword

Cardiovascular disease and cancer are the most common causes of death worldwide. They often have the same risk factors, e.g., smoking and advancing age. This tight relationship has led to the emergence of a multidisciplinary approach to patients with cancer and heart disease (termed cardio-oncology or onco-cardiology).

With increasing numbers of cancer survivors, it is not uncommon for a practicing physician to encounter a patient who has a concomitant diagnosis of both cancer and cardiovascular disease. In some patients, particularly those in older age groups, established cardiovascular disease predates the development of cancer, whereas in others, particularly Hodgkin's lymphoma and breast cancer patients, survivors develop cardiovascular disease as a result of cancer therapy (e.g., the late cardiovascular sequelae of radiation therapy or chemotherapy-induced cardiomyopathy). Most cardiovascular trials have excluded patients with cancer, and similarly most trials of cancer therapy have excluded patients with cardiovascular disease. Hence, there is little evidence-based treatment guidance for these patients.

In this atlas, the editors have compiled chapters that are related to the diagnosis and treatment of common cardiovascular diseases encountered in patients with cancer. The case-based illustrations nicely depict many of the clinical and therapeutic challenges encountered in the management of these patients. The atlas covers a wide range of topics, ranging from chemotherapy-related cardiac dysfunction to radiation-induced heart disease and cardiac tumors.

The readers will find the atlas useful for clinical practice, and it will also serve as a resource for all health care professionals caring for patients with cancer and cardiovascular disease.

Kim A. Eagle, M.D., M.A.C.C.
Albion Walter Hewlett Professor of Medicine
Director Frankel Cardiovascular Center
University of Michigan Health System
Ann Arbor, MI, USA

Patrick T. O'Gara, M.D., M.A.C.C.
Professor of Medicine, Harvard Medical School
Watkins Family Distinguished Chair in Cardiology
Brigham and Women's Hospital
Boston, MA, USA

Preface

"Variability is the law of life and as no two faces are the same, so no two bodies are alike and no two individuals react alike and behave alike under the abnormal conditions which we know as disease." Sir William Osler

Advancement in cancer detection and therapy has led to an increasing number of cancer survivors that currently exceeds 15 million in the USA. With an improvement in survival, from both cancer and cardiovascular disease, it is not uncommon for these two conditions to coexist. Cardiovascular disease sometimes precedes the diagnosis of cancer, and in other cases, cancer therapy can cause or accelerate preexisting cardiovascular diseases.

Both chemotherapy and radiation cause long-term cardiovascular side effects. Chemotherapy agents can cause a wide range of cardiotoxicity, ranging from vascular disease to cardiomyopathy, whereas radiation toxicity can cause vascular, pericardial, valvular, conduction system, and myocardial disease.

The diagnosis and management of cardiovascular disease in patients with malignancy poses complex clinical challenges. Concurrent anemia, comorbidities, fatigue, and side effects of chemotherapy frequently mask the typical symptoms of cardiovascular disease. The presence of thrombocytopenia and the risk of bleeding are a particular concern in patients who need antiplatelet agents and/or anticoagulants, e.g., those with coronary stent, atrial fibrillation, and prosthetic valve. Due to lack of well-designed large clinical trials, there is limited data available on the treatment of cardiovascular diseases in patients with cancer. With this atlas, we hope to provide a clear, case-based approach to the common clinical problems faced by the practicing clinicians.

The authors of the chapters have extensive clinical and research background in their respective fields. We are greatly indebted to them for providing us with superb clinical cases and their valuable time.

We hope that the readers will find this atlas useful for their day-to-day practice.

Houston, TX, USA — Syed Wamique Yusuf
Houston, TX, USA — Jose Banchs

Acknowledgements

To my parents, siblings, wife and daughters for their love and endless support in life. To my friends for providing unconditional help. To my teachers: Mr. Alvi, for his guidance and encouragement; Dr. Roger L. Blandford, for inspiring me to be a clinical cardiologist; Dr. J.T. Willerson, Dr. V. Lavis, Dr. F. Fuentes, Dr. H.V. Anderson, Dr. K. Lance Gould, Dr. S. Sdringola, and Late Dr. S. Ward Casscells for clinical training; Late Dr. R.M. Mishra for providing me with an opportunity to pursue clinical research; and Dr. Syed Zaki Hussain for his constant support. I would also like to thank Dr. Patrick T. O'Gara and Dr. Kim A. Eagle for their guidance and mentoring, Ms. Lauren Sutton for her secretarial support, Dr. Rizwan Karatela for providing us with the cover image, and our publisher Springer, especially Mr. Grant Weston and Mr. Andre Tournois, for their help and guidance.

Above all, this book is dedicated to our patients, without whom none of this would have been possible.

Syed Wamique Yusuf

I would like to thank my family, for their time and support.

My mentor Dr. Julio Perez, for his patience, teaching, and dedication.

I thank everyone who crossed path with me as a patient, for the privilege of sharing something so special.

Jose Banchs

Contents

Global Burden of Cancer and Cardiovascular Disease

1

Gagan Sahni and Jagat Narula

Abstract

Cancer and Cardiovascular disease [CVD] are an unholy matrimony, being inexorably linked to each other and fostering a substantial global health burden of our time.

Keywords

Cancer • Cardiovascular disease • Global burden

Cancer and Cardiovascular disease [CVD] are an unholy matrimony, being inexorably linked to each other and fostering a substantial global health burden of our time.

In 2013 there were >54 million deaths globally, of which 17 million or 32% of deaths were attributable to Cardiovascular disease [CVD] and eight million or 15% were due to cancer deaths [1]. Cancer has moved from the third leading cause of death in the industrialized world in 1990 to the second leading cause behind cardiovascular disease in 2013, owing largely due to a growing and aging global population as well as risk factors like smoking, obesity, and dietary patterns. Not surprisingly, these are common risk factors for cardiovascular disease as well, making the combined burden of disease due to CVD and cancer not only a prodigious global problem but one necessitating a mutually inclusive approach to prevention, detection and treatment.

Moreover, since the advent of more effective cancer treatments and the increasing likelihood of an earlier cancer diagnosis due to screening, the overall cancer mortality has declined since the early 2000s [2]. Of these cancer survivors, 69% will have at least a 5-year life expectancy. This implies that cancer survivors now live longer, allowing the subsequent manifestation of potential cardiac toxicities of cancer treatments [including chemotherapy and radiation], as well as an increase in the incidence of cardiovascular disease due to common risk factors such as age, lifestyle and smoking. In fact, amongst cancer survivors, > 50% of men and >40% of women above the age of 50 years will develop some cardiovascular disease during their remaining lifespan [3].

Adding to this demographic are the survivors of childhood cancers. With today's cancer therapeutics, >80% of children and adolescents who are treated for cancer become long-term survivors into adulthood in countries such as the US and UK. These numbers, of course are as dismal as 10% survivorship in developing nations. However, survivorship of these patients into adulthood poses the new challenge of early cardiovascular disease due to their childhood exposure to cardiotoxic chemo such as anthracyclines and chest directed radiation therapy. As per the Childhood Cancer Survivor Study (CCSS) cohort, the cardiac mortality in these childhood cancer survivors was sevenfold higher and a 15-fold lifetime risk of developing heart failure (HF) compared to age-matched population [4].

Other than the extended survival of cancer patients and the aging population, there has been an increase in the recognition of chemotherapy-induced cardiotoxicity, adding to the linkage between patients with cancer and their risk for cardiovascular diseases. In addition, some patients with cancer may be at a higher risk for cardiovascular complications as compared with the general population. For example, protein kinases are the most frequently mutated genes in the cancer genome, which makes them an attractive therapeutic target for chemotherapy drugs. However the use of several kinase inhibitors [KI's] have been associated with toxicities to the heart and vasculature, including acute coronary syndromes and heart failure. Ongoing genomic studies are thereby focusing on mutations in these protein kinases that

G. Sahni, M.B.B.S. • J. Narula, M.D., D.M., Ph.D., M.A.C.C., F.R.C.P. (✉)
Icahn School of Medicine, Mount Sinai Medical Center, New York, NY, USA
e-mail: jagat.narula@mountsinai.org

S.W. Yusuf, J. Banchs (eds.), *Cancer and Cardiovascular Disease*, https://doi.org/10.1007/978-3-319-62088-6_1

not only lead to tumorigenesis but also study the underlying mechanisms that drive the cardiotoxicity of these KI's [5].

Indeed, the increased use of combination chemotherapy, overall increased survival, concomitant radiation therapy and development of emerging agents with potential cardiotoxicity have led to the emergence of cancer therapeutics induced cardiotoxicity as a growing public health issue. This cardiotoxicity includes a spectrum of effects such as heart failure, angina, acute coronary syndromes, arrhythmias, hypertension, hypotension, valvulopathies and pericardial diseases. Moreover, cancer is associated with a hypercoagulable state, which increases the risk of acute thrombotic events; thus, the need for invasive evaluation and management in the cardiac catheterization laboratory rises. Unique issues can present, such as the timing of invasive cardiac interventions in relation to oncologic treatments, managing a wide range of comorbid diseases including thrombocytopenia and bleeding diathesis, paraneoplastic disease, difficulties with vascular access, coagulopathies, and a lack of prior outcome-driven data for interventions in this patient population. These challenges posed by CVD in patients with cancer often need a multi-disciplinary approach, tailor-made to each patient's risk-benefit profile as discussed amongst the cardiologist, oncologist, radiation oncologist and oncological surgeons.

Recognizing and responding to this emerging global health burden, cardiologists dedicated to the care of oncology patients with cancer therapeutics-induced cardiotoxicity and concomitant cardiovascular problems, are an emerging subspecialty called "Cardio-Oncology" or "Onco-Cardiology." Many cancer centers and tertiary care hospitals globally are now establishing dedicated Cardio-Oncology clinics where cardiovascular specialists play a dedicated role in managing heart disease in cancer patients [6]. This "super-specialization" of cardiovascular care provides efficient and timely access to cardiology services, including pre-chemotherapy cardiac risk assessment, interventions for minimizing risk, assessment of the cardiac effects of cardiotoxic chemotherapies, use of emerging imaging techniques such as strain rate measurements in echocardiography to detect early cardiotoxicity, and early treatment of heart disease should it develop. It is a multi-disciplinary platform where cardiovascular interventions are balanced with cancer therapeutics to provide the patient with the best possible oncological and cardiovascular outcomes.

References

1. GBD 2013 Mortality and Causes of Death Collaborators Global, regional, and national age-sex specific all-cause and cause-specific mortality for 240 causes of death, 1990–2013: a systematic analysis for the Global Burden of Disease Study 2013. Lancet. 2015;385(9963):117–71.
2. Cancer trends progress report. National Cancer Institute, NIH, DHHS, Bethesda, MD, January 2017. http://progressreport.cancer.gov.
3. Lloyd-Jones DM, Leip EP, Larson MG, et al. Prediction of lifetime risk for cardiovascular disease by risk factor burden at 50 years of age. Circulation. 2006;113:791–8.
4. Armstrong G, Ross J. Late Cardiotoxicity in Aging Adult Survivors of Childhood Cancer. Prog Pediatr Cardiol. 2014;36(1–2):19–26.
5. Lal H, Kolaja KL, Force T. Cancer genetics and the cardiotoxicity of the therapeutics. J Am Coll Cardiol. 2013;61:267–74.
6. Okwuosa TM, Barac A. Burgeoning Cardio-Oncology Programs challenges and opportunities for early career Cardiologists/Faculty Directors. J Am Coll Cardiol. 2015;66:1193–7.

Utility of Cardiac Ultrasound Imaging in Oncology, a Case Based Illustration

2

Jose A. Banchs

Abstract

Cardiac Ultrasound imaging (Echocardiogram) is an integral modality for the investigation of patients undergoing chemotherapy. In this chapter we briefly discuss the evolution and provide case based illustrations to exemplify the use of this modality.

Keywords

Echocardiogram • Chemotherapy • Cardiotoxicity

Several chemotherapy agents, but in particular Adriamycin, are known to cause cardiomyopathy [1, 2]. Ever since the first reports of possible cardio-toxic effects from anti-cancer agents, there has been well documented steady progress in efforts to detect and characterize this pathology in clinical practice as soon as technologically possible in the course of chemotherapy.

The earliest methods to detect cardiotoxicity utilized a combination of ECG and chest X-ray films in conjunction to phonocardiography and carotid pulse tracing with serial photography, to describe a ratio of the pre-ejection period to left ventricular ejection time [3]. Shortly afterward, a non-invasive method using a sphygmo-recording of the pulse wave delay [4]; and ultrasound imaging quickly followed in a report from the pediatric population [5]. Once cardiac imaging was established in the late 1970s and early 1980s; a number of publications supported the different available modalities [5–9], establishing left ventricular ejection fraction (LVEF) as the traditional method for initial and follow-up evaluation of ventricular function during the administration of cardio-toxic chemotherapeutic agents.

Over a short period of time, measurement of LVEF by nuclear methods (MUGA) became an established practice and was considered the gold standard for LV function assessment during chemotherapy. LVEF by radionuclide imaging proved to be sensitive, specific, and reproducible and in at least one early report when used with stress was a predictor of early cardiac toxicity [6]. LVEF, reported as a single measure, was clearly the real strength of this imaging technique.

Improvement in imaging quality, particularly in the last two decades has been noticeable in two-dimensional echocardiography. The use of second harmonic imaging [10] as well as the use of echocardiographic contrast [11] has significantly increased the accuracy of LVEF measurement with Two-dimensional echocardiography. Newer ultrasound systems are now able to achieve superior temporal and spatial resolution.

With time, 3D echocardiography has been recognized as another method for LVEF measurement that compares more favorably with the current gold standard; i.e. cardiac MRI [12] and conventional MUGA scans [13]. But measurement of LVEF as a sole indicator of cardiotoxicity has many limitations. Accurate assessment of LVEF is not only limited by image quality, or the technicality of the measurement (single beat, operator experience, volume drawing style or rules), but the ejection fraction is merely the relative volume ejected in systole, and it can be load dependent. In a variety of conditions affecting the heart, such as diabetes, coronary artery disease, amyloid infiltration, and hypertension, the LVEF measure may be well preserved until late in the course of the disease. In the case of chemotherapy-related cardiac dysfunction it has become increasingly clear that LVEF is an imperfect tool. It is only documenting that a process has indeed already changed, and maybe perhaps permanently [14, 15].

New methods for reliable non-invasive evaluation of cardiac function such as speckle tracking echocardiography

J.A. Banchs, M.D., F.A.C.C., F.A.S.E.
Department of Cardiology, University of Texas MD Anderson Cancer Center, Houston, TX, USA
e-mail: jbanchs@mdanderson.org

S.W. Yusuf, J. Banchs (eds.), *Cancer and Cardiovascular Disease*, https://doi.org/10.1007/978-3-319-62088-6_2

(STE) are now available. Speckle tracking takes full advantage of a new capacity for image acquisition at higher frame rates. This new avenue for evaluation of myocardial function has helped immensely in the understanding and the evaluation of some of these disorders just mentioned [16]. Several reports now have been published in the cancer population receiving cardio-toxic agents and the use of this particular technology in the realm of cancer therapeutics–related cardiac dysfunction (CTRCD) has been very exciting, particularly the use of longitudinal deformation measures and the global longitudinal strain value (GLS). It was first reported in 2009 that changes in tissue deformation, assessed by myocardial strain and strain rate was able to identify LV dysfunction earlier than LVEF in women undergoing treatment with trastuzumab for breast cancer [17]. Following this, two reports in 2011 have resulted in comparable findings [18, 19].

In a multi-center study, utilizing troponin and longitudinal strain measures to predict the development of cardiotoxicity (defined as a reduction of LVEF of ≥5 to <55% with symptoms of heart failure or an asymptomatic reduction of the LVEF of ≥10 to <55% in patients treated with anthracyclines and trastuzumab) it was found that patients who demonstrated decreases in longitudinal strain measures or elevations in hypersensitive troponin had a ninefold increase in risk for cardiotoxicity at 6 months compared to those with no changes in either of these markers [19]. Furthermore; LVEF alone, diastolic function parameters, and N-terminal pro–B-type natriuretic peptide did not help predict cardiotoxicity [19].

In a review including over 30 studies, it has been reported that although the best GLS to predict cardiotoxicity was not clear, an early relative change between 10 and 15% appears to have the best specificity [20]. A consensus statement on the evaluation of adult patients during and after cancer therapy suggests that based on the currently available literature, a relative percentage reduction in GLS of >15% is very likely to be abnormal, whereas a change of <8% appears not to be of clinical significance [21]. It also suggests that an abnormal GLS value should be confirmed by a repeat study. The repeat study is recommended to be performed 2–3 weeks after the initial abnormal study. It should be noted that these suggestions have been mostly reported in the breast cancer population.

If this same cardiac imaging benefit will extend to other malignancies in their treatment course remain to be seen. In practice, however, due to the seemingly low values for relative GLS % change in the early follow-up of these patients, and particularly in labs where there are systems from multiple vendors, the concern for reproducibility and consistency among vendors continues to be an issue [22].

Illustrated Case Presentation and Discussion; Use of GLS in Breast Cancer

A 63-year-old female with HER-2 positive breast cancer is seen in the clinic.

The patient had a history of hypertension for 10 years prior to the diagnosis of breast cancer, managed with low dose Lisinopril (5 mg daily). The BP on exam was 145/90 mmHg with similar BP readings on the last few visits. The baseline echocardiogram showed an LVEF of 54% measured using the biplane method of disks (MOD); the GLS was 19.6% (Fig. 2.1). It was recommended to increase the ACE-I dose and in a 2 week follow up the BP was noticeably improved to 135/81 mmHg. The patient was started on a chemotherapy regimen that included four cycles of epirubicin to be followed by 12 months of trastuzumab. A follow-up echo 3 months into trastuzumab showed a 2D and 3D LVEF of 55%, but the GLS obtained using the same imaging system and the same sonographer was 14.6% (a 26% relative drop from previous) (Fig. 2.2).

In follow-up, the GLS information and its potential implication were discussed in detail with both the patient and the oncologist. The option to start a beta-blocker or further increase the Lisinopril dose were discussed. The patient, however, declined any therapeutic changes that were suggested.

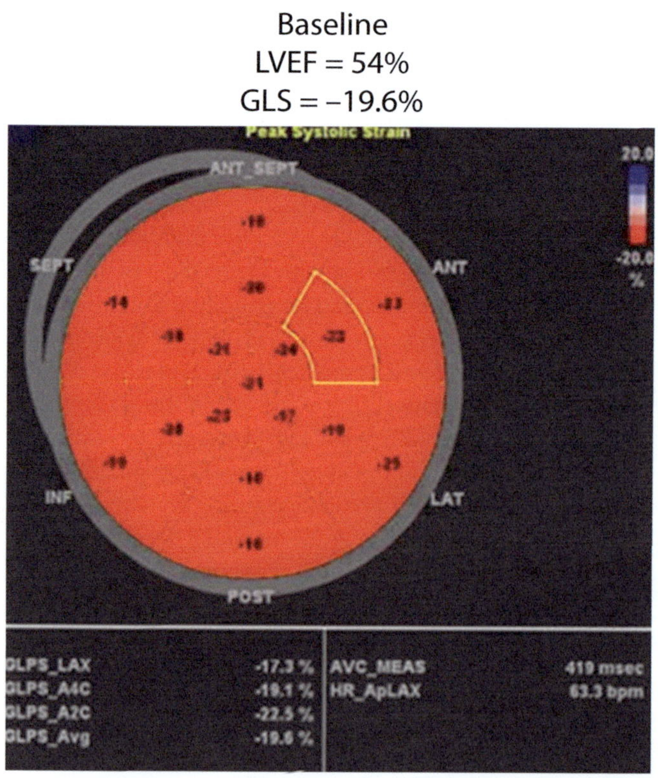

Fig. 2.1 A female with HER-2 positive breast cancer baseline GLS polar map, normal value −19.6%

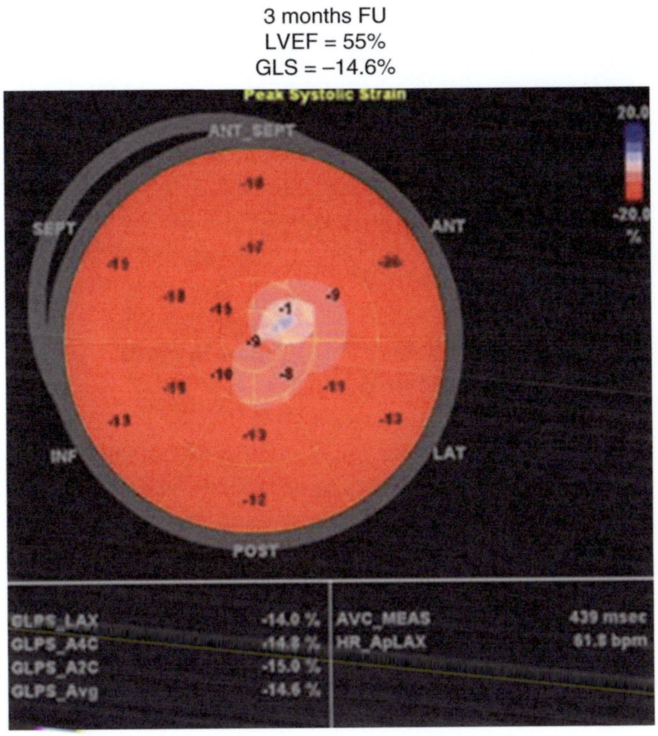

Fig. 2.2 Same patient from Fig. 2.1, a 3 month follow up GLS obtained using the same imaging system and same sonographer was 14.6%; a significant relative drop (>15% is considered significant based on multiple studies)

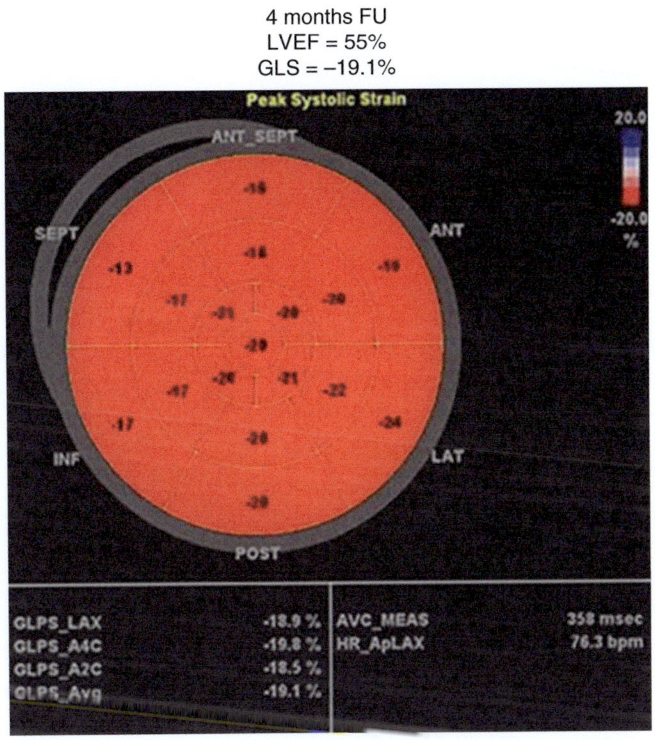

Fig. 2.3 Improved GLS 1 month later −19.1%

She was continued on trastuzumab and on follow up at 6 months, an echocardiogram with GLS, using the same imaging system and even the same sonographer was done. Clinically the patient was asymptomatic, with no abnormality in cardiac biomarkers, but the 2D LVEF was 41%, with a mild increase in the measured biplane LVESV. In this case the decision was made for a 3–4 break off trastuzumab and low dose carvedilol was added.

At 1 month follow up an echocardiogram showed improvement (EF 55% with biplane MOD, GLS 19.1%) and the patient completed her treatment from that point forward without further events (Fig. 2.3).

Illustrated Case Presentation and Discussion; GLS Utility in Enhancing Clinical Confidence

A 24 year female with acute leukemia, is treated at an outside facility with an anthracycline-containing regimen and a baseline echocardiogram is reported to have a qualitative EF of 55%. A repeat study is performed in approximately 30 days and again only qualitative measures are reported.

This time the LVEF is reported as 40–45%, and the patient receives a clinical recommendation to avoid all further cancer therapy and a consultation with advanced heart failure service is ordered. The patient's oncologist's requests a comprehensive evaluation at MD Anderson, and further chemotherapy is contemplated.

While a definitive oncologic treatment plan is being established, the patient is evaluated in our cardiology clinic; the young female is clinically essentially asymptomatic, biomarkers (BNP, TnI) are normal, with the echocardiogram showing an LVEF (measured by biplane MOD) of 46% (Fig. 2.4).

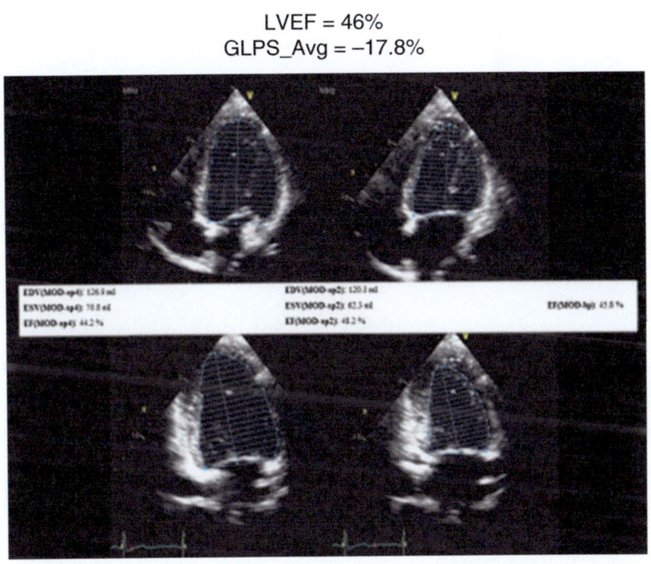

Fig. 2.4 A young female received 36 mg/m2 of Idarubicin; echo at 30 days with LVEF 46% using the biplane MoD

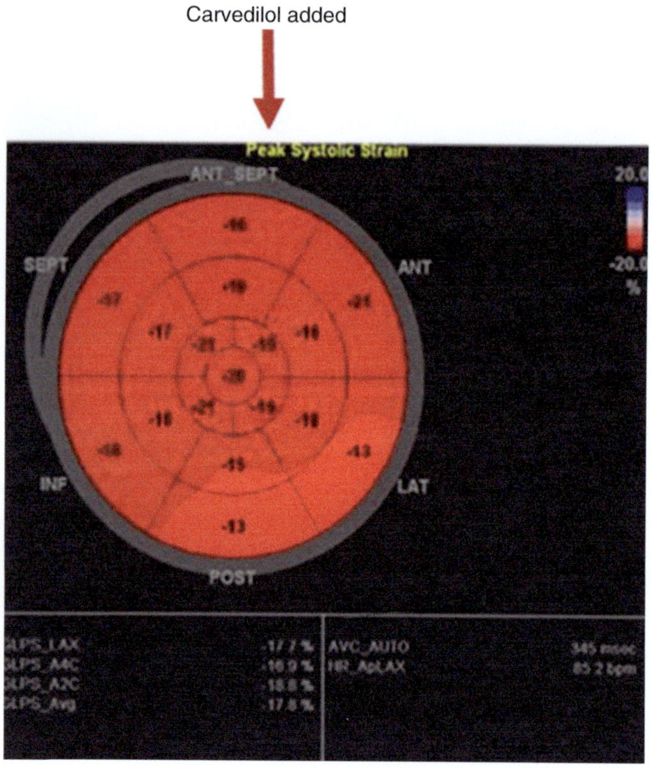

Fig. 2.5 Polar map GLS of that same visit, measured at 17.8%, almost a normal value

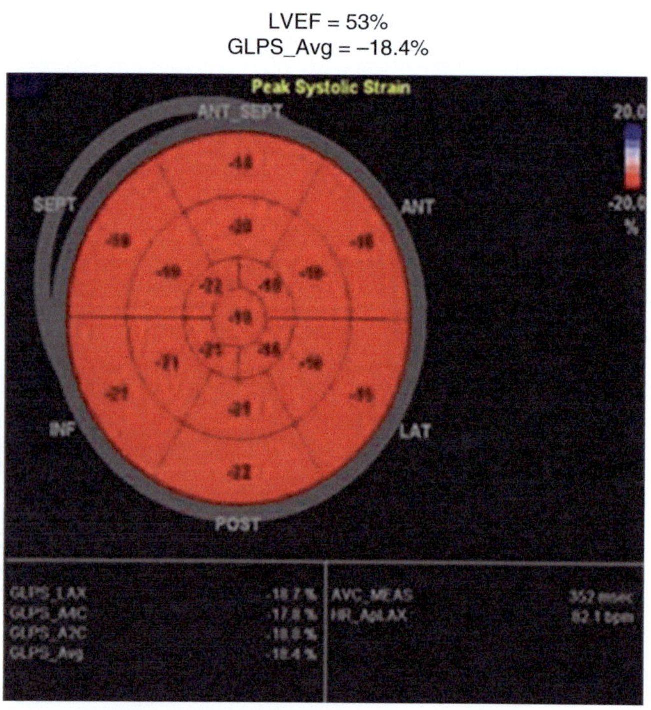

Fig. 2.6 Polar map GLS now another month later, measured at 18.4%, normal value

Using 2D speckle tracking the GLS is measured at 17.8% (Fig. 2.5), which is considered to be very close to normal.

The patient is given low dose carvedilol and on 4 week follow up the LVEF improved to 53% and the GLS was 18.4% (Fig. 2.6). The patient was able to complete her anticancer therapy without delay continued to do well clinically and subsequent cardiac imaging tests at 1 and 2 years follow up were all within normal range.

Brief Discussion; Key Points and a Note About GLS Acquisition

The first case presents the opportunity to focus on the importance of optimal BP control in all patients undergoing chemotherapy regimens that have any Cardiotoxic potential.

Our second case brings the use of the GLS measure as an additional tool to answer a clinical question about the continuation of potential cardiotoxic chemotherapy. In our experience it can represent, in conjunction with the clinical picture and other available indicators, such as biomarkers, a confidence measure when normal or within 1% point to normal.

We emphasize using the best available method of LVEF measures in this patient population during the course of therapy. As already is extensively reported in the literature, in terms of best reproducibility and inter and intra observer plus temporal variability the order is: 3D (unenhanced) > contrast 2D (biplane MOD) > unenhanced 2D (biplane MOD) [23].

We also give several key recommendations when using GLS capable systems:

1. Optimal image quality is imperative, there is a great need to visualize all 16 segments (ASE standard 16 segment model). In most systems, your GLS will be expressed using a 17+ segment model. Parallel to the two segments "contrast rule" we also apply judgment of image quality when more than two segments are not well visualized (our rule of thumb).

   Use individual judgment when a patient has a preexisting BBB on the ECG and the polar map shows a septal defect. The patient is its own "control" over time, therefore this defect, particularly when the overall kinesis and thickening of the segments appear visually fairly normal, become of less concern using this modality, in our experience.
2. Acquisition frame rate is important. Don't forget that frame rate is a number of single images per second, and we are focusing in longitudinal deformation in systole, therefore only the initial third of the cardiac cycle. Our sensing is also in a single beat, which forces us to be

extremely vigilant of quality. Think of LV apical focused images with only the necessary sector width.
3. The learning curve we have seen in our experience for a sonographer using this modality is usually conquered at the 12–16 month of experience.
4. In our experience, the GLS measure in tachycardia or in situations of irregular HR is not useful.

References

1. Kobayashi T, Nakayama R, Takatani O, Kimura K. Positive chronotropic and inotropic actions of new antitumor agent adriamycin and its cardiotoxicity–its special references to myocardial contractile force and the change of the transmembrane action potential. Jpn Circ J. 1972;36:259–65.
2. Lefrak EA, Pitha J, Rosenheim S, Gottlieb JA. A clinicopathologic analysis of adriamycin cardiotoxicity. Cancer. 1973;32:302–14.
3. Rinehart JJ, Lewis RP, Balcerzak SP. Adriamycin cardiotoxicity in man. Ann Intern Med. 1974;81:475–8.
4. Greco FA, Brereton HD, Rodbard D. Noninvasive monitoring of adriamycin cardiotoxicity by "Sphygmo-Recording" of the pulse wave delay (QKd interval). Cancer Treat Rep. 1976;60:1239–45.
5. Ramos A, Meyer RA, Korfhagen J, Wong KY, Kaplan S. Echocardiographic evaluation of adriamycin cardiotoxicity in children. Cancer Treat Rep. 1976;60:1281–4.
6. Alcan KE, Robeson W, Graham MC, Palestro C, Oliver FH, Benua RS. Early detection of anthracycline-induced cardiotoxicity by stress radionuclide cineangiography in conjunction with Fourier amplitude and phase analysis. Clin Nucl Med. 1985;10:160–6.
7. Lenzhofer R, Dudczak R, Gumhold G, Graninger W, Moser K, Spitzy KH. Noninvasive methods for the early detection of doxorubicin-induced cardiomyopathy. J Cancer Res Clin Oncol. 1983;106:136–42.
8. McKillop JH, Bristow MR, Goris ML, Billingham ME, Bockemuehl K. Sensitivity and specificity of radionuclide ejection fractions in doxorubicin cardiotoxicity. Am Heart J. 1983;106:1048–56.
9. Pauwels EK, Horning SJ, Goris ML. Sequential equilibrium gated radionuclide angiocardiography for the detection of doxorubicin cardiotoxicity. Radiother Oncol. 1983;1:83–7.
10. Senior R, Soman P, Khattar RS, Lahiri A. Improved endocardial visualization with second harmonic imaging compared with fundamental two-dimensional echocardiographic imaging. Am Heart J. 1999;138:163–8.
11. Hundley WG, Kizilbash AM, Afridi I, Franco F, Peshock RM, Grayburn PA. Administration of an intravenous perfluorocarbon contrast agent improves echocardiographic determination of left ventricular volumes and ejection fraction: comparison with cine magnetic resonance imaging. J Am Coll Cardiol. 1998;32:1426–32.
12. Chuang ML, Hibberd MG, Salton CJ, Beaudin RA, Riley MF, Parker RA, et al. Importance of imaging method over imaging modality in noninvasive determination of left ventricular volumes and ejection fraction: assessment by two- and three-dimensional echocardiography and magnetic resonance imaging. J Am Coll Cardiol. 2000;35:477–84.
13. Walker J, Bhullar N, Fallah-Rad N, Lytwyn M, Golian M, Fang T, et al. Role of three-dimensional echocardiography in breast cancer: comparison with two-dimensional echocardiography, multiple-gated acquisition scans, and cardiac magnetic resonance imaging. J Clin Oncol. 2010;28:3429–36.
14. Telli ML, Hunt SA, Carlson RW, Guardino AE. Trastuzumab-related cardiotoxicity: calling into question the concept of reversibility. J Clin Oncol. 2007;25:3525–33.
15. Cardinale D, Colombo A, Lamantia G, Colombo N, Civelli M, De Giacomi G, et al. Anthracycline-induced cardiomyopathy: clinical relevance and response to pharmacologic therapy. J Am Coll Cardiol. 2010;55:213–20.
16. Ernande L, Bergerot C, Rietzschel ER, De Buyzere ML, Thibault H, Pignonblanc PG, et al. Diastolic dysfunction in patients with type 2 diabetes mellitus: is it really the first marker of diabetic cardiomyopathy? J Am Soc Echocardiogr. 2011;24:1268–75.e1.
17. Hare JL, Brown JK, Leano R, Jenkins C, Woodward N, Marwick TH. Use of myocardial deformation imaging to detect preclinical myocardial dysfunction before conventional measures in patients undergoing breast cancer treatment with trastuzumab. Am Heart J. 2009;158:294–301.
18. Fallah-Rad N, Walker JR, Wassef A, Lytwyn M, Bohonis S, Fang T, et al. The utility of cardiac biomarkers, tissue velocity and strain imaging, and cardiac magnetic resonance imaging in predicting early left ventricular dysfunction in patients with human epidermal growth factor receptor II-positive breast cancer treated with adjuvant trastuzumab therapy. J Am Coll Cardiol. 2011;57:2263–70.
19. Sawaya H, Sebag IA, Plana JC, Januzzi JL, Ky B, Cohen V, et al. Early detection and prediction of cardiotoxicity in chemotherapy-treated patients. Am J Cardiol. 2011;107:1375–80.
20. Thavendiranathan P, Poulin F, Lim KD, Plana JC, Woo A, Marwick TH. Use of myocardial strain imaging by echocardiography for the early detection of cardiotoxicity in patients during and after cancer chemotherapy: a systematic review. J Am Coll Cardiol. 2014;63:2751–68.
21. Plana JC, Galderisi M, Barac A, Ewer MS, Ky B, Scherrer-Crosbie M, et al. Expert consensus for multimodality imaging evaluation of adult patients during and after cancer therapy: a report from the American Society of Echocardiography and the European Association of Cardiovascular Imaging. J Am Soc Echocardiogr. 2014;27:911–39.
22. Marwick TH. Consistency of myocardial deformation imaging between vendors. Eur J Echocardiogr. 2010;11(5):414–6. https://doi.org/10.1093/ejechocard/jeq006. Epub 17 Feb 2010.
23. Thavendiranathan P, Grant AD, Negishi T, Plana JC, Popović ZB, Marwick TH. Reproducibility of echocardiographic techniques for sequential assessment of left ventricular ejection fraction and volumes: application to patients undergoing cancer chemotherapy. J Am Coll Cardiol. 2013;61(1):77–84. https://doi.org/10.1016/j.jacc.2012.09.035. Epub 28 Nov 2012.

Cancer Treatment-Related Cardiotoxicity: Role of Cardiovascular Magnetic Resonance Imaging

3

Felipe Kazmirczak, Prajwal Reddy, Anne H. Blaes, and Chetan Shenoy

Abstract

Cardiomyopathy is one of the most common cardiotoxic manifestations from cancer treatment. Clinically, identifying the presence or absence of cardiomyopathy has significant implications on the management of cancer patients. Decisions regarding the continuation, temporary stopping or permanent stopping of potentially life-saving cancer treatment are made based on the presence or absence of, the etiology of (i.e., whether it is a consequence of the cancer treatment or unrelated), and the severity of cardiomyopathy. Thus, it is critically important to use an imaging test that can reliably and accurately provide these data. Cardiovascular magnetic resonance (CMR) is ideally suited for this role—it provides the ability to assess ventricular function, morphology, valvular function, perfusion and tissue characterization all in one setting.

Keywords

Cardiac magnetic resonance • Cancer treatment related cardiotoxicity • Cardiomyopathy

Assessment of Ventricular Volumes and Function to Determine the Presence or Absence, and the Severity of Cardiomyopathy

Case 1

A 50-year-old female with breast cancer T1bN0, invasive ductal carcinoma, estrogen receptor negative, HER-2 amplified status post bilateral mastectomies with reconstruction, was treated with AC (cyclophosphamide and doxorubicin) followed by paclitaxel and trastuzumab for 1 year. She was in remission for 2 years when she developed palpitations. An event monitor showed multiple episodes of non-sustained ventricular tachycardia and high premature ventricular contraction (PVC) burden. To rule out structural heart disease an echocardiogram was ordered. It showed poor acoustic windows with poor endocardial border definition. The visually estimated left ventricular ejection fraction (LVEF) was 55% (Fig. 3.1a). Reliable quantitation by Simpson's method could not be performed due to poor endocardial border definition. Ultrasound contrast was not given. Given the poor image quality on echocardiography and the frequent PVCs, a cardiovascular magnetic resonance (CMR) imaging was performed for evaluation of ventricular function and fibrosis as a substrate for her ventricular arrhythmias. The CMR showed LVEF of 66%, right ventricular ejection fraction (RVEF) of 57% and no evidence of myocardial fibrosis (Fig. 3.1b).

Discussion

In patients with suspected cancer-treatment related cardiomyopathy, CMR can help identify the presence or absence of a cardiomyopathy with high reliability and accuracy. CMR is

F. Kazmirczak • C. Shenoy (✉)
Cardiovascular Division, Department of Medicine, University of Minnesota Medical Center, 420 Delaware Street SE, MMC 508, Minneapolis, MN 55455, USA
e-mail: cshenoy@umn.edu

P. Reddy
Department of Medicine, University of Minnesota Medical Center, Minneapolis, MN, USA

A.H. Blaes
Division of Hematology, Oncology and Transplantation, Department of Medicine, University of Minnesota Medical Center, 420 Delaware Street SE, MMC 508, Minneapolis, MN 55455, USA

S.W. Yusuf, J. Banchs (eds.), *Cancer and Cardiovascular Disease*, https://doi.org/10.1007/978-3-319-62088-6_3

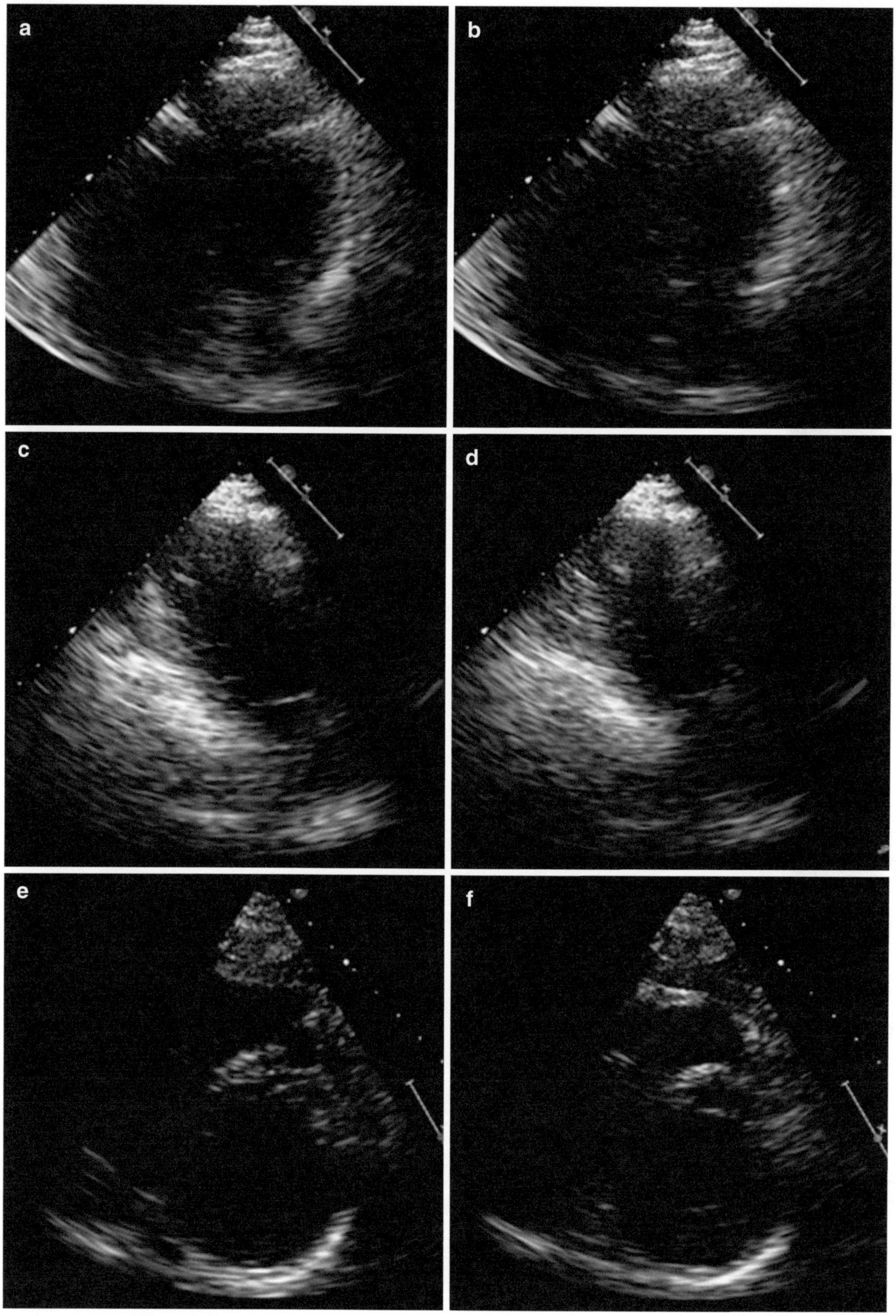

Fig. 3.1 (**a**) Echocardiogram. Poor acoustic windows with a visually estimated LVEF of 55%. a: Apical 4-chamber view at end diastole. b: Apical 4-chamber at end systole demonstrating poor acoustic windows in the setting of breast implants. c: Apical 2-chamber at end diastole. d: Apical 2-chamber at end systole. e: Parasternal short axis view at end diastole. f: Parasternal short axis view at end systole showing poor endocardial definition.

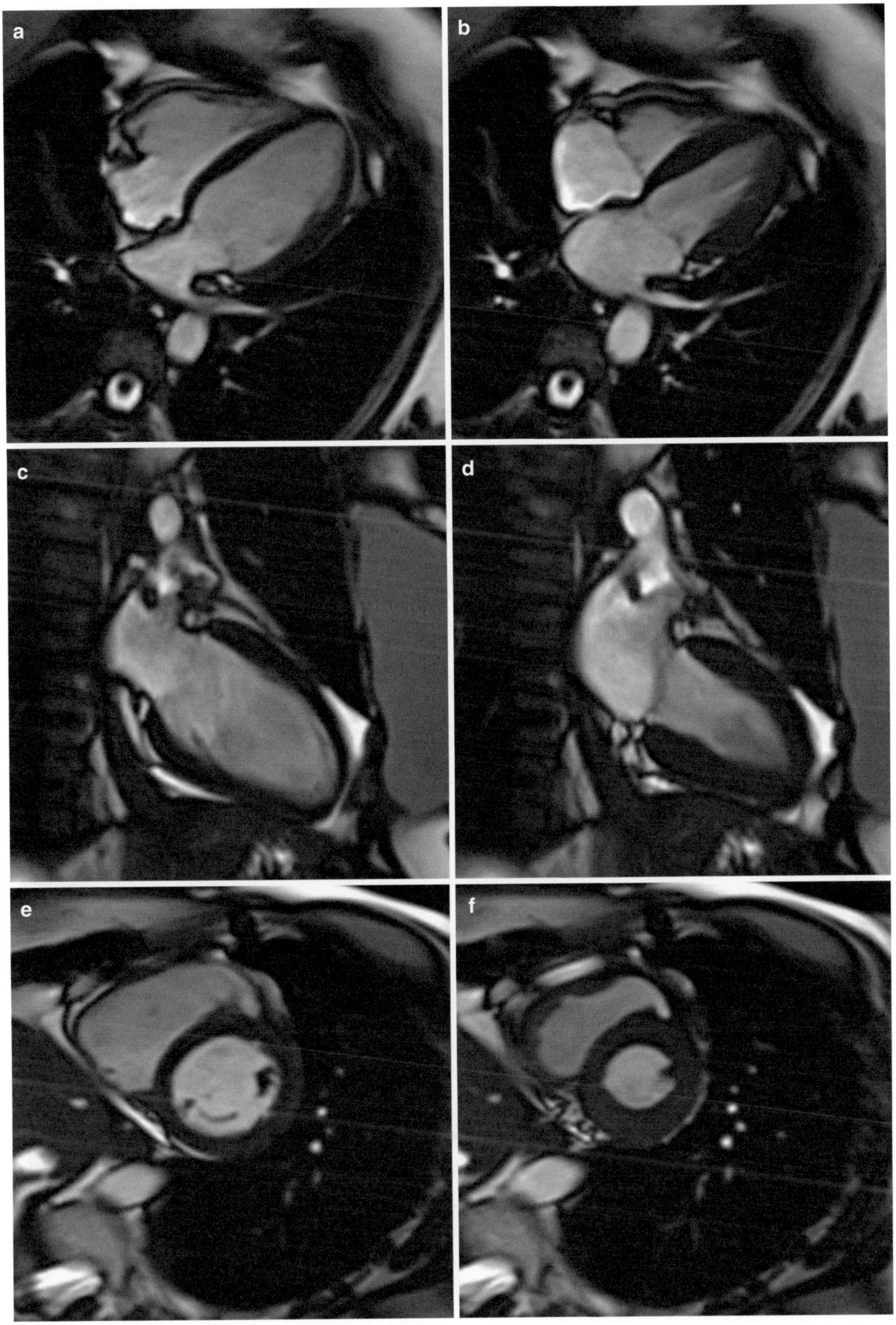

Fig. 3.1 (continued) (**b**) CMR. Same patient as in (**a**), showing an LVEF of 66%, RVEF of 57% and no myocardial fibrosis. a: 4-chamber cine image at end diastole. b: 4-chamber cine image at end systole showing normal ventricular function with LVEF of 66% and RVEF of 57%. c: 2-chamber cine image at end diastole. d: 2-chamber cine image at end systole showing normal LV function and no evidence of wall motion. e: Basal short axis cine image at end diastole. f: Basal short axis cine image at end systole showing normal ventricular function

well-accepted as the gold standard technique for assessment of left ventricular volumes, LVEF [1] and LV mass [2]. After a simple non-contrast acquisition of a 3-dimensional stack of contiguous short-axis cine images with full ventricular coverage, LV and RV volumes and masses are quantified by planimetry for each slice and summed for the whole ventricles. CMR has been demonstrated to perform better than two-dimensional echocardiography [3] in identifying cancer treatment-related cardiomyopathy. Additionally, CMR-derived LV mass has been demonstrated to be associated with major adverse cardiovascular events in patients treated with anthracyclines [4].

Case 2

A 67-year-old-female with acute myeloid leukemia (AML) treated with an anthracycline-based regimen, in remission for the past 9 years, hypertension and morbid obesity (body mass index of 48) was referred to cardiology for evaluation of shortness of breath. An echocardiogram was performed to evaluate cardiac function and showed poor acoustic windows and suboptimal image quality despite the use of ultrasound contrast. The LVEF was estimated at 40-45% (Fig. 3.2a). Given the reduced diagnostic accuracy of the echocardiogram, a stress CMR was requested to evaluate ventricular function and to evaluate for the presence of coronary artery disease. The stress CMR revealed LVEF of 67%, RVEF of 56%, normal perfusion without inducible ischemia, and no myocardial infarction or fibrosis (Fig. 3.2b).

Discussion

CMR can provide optimal image quality even in obese patients without limitations of acoustic windows. The average CMR scanner can accommodate a weight of up to 550 lb and a body girth (circumference) of 74 in. (60 cm bore diameter). Newer wide-bore scanners can accommodate up to 86 in. (70 cm bore diameter). As in this case, a single CMR study can provide a wide variety of information—ventricular and atrial size and function, the presence or absence of ischemia, the presence or absence of myocardial infarction or fibrosis, evaluation of valve disease, evaluation of the pericardium, etc.

Case 3

A 61-year-old male with lymphoma treated with an anthracycline-based regimen had a multiple gated acquisition scan (MUGA) for surveillance imaging that showed a LVEF of 47% (Fig. 3.3, Panel A and B). A CMR performed 4 days later for evaluation of the cardiomyopathy revealed a LVEF of 55% (Fig. 3.3, Panel C and D). A 61-year-old female with breast cancer treated with an anthracycline-based regimen had a MUGA for surveillance imaging that showed a LVEF of 69% (Fig. 3.3, Panel E and F). A CMR performed 7 days later for evaluation of the cardiomyopathy revealed a LVEF of 44% (Fig. 3.3, Panel G and H). Figure reproduced from Huang et al. [5].

Discussion

CMR has also been demonstrated to perform better than MUGA [5] in identifying cancer treatment-related cardiomyopathy. Because of its higher accuracy and reproducibility, and superiority over two-dimensional echocardiography and MUGA, CMR is the imaging technique of choice for longitudinal study of patients over time [6], such as cancer patients under surveillance for cardiotoxicity.

Case 4

A 61-year-old male was treated for Stage IIIB diffuse large B-cell lymphoma in 2005 with four cycles of anthracycline-based chemotherapy, attaining promptly remission. In 2014, he had recurrence and received two cycles of anthracycline-based therapy. A routine post-treatment MUGA showed an LVEF of 46% and he was referred for a CMR to confirm and further evaluate his cardiomyopathy. The CMR showed a LVEF of 50%, RVEF of 45% and no evidence of myocardial fibrosis (Fig. 3.4).

Discussion

Currently, RV function is not included in the definition of cardiotoxicity. Recent studies have described the involvement of the RV in cardiotoxicity—most often as RV dys-

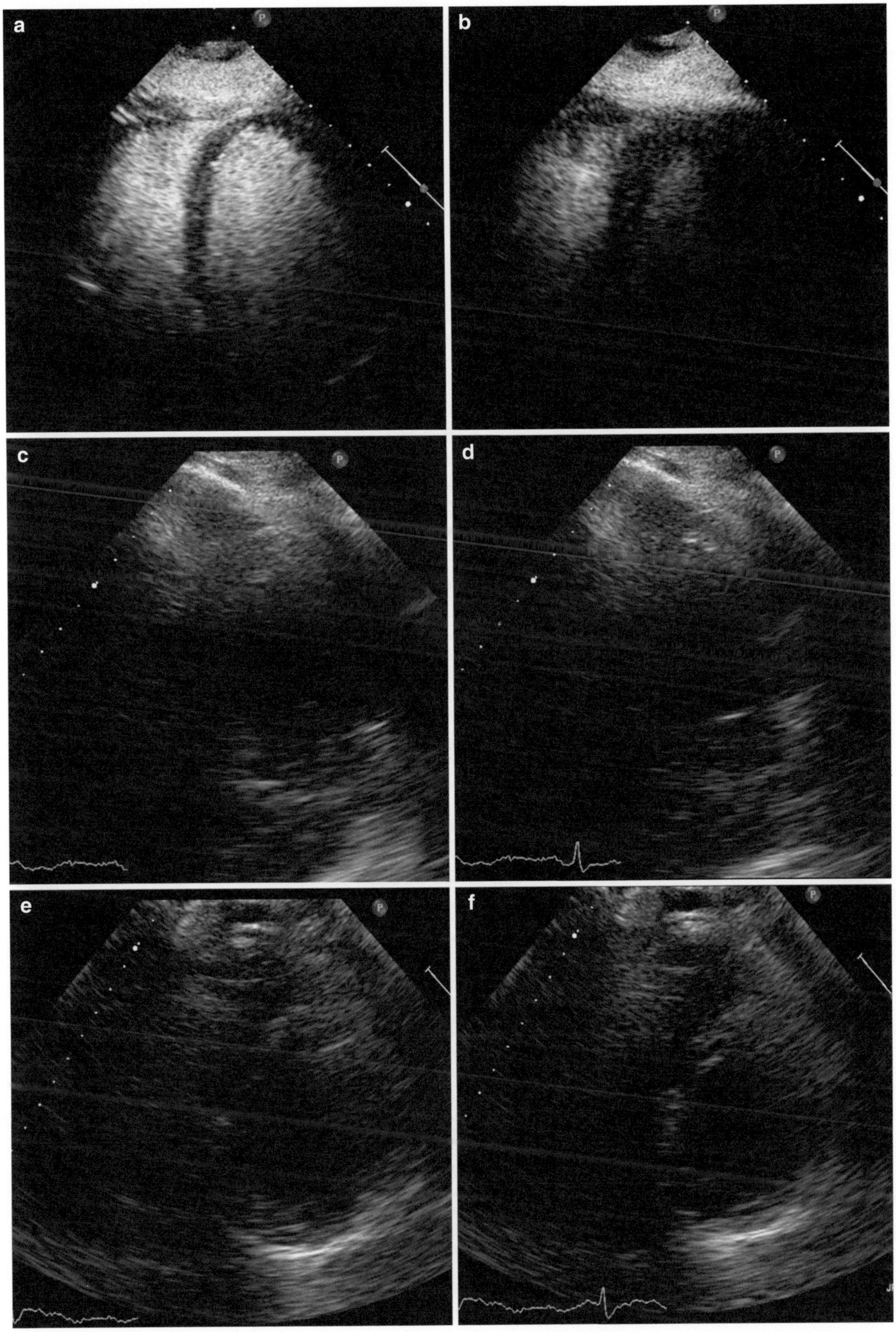

Fig. 3.2 (**a**) Echocardiogram. Poor acoustic windows with a visually estimated LVEF of 40–45%. a: Apical 4-chamber view at end diastole. b: Apical 4-chamber at end systole with contrast enhanced imaging for better endocardial definition showing poor acoustic window and inability to assess the lateral segment. c: Apical 2-chamber at end diastole with poor imaging quality. d: Apical 2-chamber at end systole with poor imaging quality. e: Parasternal short axis view at end diastole. f: Parasternal short axis view at end systole with poor endocardial definition.

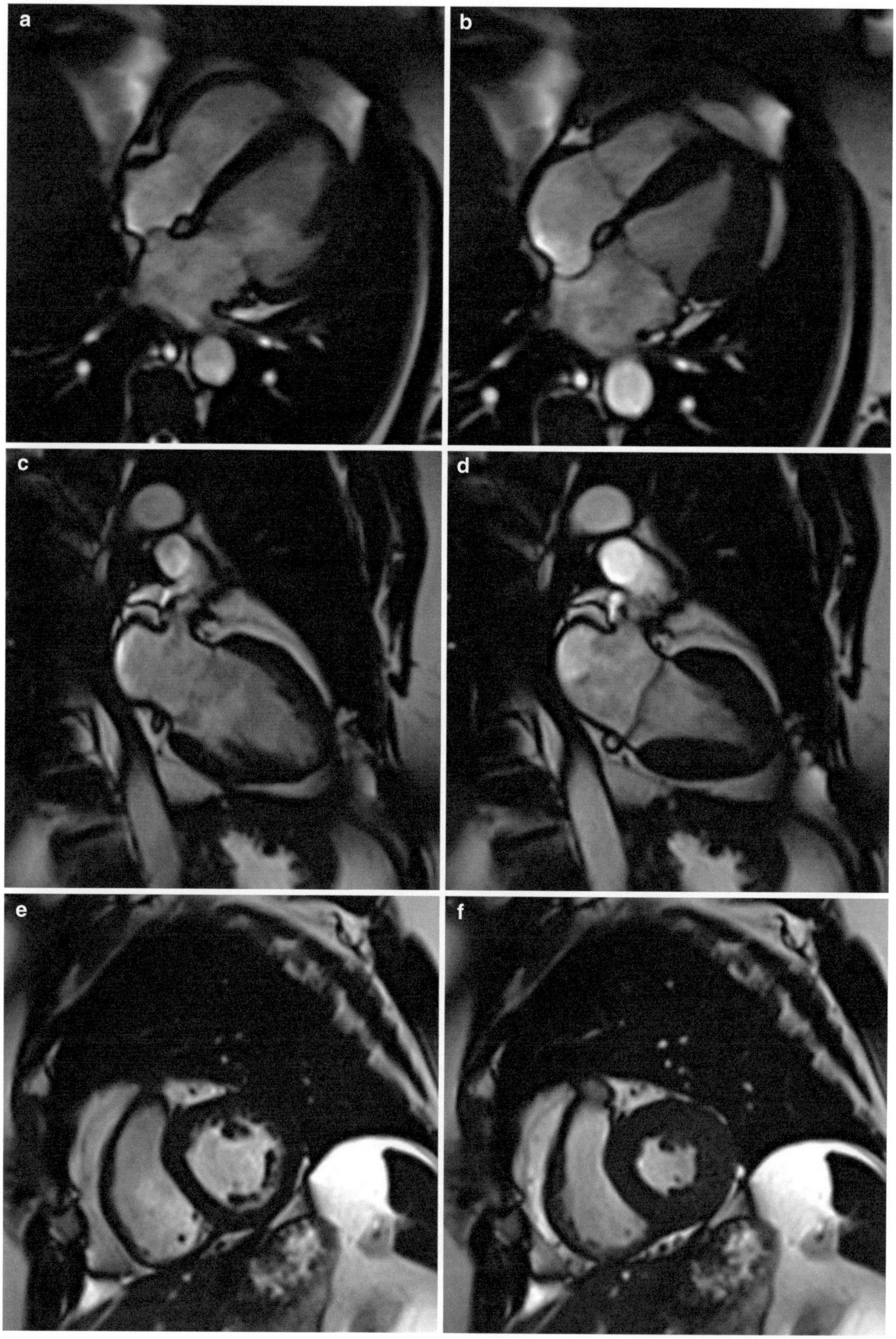

Fig. 3.2 (continued) (**b**) CMR. Same patient as in (**a**), showing normal LV and RV function and no ischemia or scar. a: 4-chamber cine image at end diastole. b: 4-chamber cine image at end systole showing clear endocardial definition and normal biventricular function with LVEF of 67% and RVEF of 56%. c: 2-chamber cine image at end diastole. d: 2-chamber cine image at end systole showing normal LV function and no evidence of wall motion. e: Basal short axis cine image at end diastole. f: Basal short axis cine image at end systole showing normal biventricular function

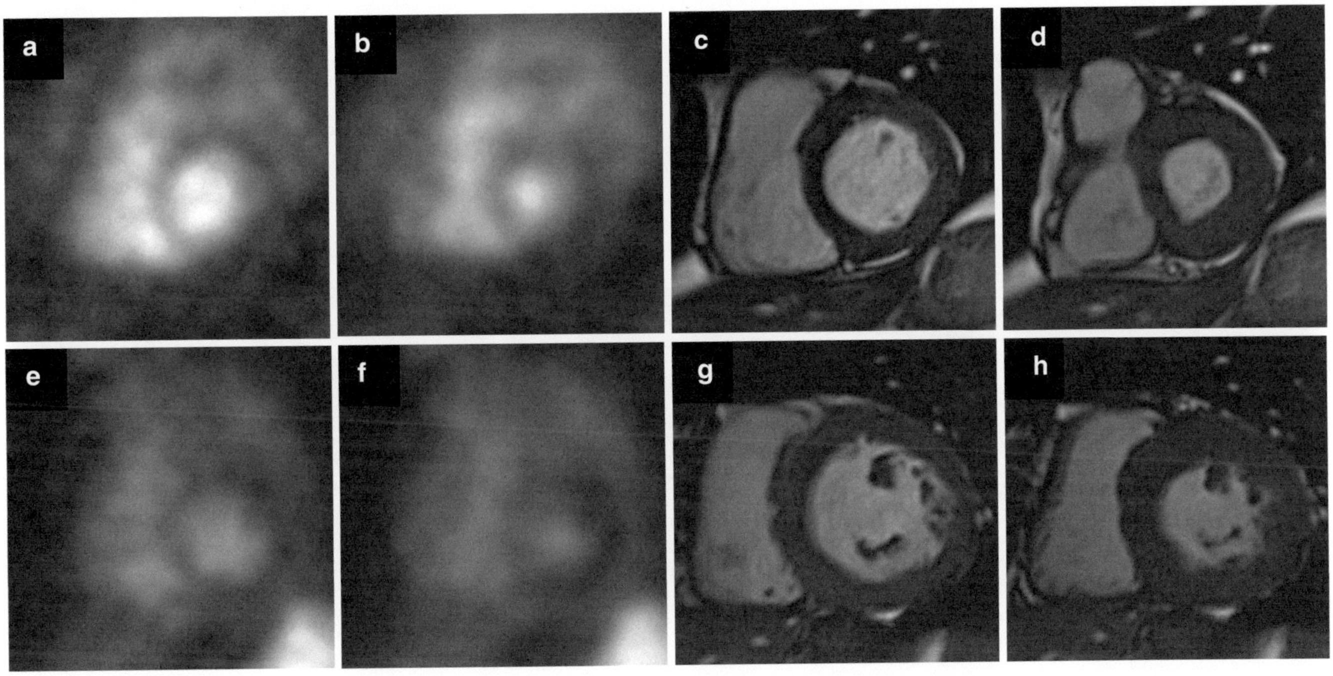

Fig. 3.3 Comparative Images of MUGA scan and CMR. (**a**) MUGA image at end diastole for the first patient. (**b**) MUGA image at end systole for the first patient. (**c**) CMR short axis cine image at end diastole for the first patient. (**d**) CMR short axis cine image at end systole for the first patient. (**e**) MUGA image at end diastole for the second patient. (**f**) MUGA image at end systole for the second patient. (**g**) CMR short axis cine image at end diastole for the second patient. (**h**) CMR short axis cine image at end systole for the second patient. Reproduced with permission from Huang et al. [5]

function [7–13]. However, most of these studies used echocardiography as the imaging modality to evaluate the RV [9–13]. Echocardiography of the RV is more difficult and less reliable than that of the LV because of two main reasons: first, the RV has a highly variable shape with relatively thin free wall and with heavy trabeculations, and second, the RV is in the near field of parasternal echocardiographic windows, and may be obscured by ribs, sternum, or the lungs in apical views [14]. CMR does not have these limitations and is the preferred modality for evaluation of right ventricular size and function. Studies on the prognostic value of right ventricular function assessed using CMR are currently underway.

Identifying the Etiology of Cardiomyopathy in Patients with Suspected Cancer Treatment-Related Cardiomyopathy

Case 5

A 66-year-old male with Stage IIB diffuse large B-cell lymphoma received eight cycles of anthracycline-based chemotherapy. Surveillance imaging with MUGA 5 years later showed severe cardiomyopathy. A CMR showed severe left ventricular dysfunction with a LVEF of 15% and no evidence of late gadolinium enhancement (LGE) suggestive of anthracycline-related cardiotoxicity (Fig. 3.5a). He subsequently had cardiac transplantation 1 year later and pathology of the explanted native heart confirmed the diagnosis of anthracycline-related cardiomyopathy.

Discussion

CMR is uniquely suited to differentiate between ischemic and non-ischemic cardiomyopathies, and to help identify the type of non-ischemic cardiomyopathy [15] (Fig. 3.5b). Knowledge of the type and etiology of the cardiomyopathy helps guide management and provides valuable prognostic insights. In addition to differentiating between ischemic and non-ischemic cardiomyopathy, CMR can help determine the specific etiology of non-ischemic cardiomyopathy in many cases with accurate diagnosis leading to disease guided therapy.

Case 6

A 71-year-old male with hypertension was diagnosed with acute myeloid leukemia and treated with induction chemotherapy idarubicin and cytarabine. His course was complicated by volume overload and heart failure. A CMR showed LVEF 56%, RVEF 67% and moderate concentric LV hypertrophy with maximal wall thickness of 1.7 cm. There was no LGE to suggest the presence of myocardial infarction or fibrosis (Fig. 3.6). Overall, the CMR findings were consistent with hypertensive cardiomyopathy, which fit with the patient history of long-standing poorly-controlled hypertension. He underwent bone marrow transplantation 6 months later. Unfortunately, he had early relapse 100 days after transplant with substantial decline in his functional status, was referred to hospice and expired 3 months after the bone marrow transplantation.

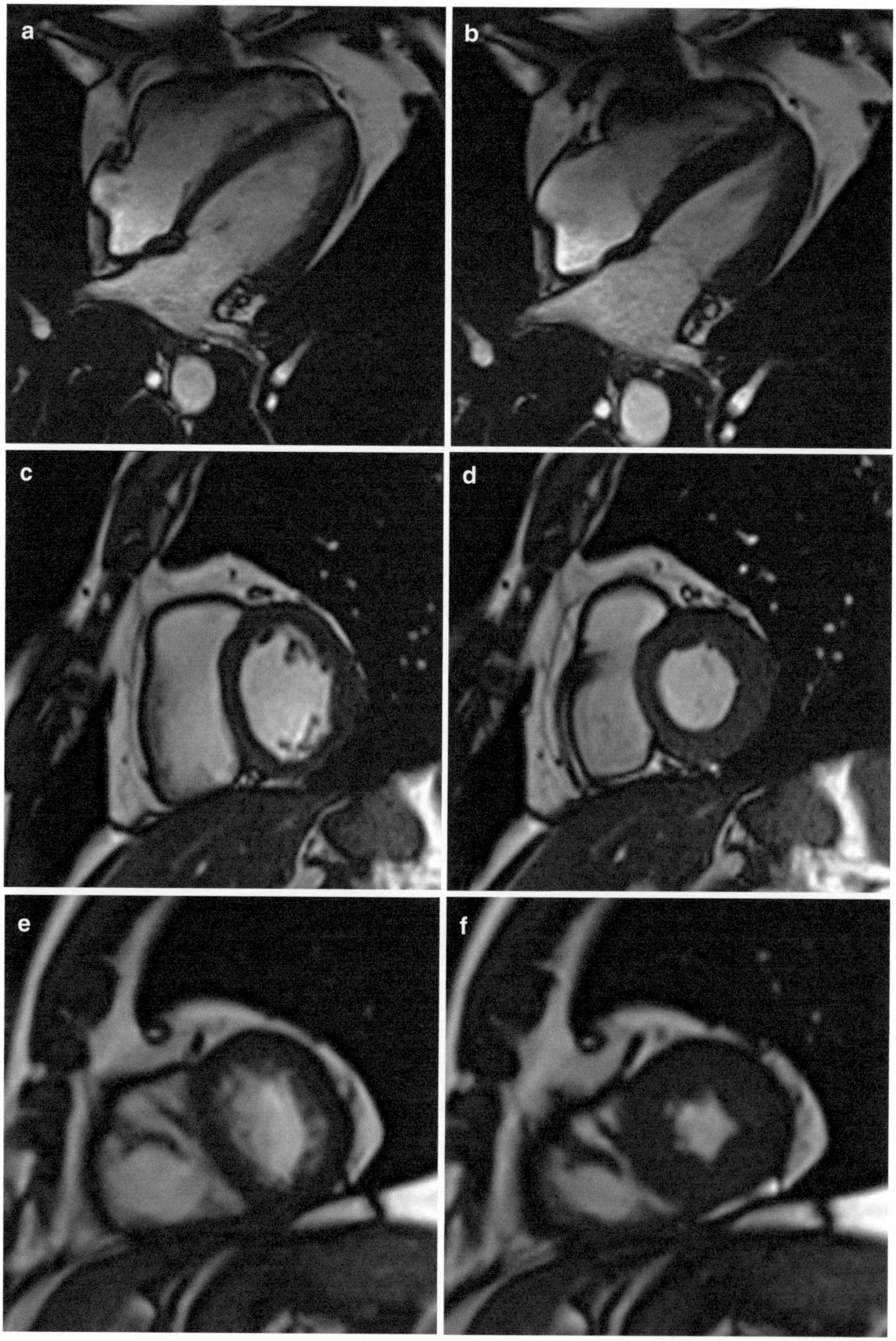

Fig. 3.4 CMR showing an LVEF of 50%, RVEF of 45% and no myocardial scar. a: 4-chamber cine image at end diastole. b: 4-chamber cine image at end systole showing reduced RV function compared to LV function. c: Basal short axis cine image at end diastole. d: Basal short axis cine image at end systole showing reduced RV function compared to LV function. e: Mid short axis cine image at end diastole. f: Mid short axis cine image at end systole showing reduced RV function compared to LV function

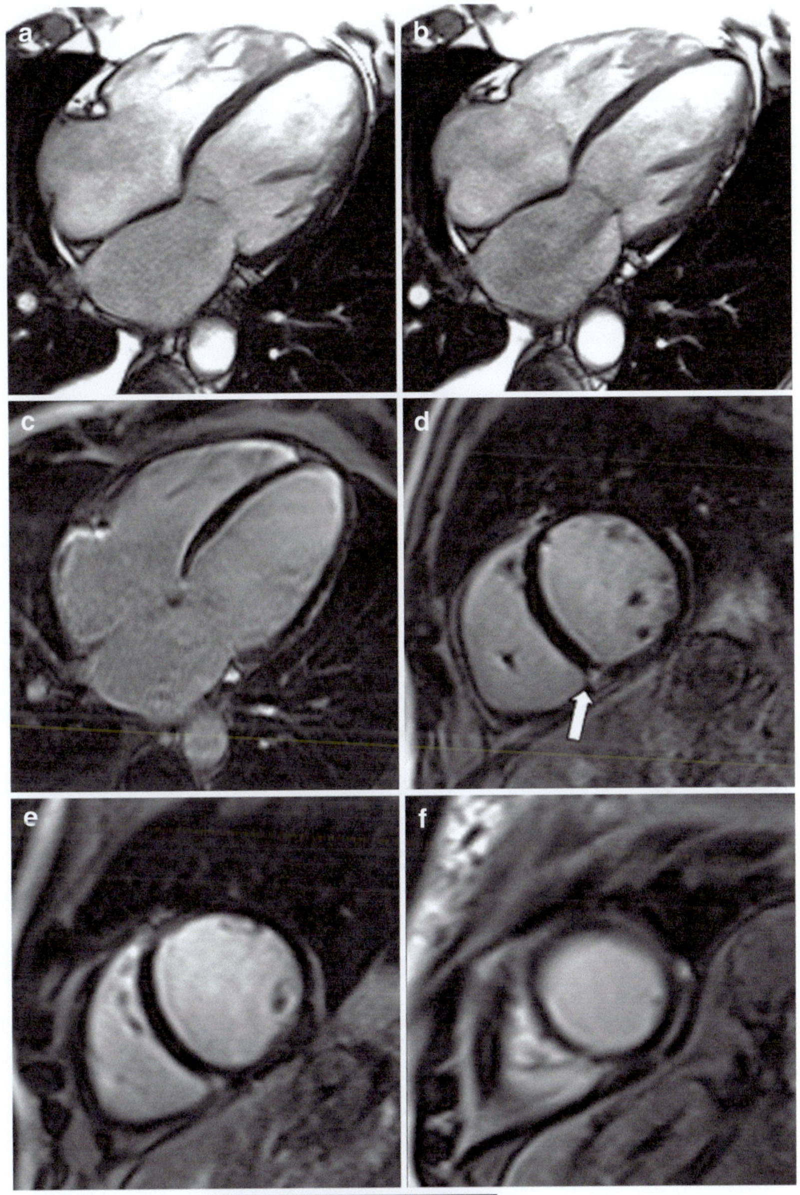

Fig. 3.5 (**a**) CMR showing biventricular dysfunction and no LGE, suggestive of anthracycline related cardiomyopathy. a: 4-chamber cine image at end diastole. b: 4-chamber cine image at end systole showing poor LV function and central mitral regurgitation. c: 4-chamber LGE image showing no evidence of scar. d: Basal short axis LGE image showed RV insertion site (*arrow*) LGE, a non-specific finding shared by several cardiomyopathies. e: Mid short axis LGE image showing no evidence of scar. f. Apical short axis LGE image showing no evidence of scar

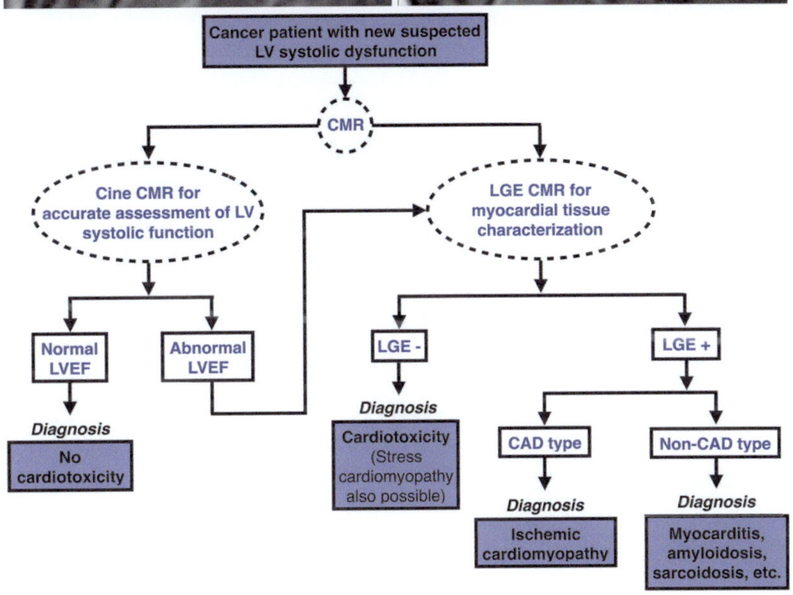

Fig. 3.5 (**b**) Algorithm for the use of CMR in identifying the etiology of cardiomyopathy in a cancer patient with newly diagnosed LV systolic dysfunction

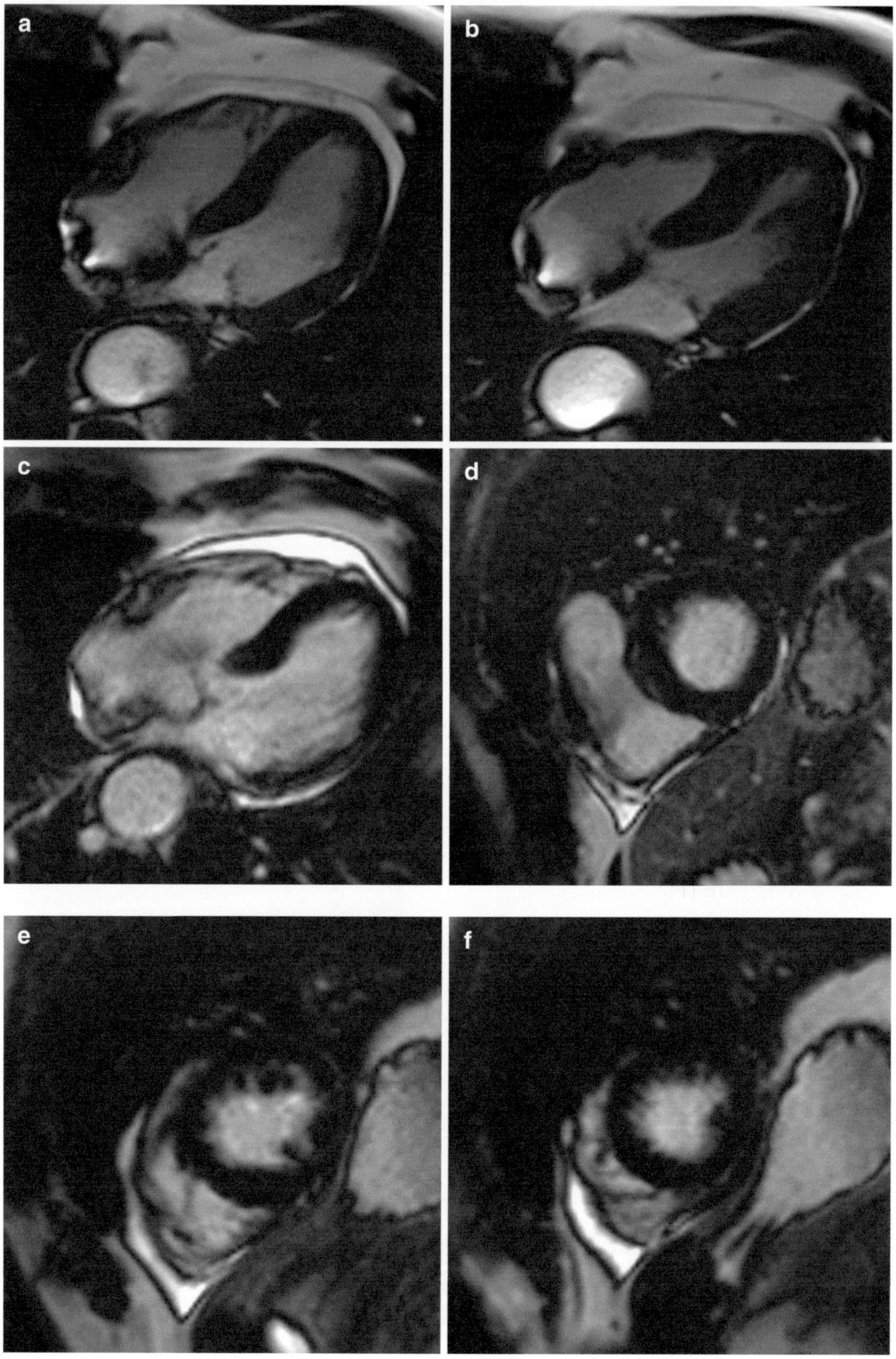

Fig. 3.6 CMR in a patient with hypertensive cardiomyopathy. a: 4-chamber cine image at end diastole. b: 4-chamber cine image at end systole showing normal ventricular function and LV hypertrophy. c: 4-chamber LGE image showing no scar. d: Basal short axis LGE image showing no scar. e: Mid short axis LGE image showing no scar. f: Apical short axis LGE image showing no scar

Discussion

In addition to differentiating between ischemic and non-ischemic cardiomyopathy, CMR can help determine the specific etiology of non-ischemic cardiomyopathy in many cases. This is, again, key to patient treatment and prognosis. For instance, beta-blockers are beneficial in some forms of non-ischemic cardiomyopathy (e.g. idiopathic dilated cardiomyopathy) but not others (e.g. cardiac amyloidosis). The prognosis also varies significantly depending on the underlying cause of non-ischemic cardiomyopathy—patients with idiopathic dilated cardiomyopathy have better survival than those with infiltrative myocardial diseases [16]. Hypertensive heart disease typically demonstrates left ventricular hypertrophy, sometimes with mild patchy areas of typically mid-myocardial LGE due to focal regions of accentuated interstitial fibrosis. Stress cardiomyopathy typically has no LGE. Cardiac amyloidosis has a spectrum from global sub-endocardial to global transmural LGE.

Case 7

A 49-year-old female with breast cancer was treated with mastectomy and anthracycline-based and paclitaxel chemotherapy. She also had biopsy proven pulmonary sarcoidosis and severe pre-capillary pulmonary hypertension. Four months later, she presented with shortness of breath and underwent a CMR that showed LVEF 47% and RVEF 35%. There was no LGE (Fig. 3.7). Based on this, the etiology of the cardiomyopathy was determined to be cardiotoxicity from prior chemotherapy treatment and not cardiac sarcoidosis.

Discussion

Etiologies of non-ischemic cardiomyopathy in which LGE is typically absent include idiopathic dilated, familial, stress, peripartum, or toxic (alcohol or cancer treatment-related) cardiomyopathies [15]. Thus, in a patient with suspected cancer treatment-related cardiotoxicity, the presence of a cardiomyopathy without LGE points towards cancer treatment as the likely etiology of the cardiomyopathy.

Case 8

A 55-year-old female with stage I breast cancer was treated with left modified radical mastectomy and anthracycline-based regimen, and then completed 5 years of tamoxifen therapy without evidence of recurrence. Surveillance echocardiography showed LVEF 45% with regional wall motion abnormalities. CMR was ordered for the evaluation of cardiomyopathy and showed LVEF of 25% and RVEF of 58%. It also showed LGE in a non-ischemic pattern involving multiple segments in epicardial and transmural patterns, which was consistent with cardiac sarcoidosis (Fig. 3.8).

Discussion

LGE CMR allows a direct assessment of myopathic processes and the pathophysiology underlying ischemic and various types of non-ischemic cardiomyopathies [15]. Cardiomyopathies often manifest with distinct locations and patterns of LGE and a pattern-recognition approach based on the visualization of LGE helps in identifying the specific etiology in most cases.

Cancer patients treated with potentially cardiotoxic treatments may also have other co-existing cardiac conditions that may be identified based on the LGE location and pattern. Cardiac sarcoidosis is diagnosed based on the presence of late gadolinium enhancement typically in a non-ischemic pattern with multiple foci of involvement manifesting as skip lesions and asymmetric depth of involvement between various lesions in the myocardium. Involvement of the RV side of the interventricular septum is seen in >80% of cases and in a patient with extra-cardiac sarcoidosis is highly suggestive of cardiac sarcoidosis.

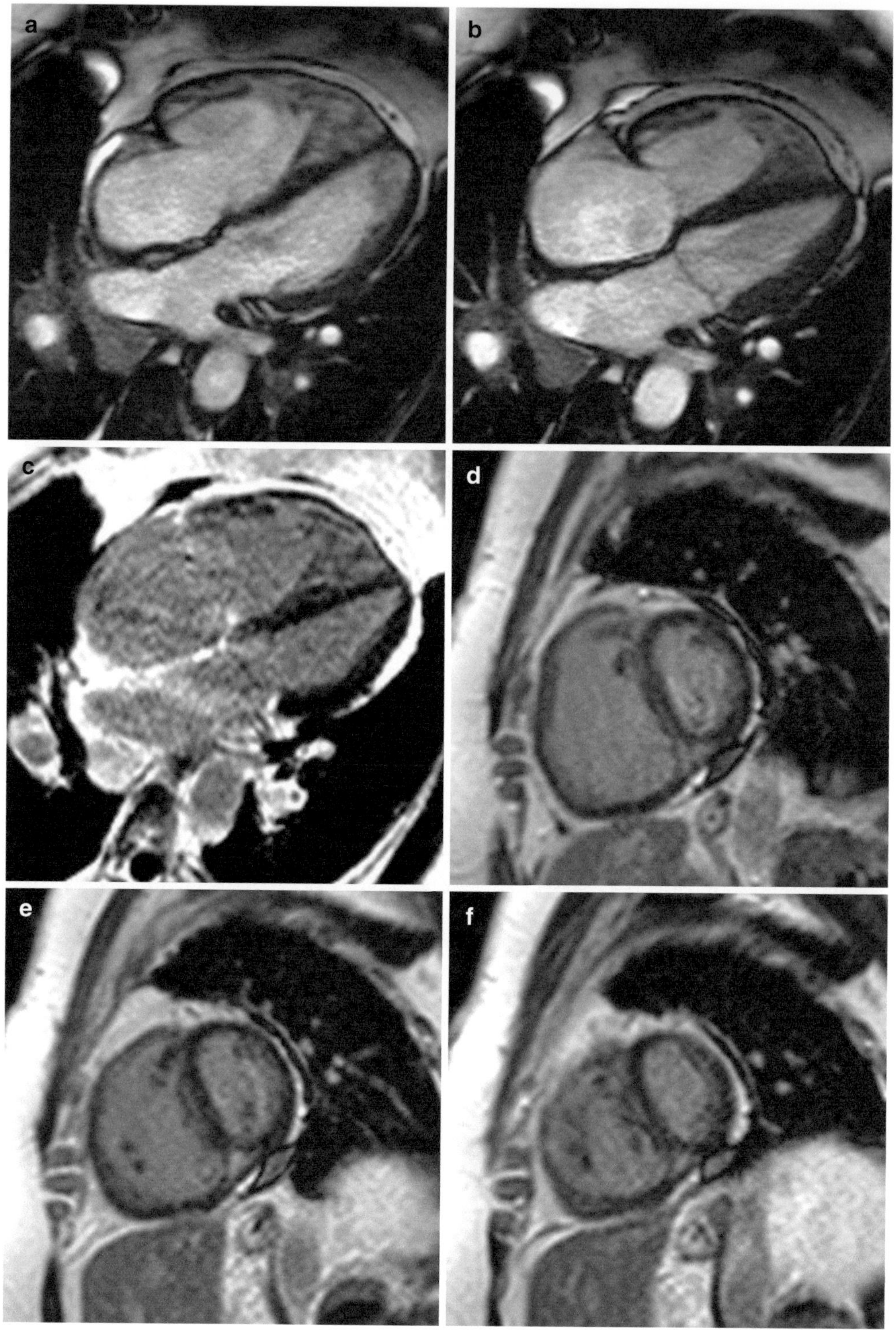

Fig. 3.7 CMR showing reduced LV and RV function. a: 4-chamber cine image at end diastole. b: 4-chamber cine image at end systole showing mildly reduced LVEF, septal bowing, dilated RV and moderately reduced RVEF. c: 4-chamber LGE image showing no scar. d: Basal short axis LGE image showing no scar. e: Mid short axis LGE image showing no scar. f: Apical short axis LGE image showing no scar

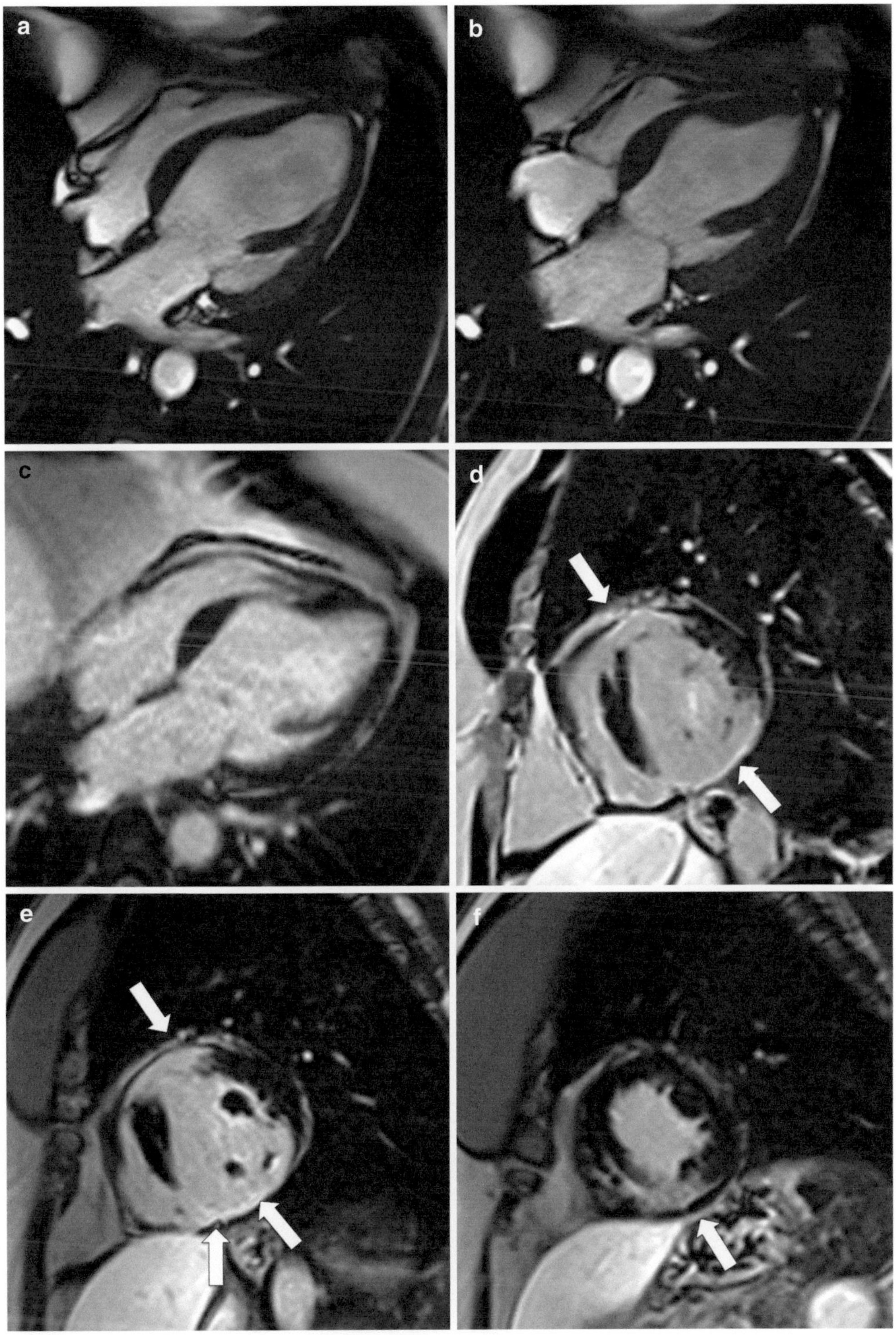

Fig. 3.8 CMR, showing findings suggestive of cardiac sarcoidosis. a: 4-chamber cine image at end diastole. b: 4-chamber cine image at end systole showing severely reduced LVEF and asymmetrical mid-septal thinning. c: 4-chamber LGE image showing LGE in the mid-septal segment. d: Basal short axis LGE image showing two areas of transmural LGE in the anterior and inferior segments. There is also involvement of the superior portion of the RV free wall. e: Mid short axis LGE image showing similar findings as above. f: Apical short axis LGE image showing septal mid-wall and inferior epicardial LGE

Case 9

A 61-year-old-male with metastatic esophageal cancer, on palliative chemotherapy with oxaliplatin, 5-fluorouracil, and folinic acid, presented with bigeminy on ECG. A CMR showed LVEF of 50%, RVEF of 50% and subendocardial LGE in the basal inferior and inferolateral segments consistent with prior myocardial infarctions in the right coronary artery and left circumflex coronary artery territories (Fig. 3.9).

Discussion

CAD is not uncommon among cancer patients since both cancer and CAD are associated with older age. The ischemic pattern of LGE from CAD always involves the subendocardium (i.e., it is subendocardial or transmural), and it is in a region consistent with the perfusion territory of an epicardial coronary artery. Ischemic cardiomyopathy is associated with reduced survival compared with non-ischemic cardiomyopathy [16].

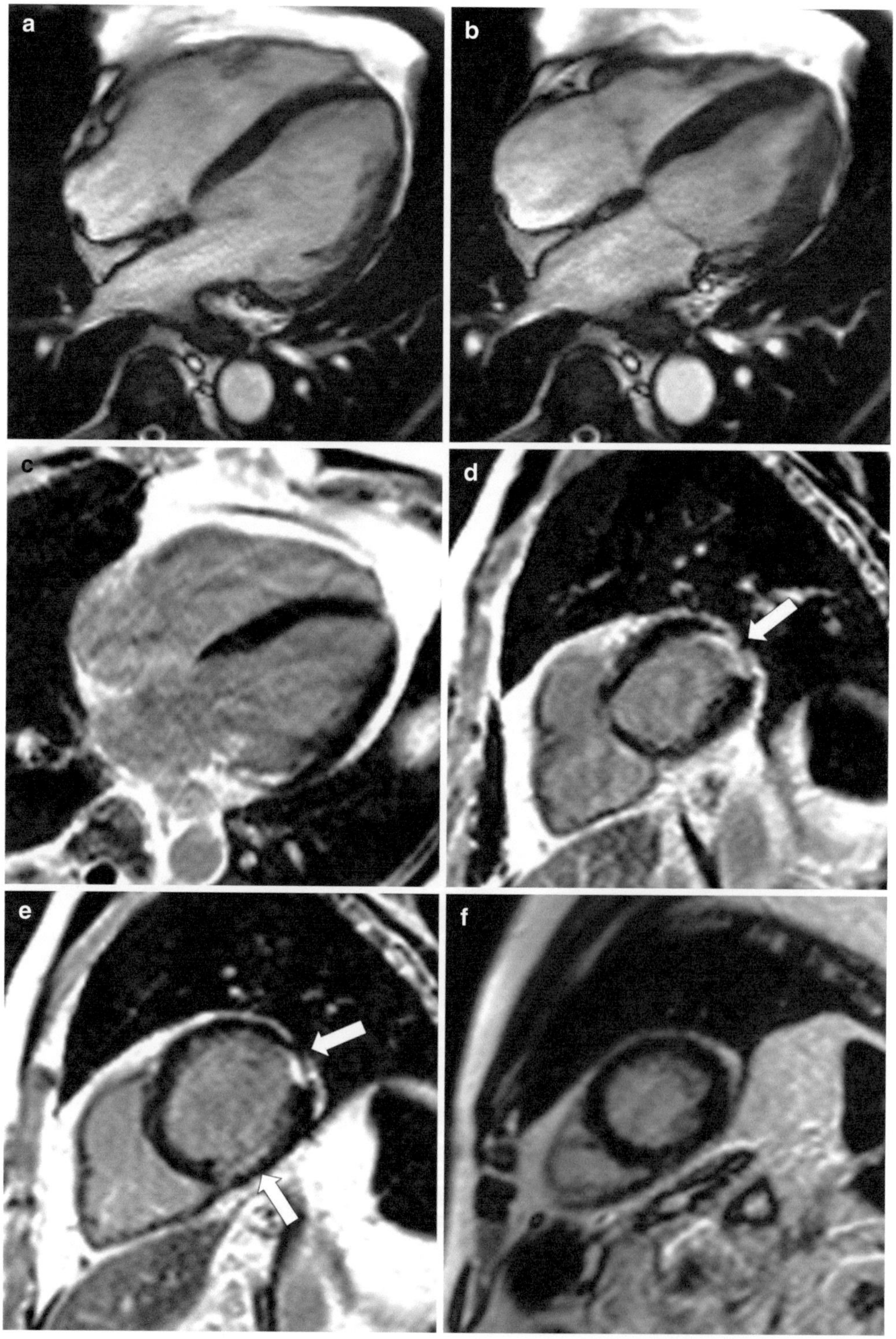

Fig. 3.9 CMR, showing ischemic pattern of LGE due to underlying coronary artery disease (CAD). a: 4-chamber cine image at end diastole. b: 4-chamber cine image at end systole showing mildly reduced LVEF and normal RVEF. c: 4-chamber LGE image showing sub-endocardial LGE in the basal lateral segment. d: Basal short axis LGE image showing sub-endocardial LGE in the anterolateral segment. e: Mid short axis LGE image showing sub-endocardial LGE in the anterolateral and inferior segments. f: Apical short axis LGE image showing no LGE

Case 10

An 80-year-old-female with CAD treated with percutaneous coronary intervention to the right coronary artery 10 years ago and moderate aortic stenosis had breast cancer treated with left mastectomy and trastuzumab therapy. The initial plan for chemotherapy was 12 months of trastuzumab, but therapy was stopped during the tenth month due to an abnormal MUGA that showed a LVEF of 43%. A CMR was ordered to evaluate the etiology of cardiomyopathy and it showed LVEF of 53% and basal inferior LGE in a subendocardial pattern in the right coronary artery territory, consistent with a myocardial infarction in the RCA territory (Fig. 3.10). While CMR showed a myocardial infarction, the LVEF was not as low as demonstrated by the MUGA, and the patient was able to resume the trastuzumab therapy to complete 12 months of therapy without any further incidents.

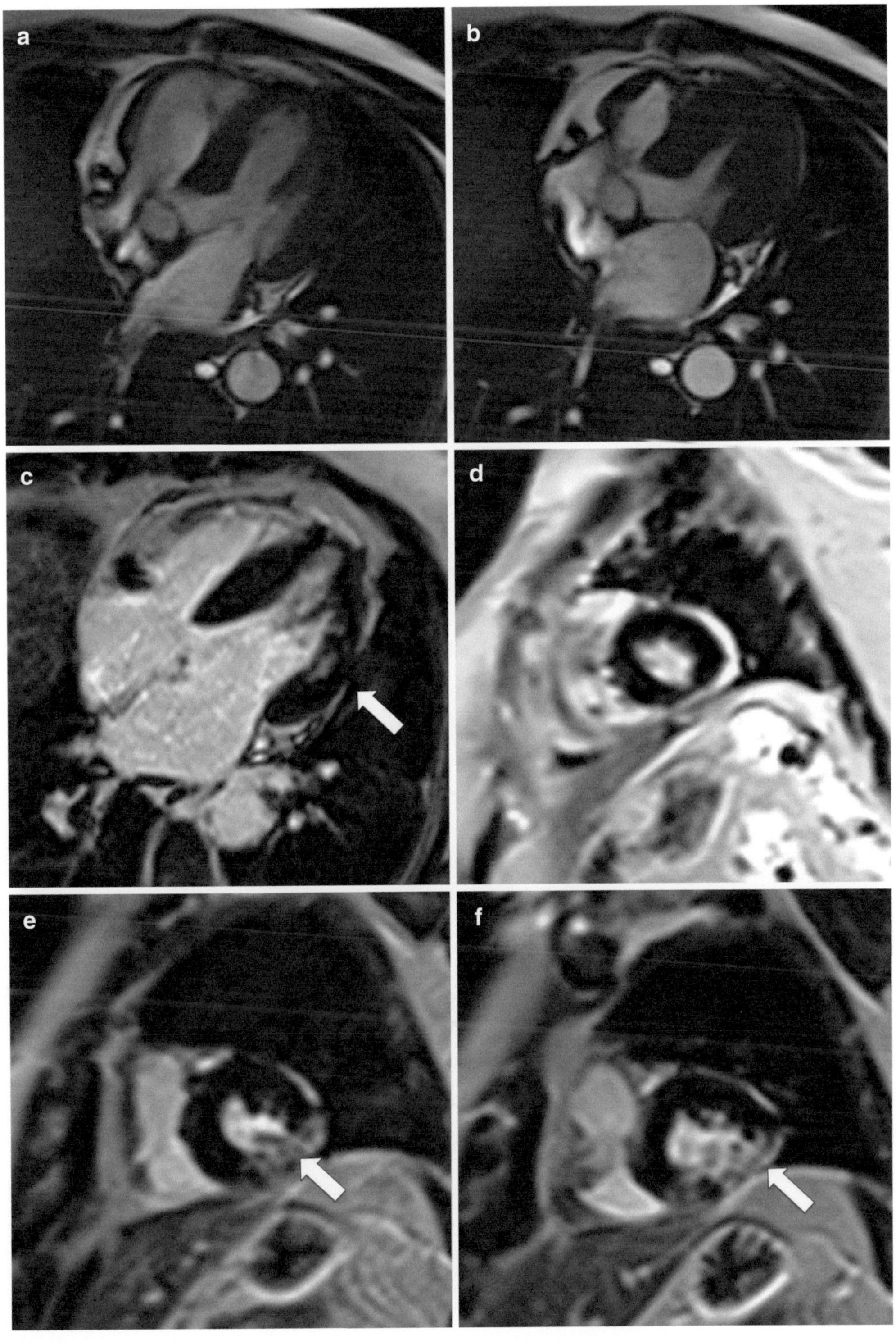

Fig. 3.10 CMR showing myocardial infarction in the RCA territory. a: 4-chamber cine image at end diastole. b: 4-chamber cine image at end systole showing a LVEF of 53%. c: 4-chamber LGE image showing sub-endocardial LGE in the mid inferolateral segment. d: Basal short axis LGE image showing and no scar. e: Mid short axis LGE image showing transmural LGE in the inferior and inferolateral segments. f: Apical short axis LGE image showing LGE in the inferior and lateral segments

Discussion

Pre-existing CAD is a risk factor for anthracycline and trastuzumab-related cardiotoxicity. Pre-treatment evaluation by CMR in high-risk patients can identify patients with myocardial scar from myocardial infarction or other causes, which predicts a higher risk for subsequent cardiotoxicity.

Case 11

A 70-year-old-female had Hodgkin lymphoma 40 years ago treated with anthracycline-based chemotherapy and mantle radiation therapy. Echocardiography revealed an abnormal LVEF that led to a CMR. The CMR showed LVEF of 44%, RVEF of 54%, moderate aortic insufficiency, mitral stenosis, mild mitral insufficiency and mild tricuspid insufficiency (Fig. 3.11). Figure 3.11, shows the mitral valve disease in this patient.

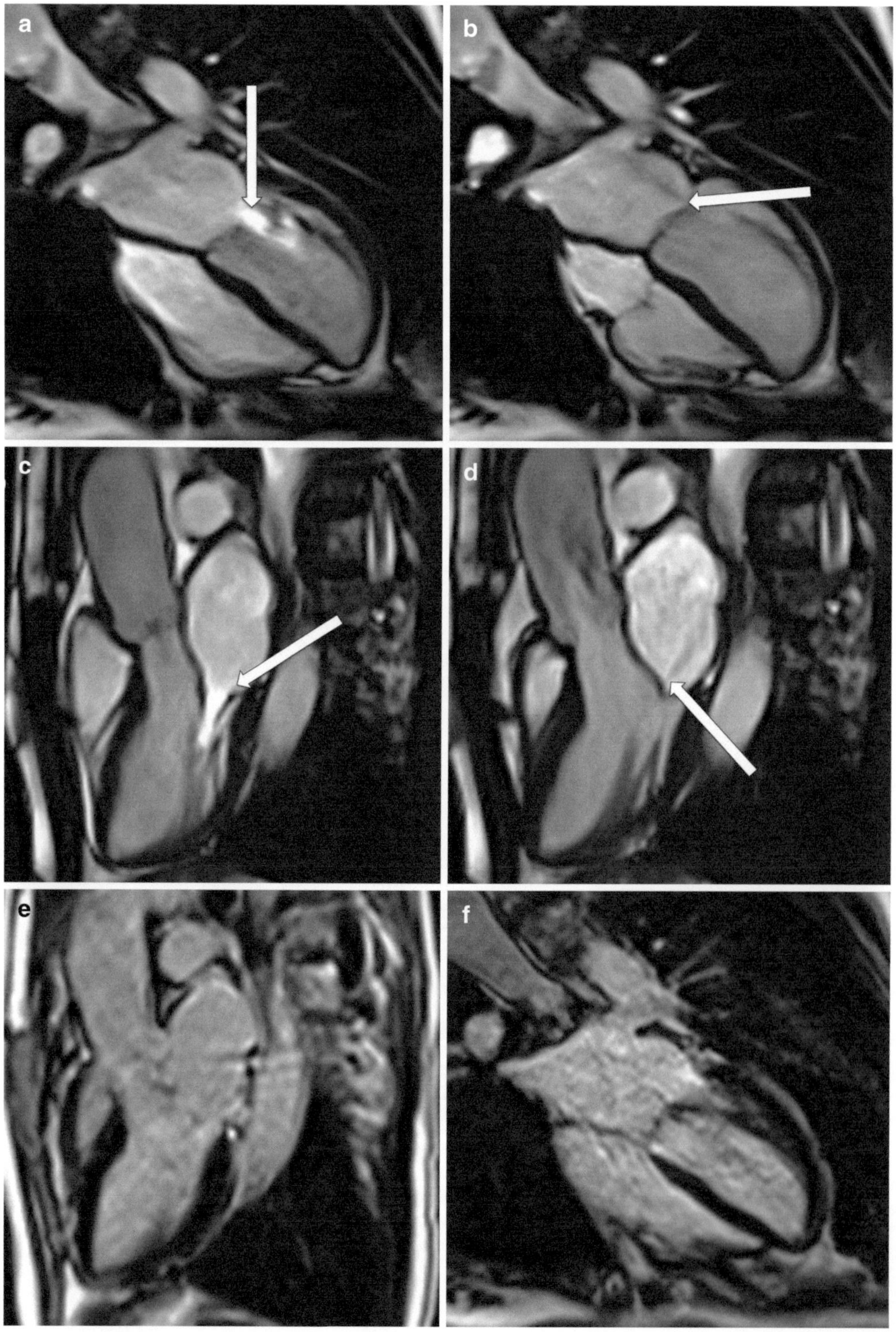

Fig. 3.11 CMR, showing valvular disease. a: 4-chamber cine image at early diastole showing flow acceleration across the mitral valve consistent with mitral stenosis. b: 4-chamber cine image at mid systole showing a regurgitant jet across the mitral valve consistent with mitral regurgitation. c: 3-chamber cine image at early diastole showing flow acceleration across the mitral valve consistent with mitral stenosis. d: 3-chamber cine image at mid systole showing a regurgitant jet across the mitral valve consistent with mitral regurgitation. e: 3-chamber LGE image showing no fibrosis f: 4-chamber LGE image showing no fibrosis

Discussion

While echocardiography is the first-line modality for evaluation of valvular dysfunction, CMR can also provide information on the presence or absence of valvular heart disease, and the severity of the valvular dysfunction using flow CMR [17].

Case 12

A 54-year-old female with myelodysplastic syndrome that progressed to acute myeloid leukemia, treated with bone marrow transplantation with subsequent relapse was being treated with a regimen that included brentuximab, an antibody-drug conjugate, when she was referred to cardiology for evaluation because a troponin was checked prior to haplo-natural killer cell therapy and was found to be elevated. The CMR showed LVEF of 53%, RVEF of 53% and epicardial LGE in the basal lateral and inferior segments, consistent with myocarditis (Fig. 3.12).

Discussion

Potential etiologies of cardiomyopathy that may be more prevalent in cancer patients than the general population include

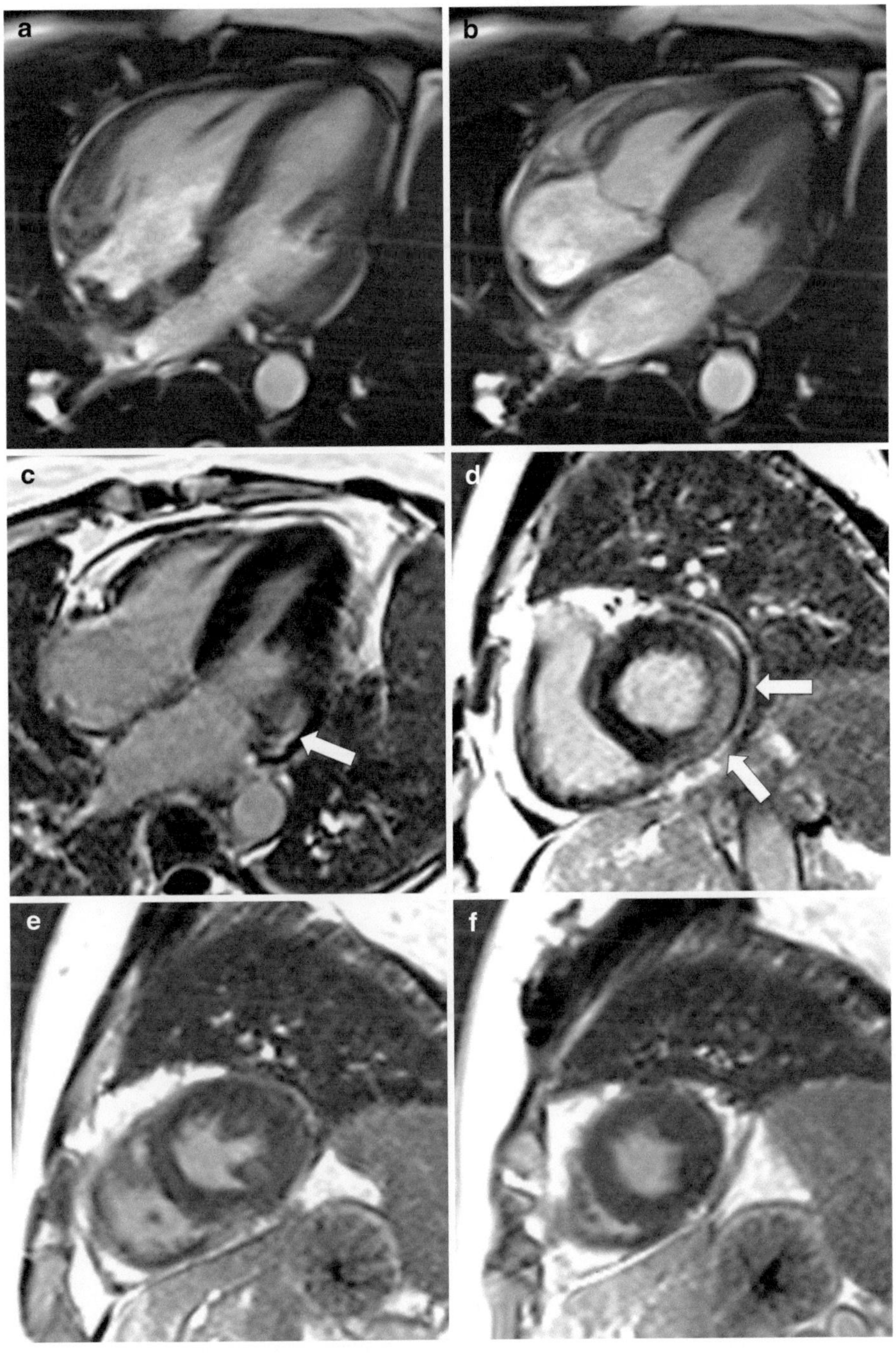

Fig. 3.12 Cardiac Magnetic Resonance (CMR) imaging, showing Myocardits: a: 4-chamber cine image at end diastole. b: 4-chamber cine image at end systole showing mildly reduced LVEF and RVEF of 53%. c: 4 chamber LGE image showing epicardial LGE in the basal lateral segment. d: Basal short axis LGE image showing epicardial LGE in the lateral and inferior segments. e: Mid short axis LGE image showing no scar. f: Apical short axis LGE image showing no scar

myocarditis, as a toxic manifestation of cyclophosphamide [18] or more recently, of immune checkpoint inhibitors [19], stress cardiomyopathy and cardiac amyloidosis. Myocarditis typically has an epicardial, multifocal pattern of LGE, with mid-myocardial LGE also prevalent. Stress cardiomyopathy typically has no LGE. Cardiac amyloidosis has a spectrum from global sub-endocardial to global transmural LGE.

Identification of Intracardiac Thrombus

Case 13

A 52-year-old male with diffuse large B-cell lymphoma treated with anthracycline-based chemotherapy was found to have abnormal LVEF on surveillance echocardiography. A CMR performed for further evaluation of the cardiomyopathy revealed LVEF of 25%, RVEF of 36% and no LGE, consistent with a non-ischemic cardiomyopathy, likely anthracycline-related cardiotoxicity. Also noted was a LV apical thrombus measuring 1.7 cm × 1.5 cm × 1.1 cm (Fig. 3.13).

Discussion

Cancer patients are at an increased risk for intracardiac thrombi due to the frequent use of central venous catheters and the hypercoagulable milieu associated with cancer.

CMR is very sensitive for identification of intracardiac thrombus and LGE CMR using the "long inversion time"

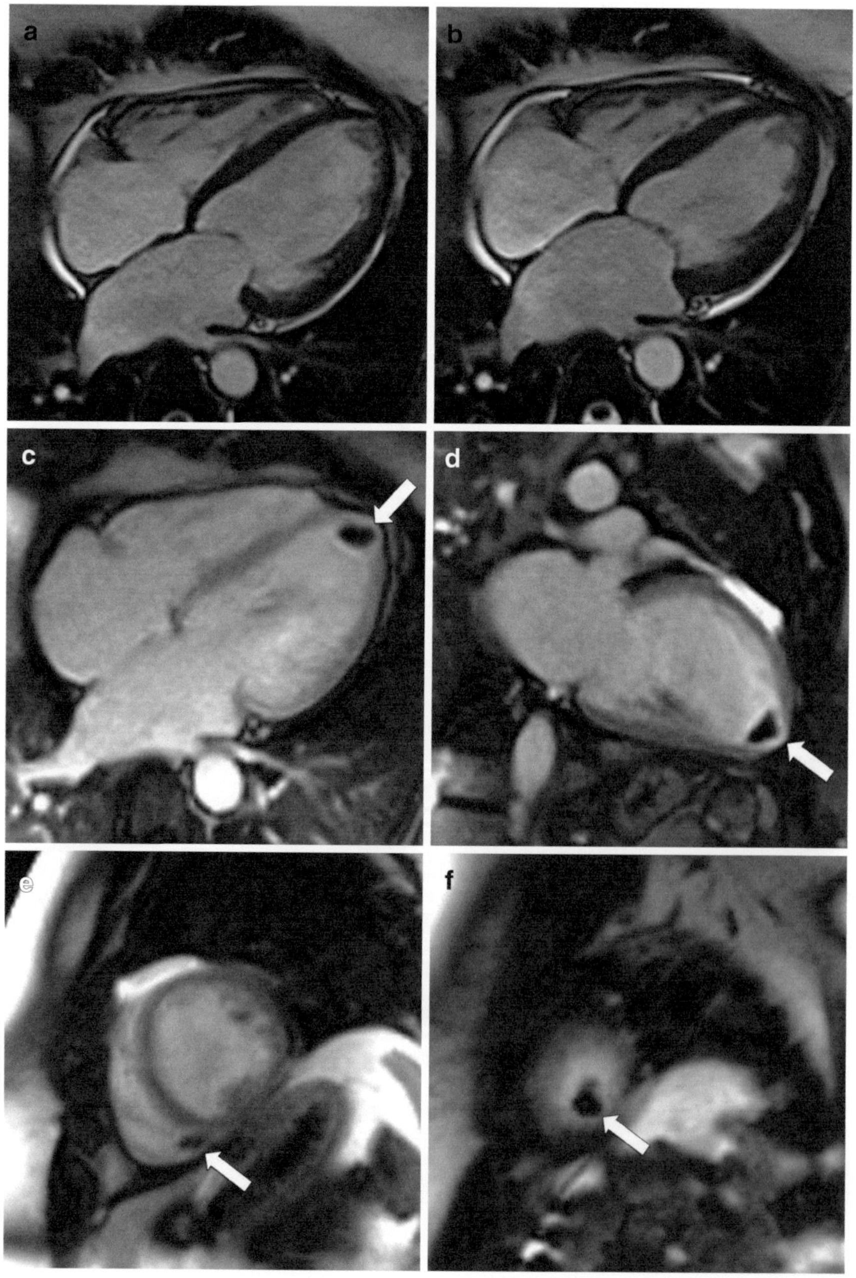

Fig. 3.13 CMR, showing findings of non-ischemic cardiomyopathy with intra-cardiac and LV apical thrombus. a: 4-chamber cine image at end diastole. b: 4-chamber cine image at end systole showing severely reduced LVEF and moderately reduced RVEF. c: 4-chamber long-TI LGE image showing an apical thrombus measuring 1.7 cm × 1.5 cm × 1.1 cm. d: 2-chamber long-TI LGE image showing the apical thrombus. e: Mid short axis long-TI LGE image showing a small inferior RV thrombus. f: Apical short axis long-TI LGE image showing the apical LV thrombus

technique is now considered the gold standard for evaluation of intracardiac thrombus [20, 21].

Case 14

A 35-year-old-male with Hodgkin lymphoma was treated with an anthracycline-based regimen, and eventually underwent autologous stem cell transplantation. A CMR was performed after abnormal LV function was noted on echocardiogram and showed LVEF of 40%, RVEF of 48% and a non-mobile mass (thrombus) attached to the inferior right atrial wall near the junction of the right atrium and the inferior vena cava, measuring 2.3 cm × 1.7 cm × 1.6 cm in close proximity to the tip of a catheter in the right atrium (Fig. 3.14).

Discussion

Due to CMR's ability to characterize tissue accurately, it can distinguish between cardiac tumors, foreign bodies such as catheters and cardiac thrombi with high precision.

Emerging Applications of CMR

Case 15

A patient with breast cancer receiving adjuvant trastuzumab therapy was referred with concern of cardiotoxicity. The LVEF by CMR was 54%. Myocardial strain analysis was performed using a feature-tracking algorithm. The peak

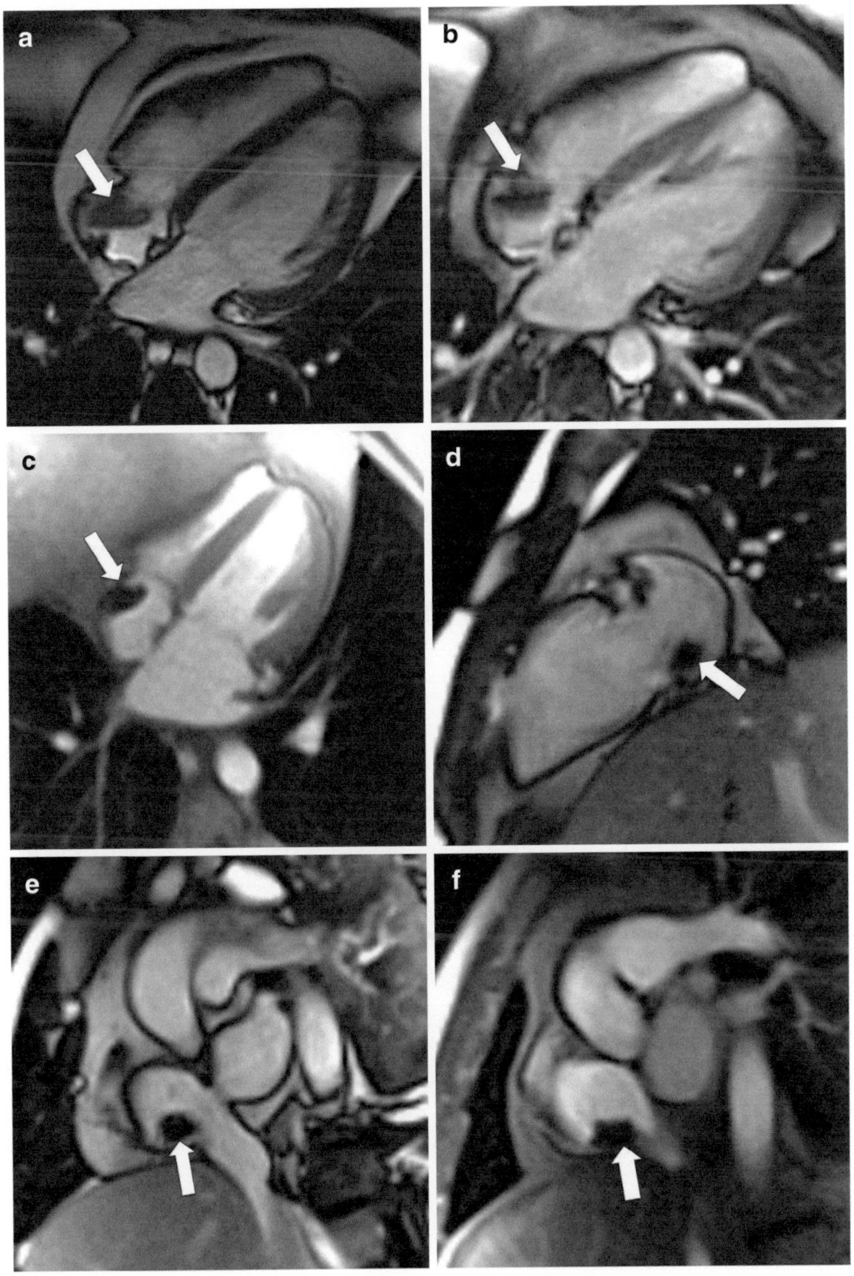

Fig. 3.14 CMR, showing a non-mobile mass attached to the right atrial wall. a: 4-chamber cine image at end diastole showing a mass in the right atrium. b: 4-chamber cine image at end systole showing mildly reduced LVEF and mildly reduced RVEF. c: 4-chamber long-TI LGE image showing a right atrial thrombus measuring 2.3 cm × 1.7 cm × 1.6 cm. d: 2-chamber long TI LGE image showing the right atrial thrombus. E: Short axis long TI LGE image at the level of the right atrium and inferior vena cava junction showing the right atrial thrombus. f: Short axis long TI LGE image at the level of the right atrium showing the right atrial thrombus

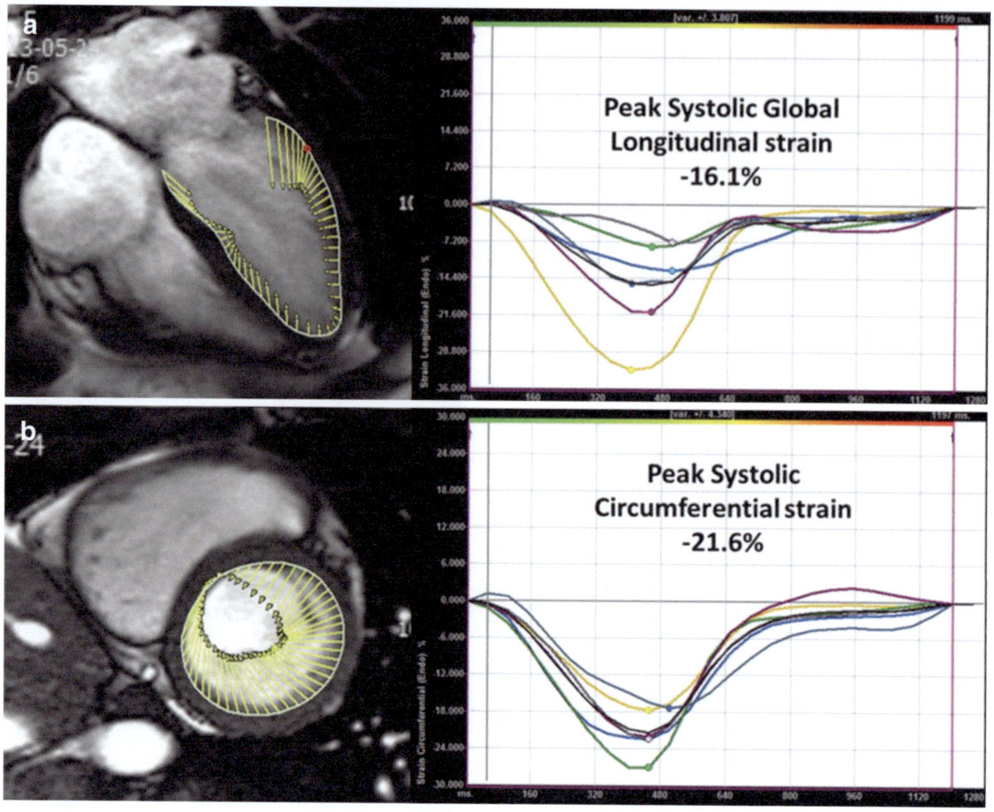

Fig. 3.15 Myocardial strain analysis. a: Assessment of longitudinal strain from a 4-chamber cine image. b: Assessment of circumferential strain from a short axis cine image (reproduced with permission from Thavendiranathan et al. [22])

systolic global longitudinal strain was mildly reduced (Fig. 3.15; top panel), whereas circumferential strain was in the normal range (Fig. 3.15; bottom panel). Yellow arrows (left) represent velocity vectors; curves represent strain measurements in each of the myocardial segments (six segments) and a global curve (black). Figure and descriptions reproduced with permission from Thavendiranathan et al. [22].

Discussion

Early reduction in myocardial strain or strain rate using echocardiography has been shown to predict subsequent cardiotoxicity. Similarly, CMR-based techniques evaluating strain are currently being studied for the early identification of injury and prediction of subsequent cardiotoxicity [22].

Case 16

A 50-year-old female with breast cancer received T_1 mapping as part of a clinical study for the prediction of cardiotoxicity using CMR. The LVEF and RVEF were normal and the LGE images showed no fibrosis. The ECV was normal at 29% (Fig. 3.16).

Discussion

T_1 mapping is a relatively new technique that can be used to detect subclinical pathophysiologic processes that influence cardiac function, manifesting as an increase in extracellular volume (ECV). Potential mechanisms for increase in the ECV after anthracycline therapy include inflammation and edema (in the short-term) and interstitial fibrosis (in the short and long terms). This technique holds great promise for advances in the prediction, early diagnosis and prognostication of cancer treatment-related cardiomyopathy [23–25].

Case 17

A 62-year-old female with breast cancer had aortic stiffness evaluation by CMR as part of a clinical study for the prediction of cardiotoxicity using CMR (Fig. 3.17). Both aortic distensibility and aortic pulse wave velocity were normal.

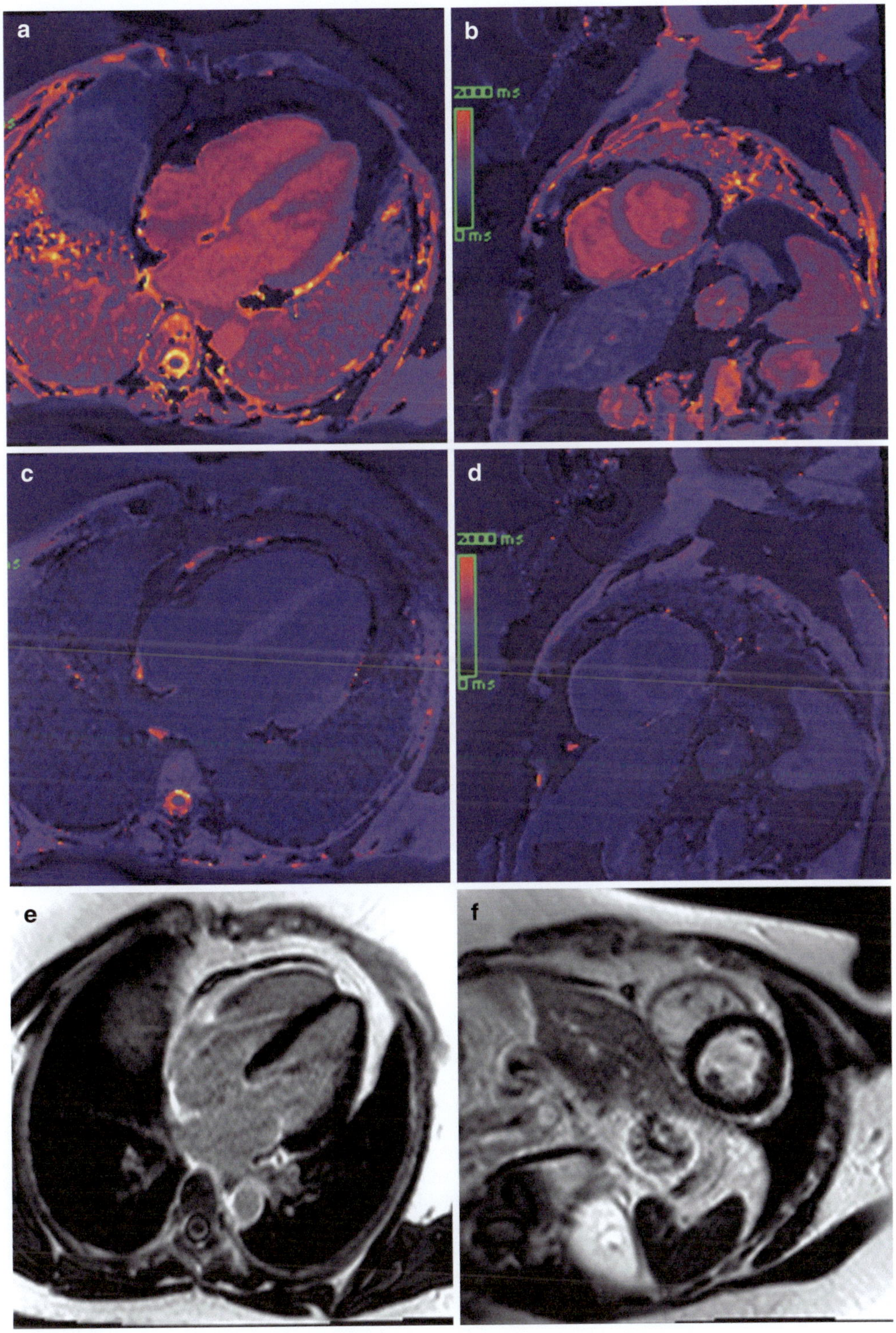

Fig. 3.16 CMR with T_1 mapping. a: Color map of 4-chamber image for pre-contrast T_1 mapping. b: Color map of mid short axis image for pre-contrast T_1 mapping. c. Color map of 4-chamber image for post-contrast T_1 mapping. d: Color map of mid short axis image for post-contrast T_1 mapping. e: 4-chamber LGE image showing no scar. f: Mid short axis LGE image showing no scar

Discussion

In two studies examining the impact of anthracycline therapy on aortic stiffness measured by CMR, patients receiving anthracyclines for breast or hematologic malignancies had a significant increase in pulse wave velocity and decrease in ascending aortic distensibility between baseline and 4 and 6 months [26, 27]. These studies demonstrate that aortic stiffness has the potential to be used as an early predictor of cardiotoxicity.

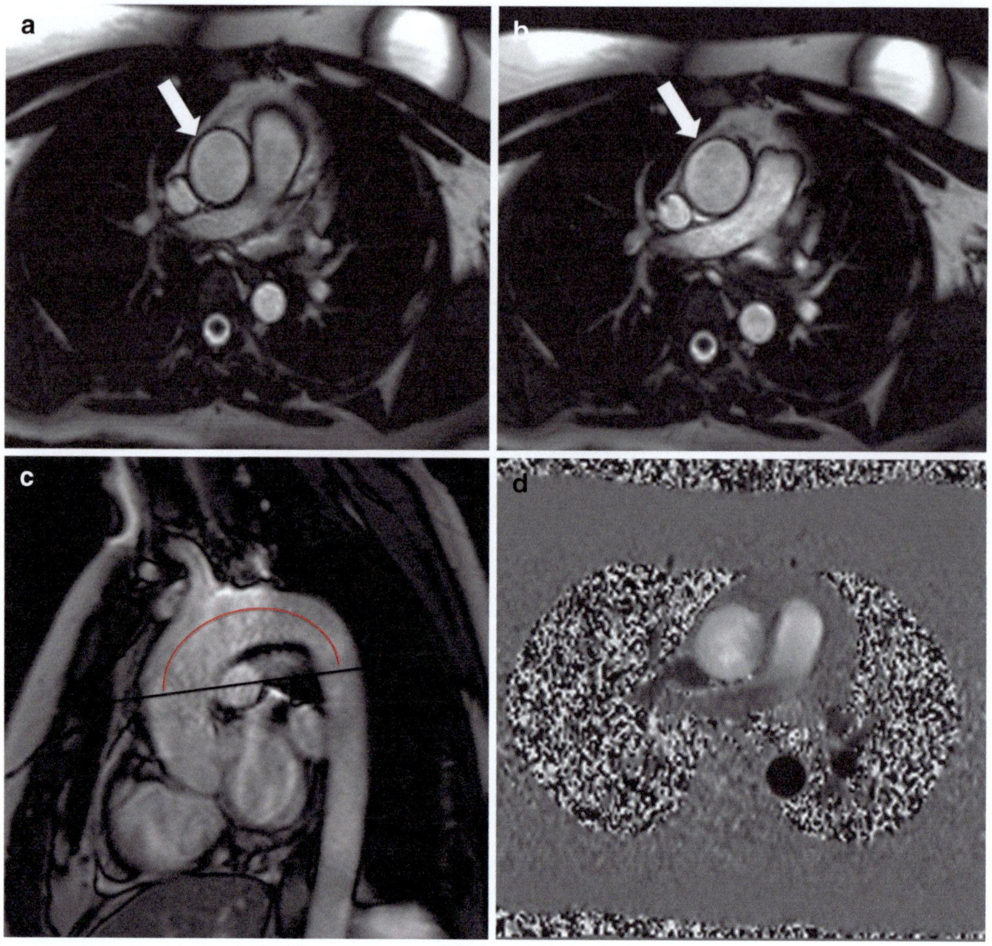

Fig. 3.17 Aortic stiffness evaluation by Cardiac magnetic resonance (CMR) imaging. a: Axial cine image of the ascending and descending aorta in diastole. b: Axial cine image of the ascending and descending aorta in systole demonstrating aortic distensibility. c: Measurement of the distance between ascending and descending thoracic aorta by tracing the centerline of the aortic lumen for calculation of aortic pulse wave velocity. d: Flow CMR image across the ascending and descending aorta at the level of the pulmonary artery for calculation of aortic pulse wave velocity

References

1. Bellenger NG, Burgess MI, Ray SG, et al. Comparison of left ventricular ejection fraction and volumes in heart failure by echocardiography, radionuclide ventriculography and cardiovascular magnetic resonance; are they interchangeable? Eur Heart J. 2000;21:1387–96.
2. Farber NJ, Reddy ST, Doyle M, et al. Ex vivo cardiovascular magnetic resonance measurements of right and left ventricular mass compared with direct mass measurement in excised hearts after transplantation: a first human SSFP comparison. J Cardiovasc Magn Reson. 2014;16:74.
3. Armstrong GT, Plana JC, Zhang N, et al. Screening adult survivors of childhood cancer for cardiomyopathy: comparison of echocardiography and cardiac magnetic resonance imaging. J Clin Oncol. 2012;30:2876–84.
4. Neilan TG, Coelho-Filho OR, Pena-Herrera D, et al. Left ventricular mass in patients with a cardiomyopathy after treatment with anthracyclines. Am J Cardiol. 2012;110:1679–86.
5. Huang H, Nijjar PS, Misialek JR, et al. Accuracy of left ventricular ejection fraction by contemporary multiple gated acquisition scanning in patients with cancer: comparison with cardiovascular magnetic resonance. J Cardiovasc Magn Reson. 2017;19:34.
6. Pennell DJ. Cardiovascular magnetic resonance. Circulation. 2010;121:692–705.
7. Ylanen K, Poutanen T, Savikurki-Heikkila P, Rinta-Kiikka I, Eerola A, Vettenranta K. Cardiac magnetic resonance imaging in the evaluation of the late effects of anthracyclines among long-term survivors of childhood cancer. J Am Coll Cardiol. 2013;61:1539–47.
8. Grover S, Leong DP, Chakrabarty A, et al. Left and right ventricular effects of anthracycline and trastuzumab chemotherapy: a prospective study using novel cardiac imaging and biochemical markers. Int J Cardiol. 2013;168:5465–7.
9. Calleja A, Poulin F, Khorolsky C, et al. Right ventricular dysfunction in patients experiencing cardiotoxicity during breast cancer therapy. J Oncol. 2015;2015:609194.
10. Christiansen JR, Massey R, Dalen H, et al. Right ventricular function in long-term adult survivors of childhood lymphoma and acute lymphoblastic leukaemia. Eur Heart J Cardiovasc Imaging. 2016;17:735–41.
11. Boczar KE, Aseyev O, Sulpher J, et al. Right heart function deteriorates in breast cancer patients undergoing anthracycline-based chemotherapy. Echo Res Pract. 2016;3:79–84.
12. Murbraech K, Holte E, Broch K, et al. Impaired right ventricular function in long-term lymphoma survivors. J Am Soc Echocardiogr. 2016;29:528–36.
13. Abdar Esfahani M, Mokarian F, Karimipanah M. Alterations in the echocardiographic variables of the right ventricle in asymptomatic patients with breast cancer during anthracycline chemotherapy. Postgrad Med J. 2017;93:271–4.
14. Ostenfeld E, Flachskampf FA. Assessment of right ventricular volumes and ejection fraction by echocardiography: from geometric approximations to realistic shapes. Echo Res Pract. 2015;2:R1–11.
15. Senthilkumar A, Majmudar MD, Shenoy C, Kim HW, Kim RJ. Identifying the etiology: a systematic approach using delayed-

enhancement cardiovascular magnetic resonance. Heart Fail Clin. 2009;5:349–67, vi.
16. Felker GM, Thompson RE, Hare JM, et al. Underlying causes and long-term survival in patients with initially unexplained cardiomyopathy. N Engl J Med. 2000;342:1077–84.
17. Zoghbi WA, Adams D, Bonow RO, et al. Recommendations for noninvasive evaluation of native valvular regurgitation: a report from the American Society of Echocardiography Developed in Collaboration with the Society for Cardiovascular Magnetic Resonance. J Am Soc Echocardiogr. 2017;30(4):303–71.
18. Yeh ET, Bickford CL. Cardiovascular complications of cancer therapy: incidence, pathogenesis, diagnosis, and management. J Am Coll Cardiol. 2009;53:2231–47.
19. Johnson DB, Balko JM, Compton ML, et al. Fulminant myocarditis with combination immune checkpoint blockade. N Engl J Med. 2016;375:1749–55.
20. Weinsaft JW, Kim HW, Shah DJ, et al. Detection of left ventricular thrombus by delayed-enhancement cardiovascular magnetic resonance prevalence and markers in patients with systolic dysfunction. J Am Coll Cardiol. 2008;52:148–57.
21. Kitkungvan D, Nabi F, Ghosn MG, et al. Detection of LA and LAA thrombus by CMR in patients referred for pulmonary vein isolation. JACC Cardiovasc Imaging. 2016;9:809–18.
22. Thavendiranathan P, Wintersperger BJ, Flamm SD, Marwick TH. Cardiac MRI in the assessment of cardiac injury and toxicity from cancer chemotherapy: a systematic review. Circ Cardiovasc Imaging. 2013;6:1080–91.
23. Jordan JH, Vasu S, Morgan TM, et al. Anthracycline-associated T1 mapping characteristics are elevated independent of the presence of cardiovascular comorbidities in cancer survivors. Circ Cardiovasc Imaging. 2016;9:e004325.
24. Jordan JH, D'Agostino RB Jr, Hamilton CA, et al. Longitudinal assessment of concurrent changes in left ventricular ejection fraction and left ventricular myocardial tissue characteristics after administration of cardiotoxic chemotherapies using T1-weighted and T2-weighted cardiovascular magnetic resonance. Circ Cardiovasc Imaging. 2014;7:872–9.
25. Melendez GC, Hundley WG. Is myocardial fibrosis a new Frontier for discovery in cardiotoxicity related to the administration of anthracyclines? Circ Cardiovasc Imaging. 2016;9:e005797.
26. Drafts BC, Twomley KM, D'Agostino R Jr, et al. Low to moderate dose anthracycline-based chemotherapy is associated with early noninvasive imaging evidence of subclinical cardiovascular disease. JACC Cardiovasc Imaging. 2013;6:877–85.
27. Chaosuwannakit N, D'Agostino R Jr, Hamilton CA, et al. Aortic stiffness increases upon receipt of anthracycline chemotherapy. J Clin Oncol. 2010;28:166–72.

4 Imaging to Diagnose Myocarditis, Cardiomyopathy, Tumor and Thrombus

Sujethra Vasu and W. Gregory Hundley

Abstract

Patients with cancer and concomitant cardiovascular disease frequently need various imaging investigations to arrive at a correct diagnosis.

In this chapter we provide some illustrative cases and briefly discuss the pertinent imaging findings in patients with myocarditis, myocardial infarction, cardiac mass and cardiomyopathy.

Keywords

Myocarditis • Cardiomyopathy • Cardiac mass

Case 1: What Is the Reason for the Elevated Troponin?

(a) A 48 year old man with limited stage small cell lung cancer, receiving chemotherapy presented with chest pain. The 12 lead ECG was normal but the troponin was elevated to 13.0 ng/L Left ventricular (LV) systolic function was normal with an LV ejection fraction (EF) of 55%. Due to normal ECG and clinical presentation the possibility of myocarditis was raised. A cardiac magnetic resonance (CMR) imaging was done, which showed distal left anterior descending (LAD) artery territory infarction without significant ischemia in the remaining LAD territory (Figs. 4.1 and 4.2). A diagnosis of myocardial infarction was made and patient discharged on aspirin, statin and ACE inhibitors. A coronary angiogram was not done given the inability to continue uninterrupted dual antiplatelet therapy.

(b) A 21 year old male, with symptoms suggestive of an upper respiratory illness presented with acute chest pain and was found to have troponin elevation to 32 ng/mL. Coronary CT angiography (CTA) was done which confirmed normal origin of coronary arteries and no evidence of coronary artery disease. CMR was done to assess for myocarditis, which showed findings consistent with myocarditis (Fig. 4.3). Below are short axis images which showed subepicardial scar involving the inferolateral and anterolateral segments. Both these segments also had markedly elevated T2 values suggesting this is an acute process (T2 values of 70 ms, normal 45–50 ms).

Teaching points

1. CMR is valuable in identifying infarct pattern from myocarditis. This has therapeutic implications particularly in cancer patients who have high bleeding risks.
2. Myocardial infarction produces a pattern which is either subendocardial or transmural scar. Due to the wave front phenomenon of myocardial injury, the subendocardium is most sensitive to ischemia and is susceptible to infarction. In contrast other myocardial processes that do not involve coronary involvement lead to "subepicardial" scar patterns and furthermore not confined to a coronary territory. T2 mapping has been established as a method to identify acute myocarditis and has been validated in studies that have also used endomyocardial biopsy to establish diagnoses of myocarditis [1, 2].

S. Vasu, M.B.B.S. (✉) • W.G. Hundley, M.D., F.A.C.C., F.A.H.A.
Section on Cardiology, Wake Forest University School of Medicine, Winston-Salem, NC 27157, USA
e-mail: svasu@wakehealth.edu

S.W. Yusuf, J. Banchs (eds.), *Cancer and Cardiovascular Disease*, https://doi.org/10.1007/978-3-319-62088-6_4

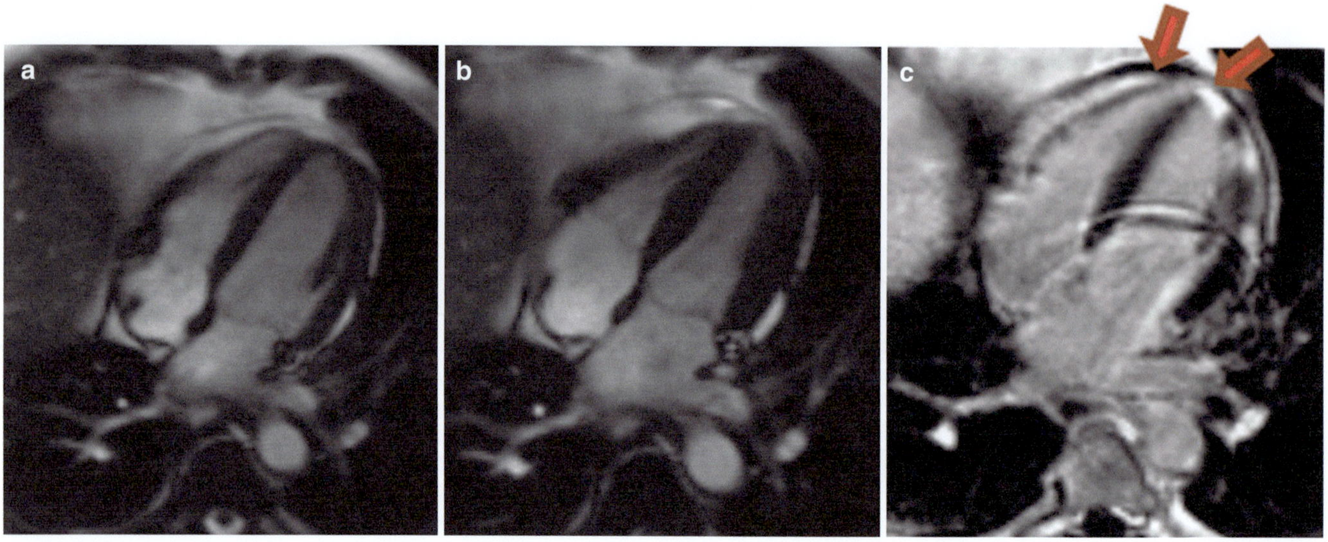

Fig. 4.1 (**a**) (Diastolic frame) and (**b**) (Systolic frame): Apical 4 chamber view of the heart shows normal wall thickening of the all segments. Figure (**c**) shows focal myocardial infarction of the apical anterolateral wall (*red arrows*)

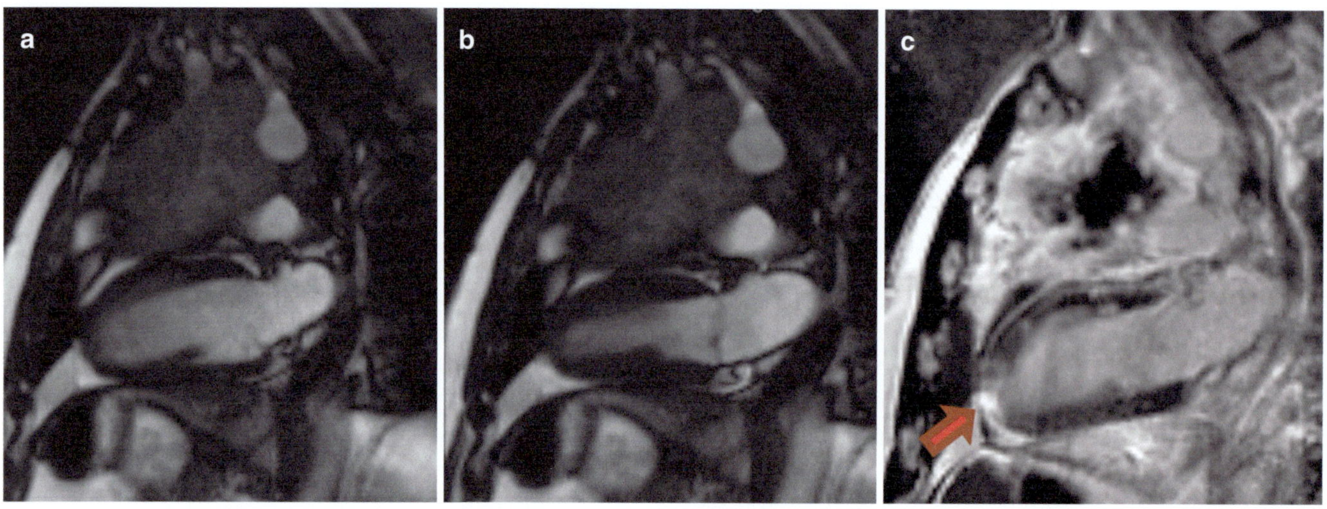

Fig. 4.2 (**a**) (Diastolic frame) and (**b**) (Systolic frame): Apical 2 chamber view of the heart shows normal wall thickening of the all segments. Figure (**c**) shows focal myocardial infarction of the apical anterior wall (*red arrow*)

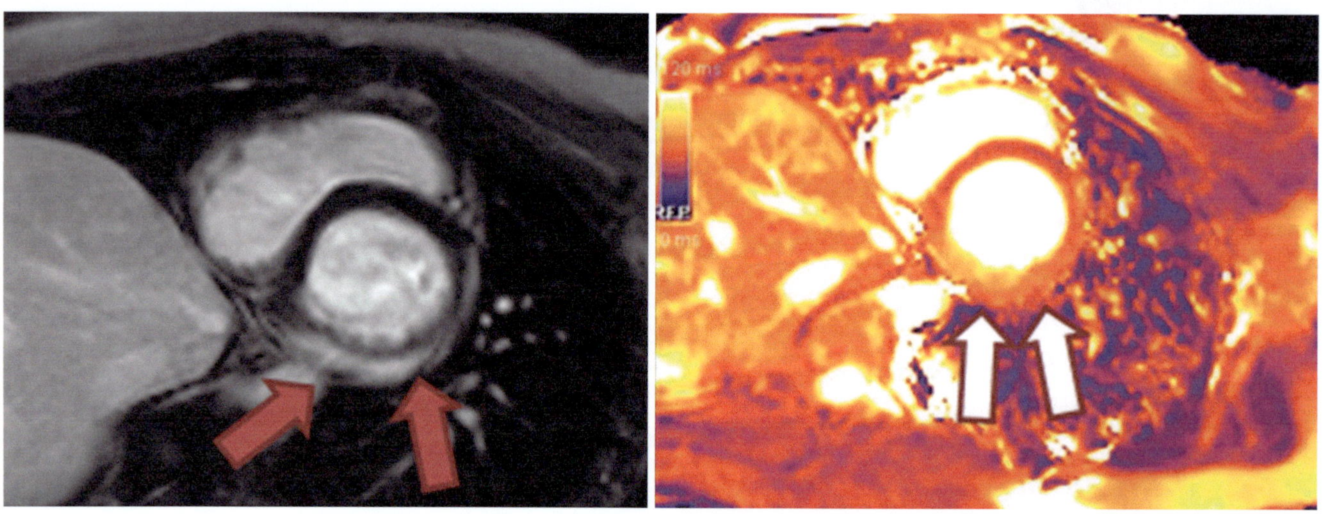

Fig. 4.3 CMR showing findings of Myocarditis. Short axis images showing subepicardial scar involving the inferolateral and anterolateral segments. Both these segments also had markedly elevated T2 values suggesting this is an acute process, (T2 values of 70 ms, normal 45–50 ms)

Case 2: What Is This Mass?

A 59 year old female, with history of atrial fibrillation, mitral regurgitation and a rapidly growing mass in the left forearm presented with worsening fatigue. In the emergency department a CT angiogram was done which revealed two left atrial masses. A transthoracic echocardiogram (TTE) showed a hypoechoic mobile mass in the left atrium, which was 2.8 × 2.5 cm in size (Fig. 4.4). A cardiac MRI was done to differentiate between tumor and thrombus. The cardiac MRI showed two masses, one in the left atrial appendage and the other in the left atrium (Figs. 4.5 and 4.6). The left atrial mass was bright on T2 weighted images, bright on fat saturation, with no evidence of perfusion. Also on post contrast delayed enhancement imaging, it was hypointense. Further confirmation of thrombus was noted, with T1 time of 600 ms. Given the appearance of the bright mass on steady state free precession images (SSFP) images, cystic transformation of a thrombus was the most likely explanation. Further workup including a biopsy of the lesion in her forearm was recommended, but the patient declined.

Teaching points

1. CMR is valuable in identifying whether a mass is a tumor or a thrombus. It can also easily distinguish benign tumors such as lipomas. Using a variety of techniques from T1 and T2 characterization, perfusion and dynamic changes after contrast administration along with T1 and T2 mapping, we can accurately characterize a mass.

Using contrast echocardiography, a filling defect confirms a mass. A mass in the setting of adjacent myocardial akinesis is most likely to be a thrombus. However using MRI, the tissue characteristics of the mass i.e. fat, cyst or thrombus can be accurately assessed using T1 and T2 weighted sequences and its change after gadolinium administration provides clues regarding perfusion of the mass [3]. MRI can demonstrate the lack of vascular perfusion of a thrombus using first pass perfusion sequences. In addition, T2 and T1 mapping can identify thrombi based on tissue characterization. For example, an inversion time, to null thrombus specifically, i.e. 600 ms, in a delayed enhancement image, can accurately differentiate thrombus from other masses i.e. myxoma [4].

Case 3: What Is the Reason for the Persistent Lower Extremity Edema?

A 34 year old man with 6 months of abdominal bloating, diarrhea initially diagnosed as irritable bowel syndrome but eventually found to have stage 4 neuroendocrine tumor of the pancreas with liver metastasis and presented to the clinic with progressive lower extremity swelling. Examination revealed a holosystolic murmur in the tricuspid area, which increased with inspiration. A TTE showed moderate tricuspid regurgitation and normal RV size and function, with significant increase in the tricuspid regurgitation relative to a TTE done 6 months ago (Figs. 4.7, 4.8 and 4.9). He also had

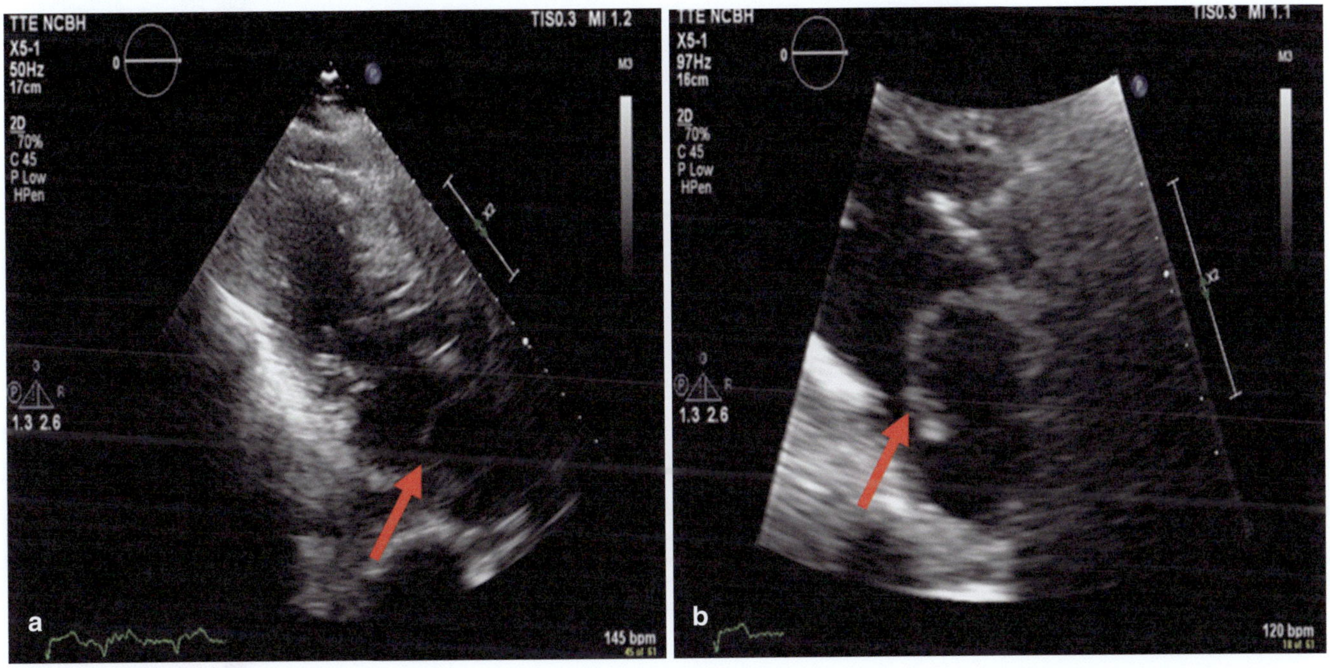

Fig. 4.4 (**a**) (Apical 3 chamber) and (**b**) (Magnified frame of the prior image). The images show a cystic mass in the left atrium. The *red arrow* points to the mass

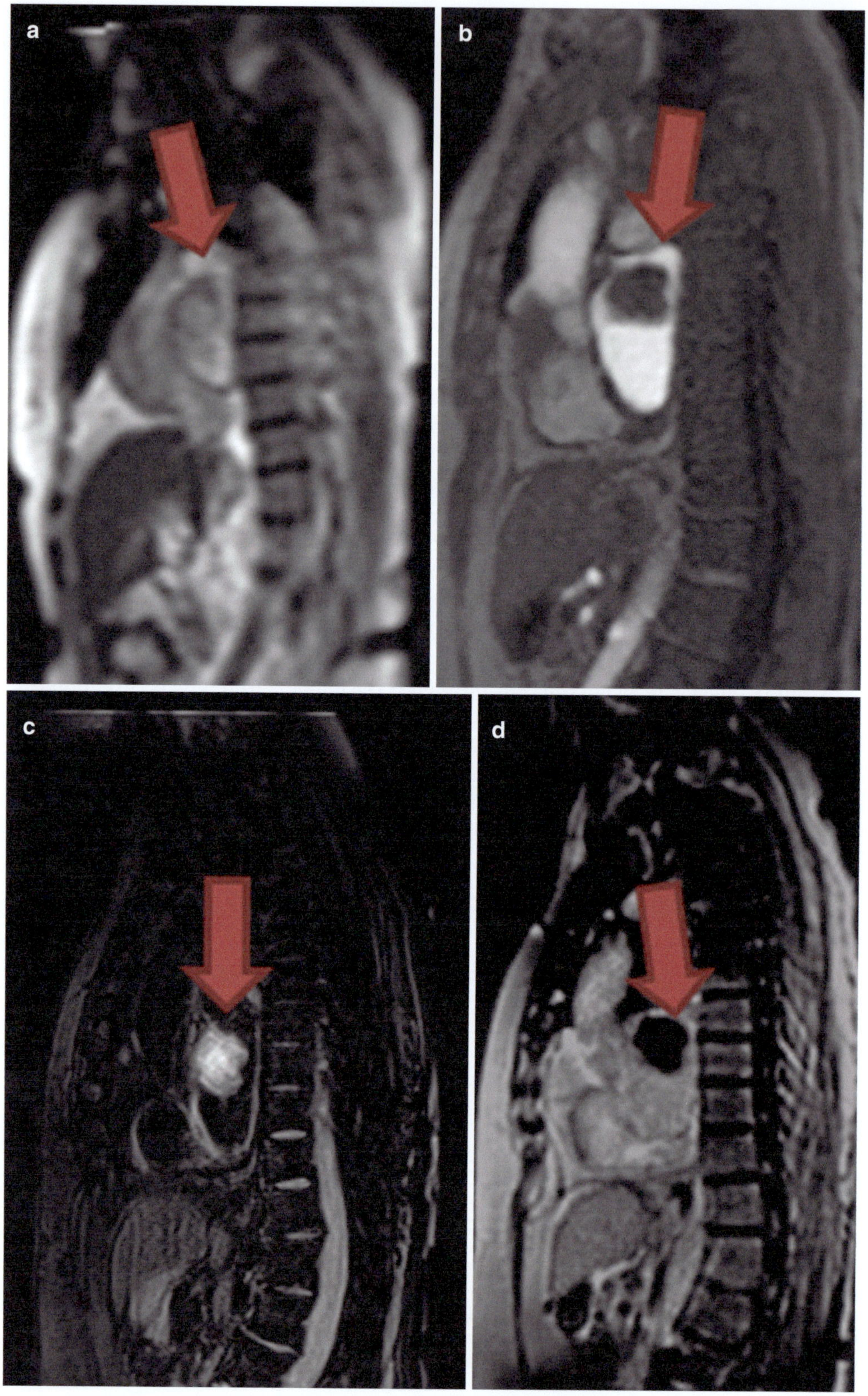

Fig. 4.5 (**a** and **b**) Cardiac MRI images of the left atrium in a sagittal plane are shown. Figure (**a**) shows the cystic mass in a cine image. Figure (**b**) shows the lack of perfusion during first pass gadolinium administration. (**c** and **d**) Cardiac MRI images of the left atrium in a sagittal plane are shown. Figure (**c**) shows the bright mass on a T2 weighted image, suggestive of a thrombus. Figure (**d**) shows the hypointense mass on a post contrast delayed enhancement image. T1 times assessed by T1 mapping were 600 ms consistent with thrombus (not shown)

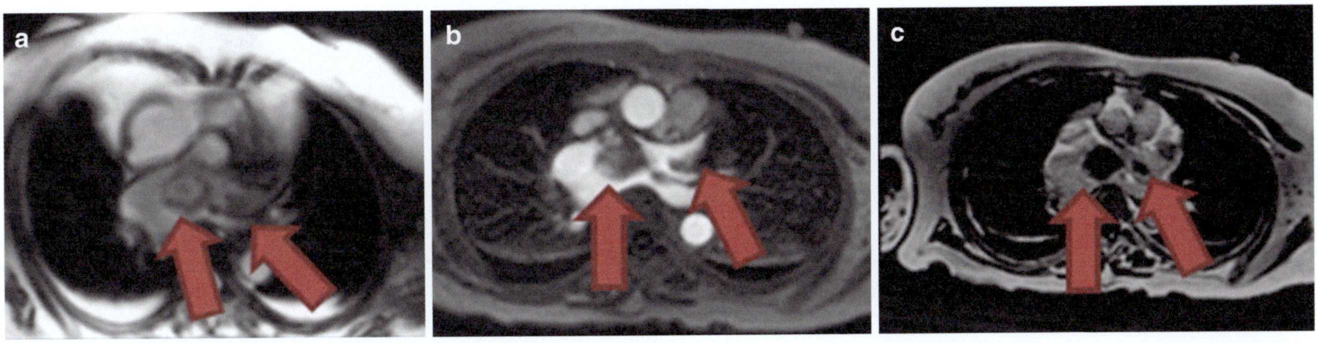

Fig. 4.6 (**a**–**c**) Cardiac MRI images of the left atrium in an axial plane are shown. (**a**) Shows the bright mass, large mass inside the left atrium and a smaller mass within the left atrial appendage, on a cine image. (**b**) Shows the lack of perfusion during first pass gadolinium administration of both the left atrial and the appendage masses. (**c**) Shows the hypointense masses on a post contrast delayed enhancement image

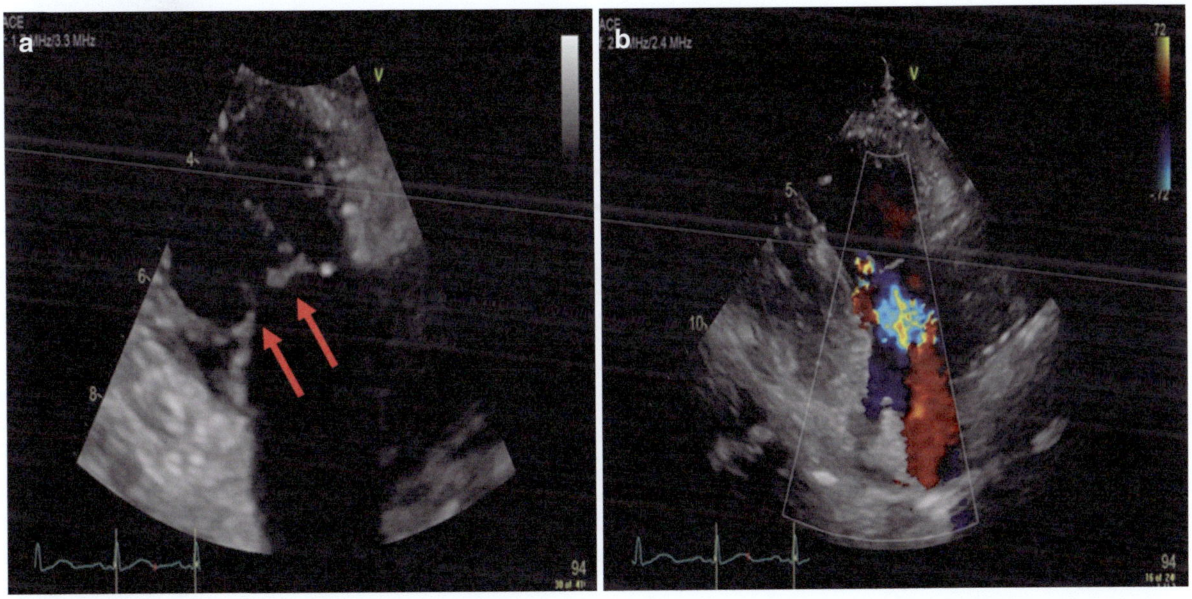

Fig. 4.7 (**a**) (Systolic frame) shows noncoaptation of the tricuspid valve (*red arrows*) and (**b**) shows moderate turbulent tricuspid regurgitation

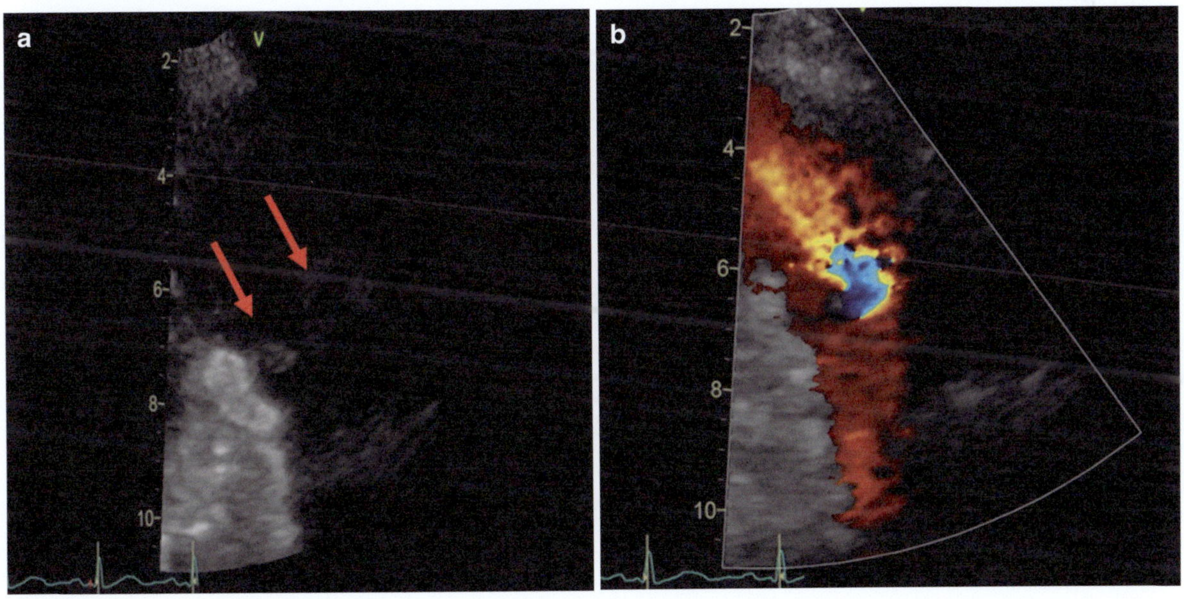

Fig. 4.8 (**a**) (Diastolic frame) shows noncoaptation of the pulmonic valve (*red arrows*) and Figure (**b**) shows moderate turbulent pulmonic regurgitation

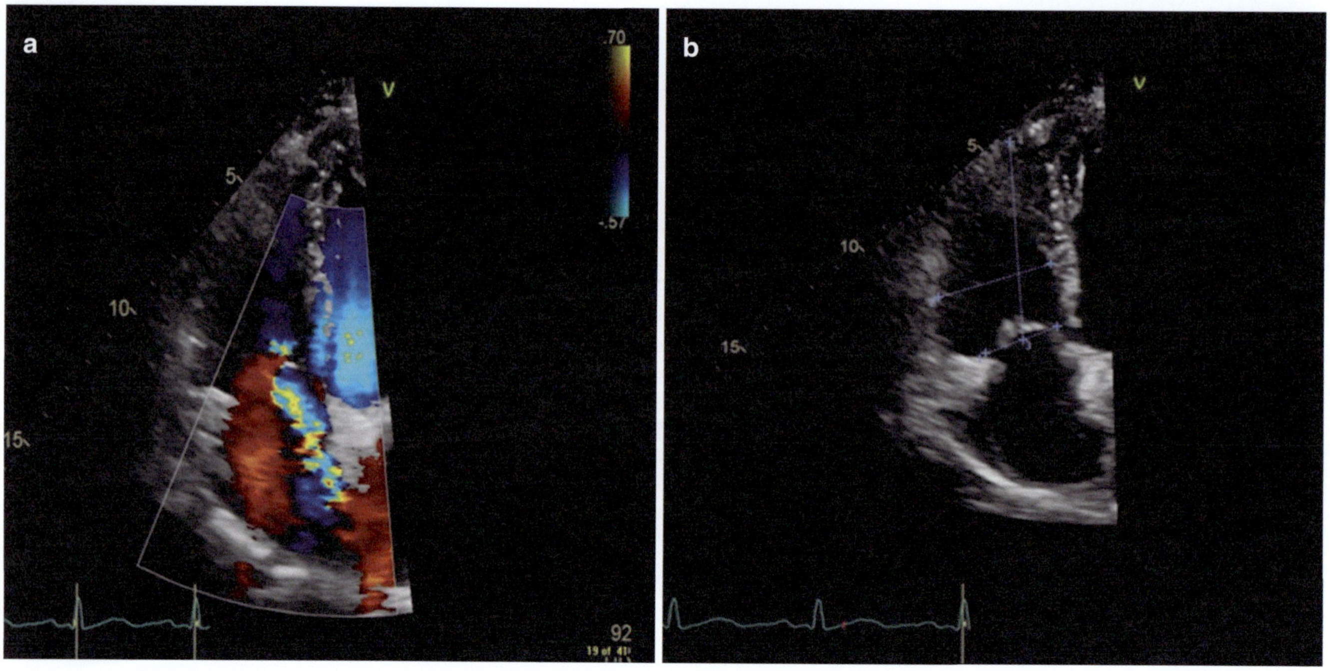

Fig. 4.9 (**a**) Shows turbulent jet of tricuspid regurgitation. Figure (**b**) shows normal Right ventricular size. Right ventricular function was also normal (not shown)

moderate pulmonic regurgitation. He had a history of markedly elevated 5 HIAA, >5000 and was receiving somatostatin. Although he initially responded to diuresis, he developed refractory lower extremity swelling. Hypoalbuminemia and IVC compression were ruled out. He developed progressive severe tricuspid regurgitation and required tricuspid valve replacement.

Teaching points

1. Carcinoid heart disease is a rare entity. It can however cause debilitating symptoms of peripheral venous congestion and edema. Prompt identification is critical and symptomatic management is the norm. However in selected patients where primary tumor is well controlled, tricuspid valve replacement is done.

Case 4: Unusual Etiology of Cardiomyopathy While Receiving Chemotherapy

A 79 year old female, with inflammatory breast cancer, and normal LV systolic function at baseline had finished receiving two cycles of Adriamycin. She had profound fatigue, was found to be anemic with a Hgb of 6 for which she received 2 units of PRBCs. Within 4 h of transfusion, she returned to the emergency department (ED) with acute dyspnea, orthopnea and chest pain. She was in florid heart failure with fluid overload. A 12 lead ECG showed a new LBBB with elevated troponin of 4.0 ng/L. A TTE demonstrated basal hyperkinesis with mid to distal akinesis (Figs. 4.10 and 4.11). A clinical diagnosis of cardiomyopathy/heart failure due to adrimaycin and concomitant NSTEMI was made and a coronary angiogram was done, which did not show any significant disease. A TTE demonstrated basal hyperkinesis with mid to distal akinesis. A diagnosis of stress (Takotsubo) cardiomyopathy was made and medical therapy was instituted which included a low dose beta blocker. On follow up in the clinic the patient was symptomatically markedly improved with no heart failure symptoms and a repeat TTE 2 weeks later revealed, normal LV systolic function with normal wall motion (Figs. 4.12 and 4.13). Diagnosis was stress cardiomyopathy and not related to anthracycline use.

Characteristic LV gram and global longitudinal strain polar map (from other patients with stress (Takotsubo) cardiomyopathy) are shown in Figs. 4.14 and 4.15 respectively.

Teaching points

1. While anthracycline mediated cardiomyopathy is the most common etiology of cardiomyopathy in cancer patients exposed to this drug, the specific pattern of stress cardiomyopathy should warrant suspicion of stress cardiomyopathy. In patients not receiving cardiotoxic chemotherapy, stress cardiomyopathy should be entertained

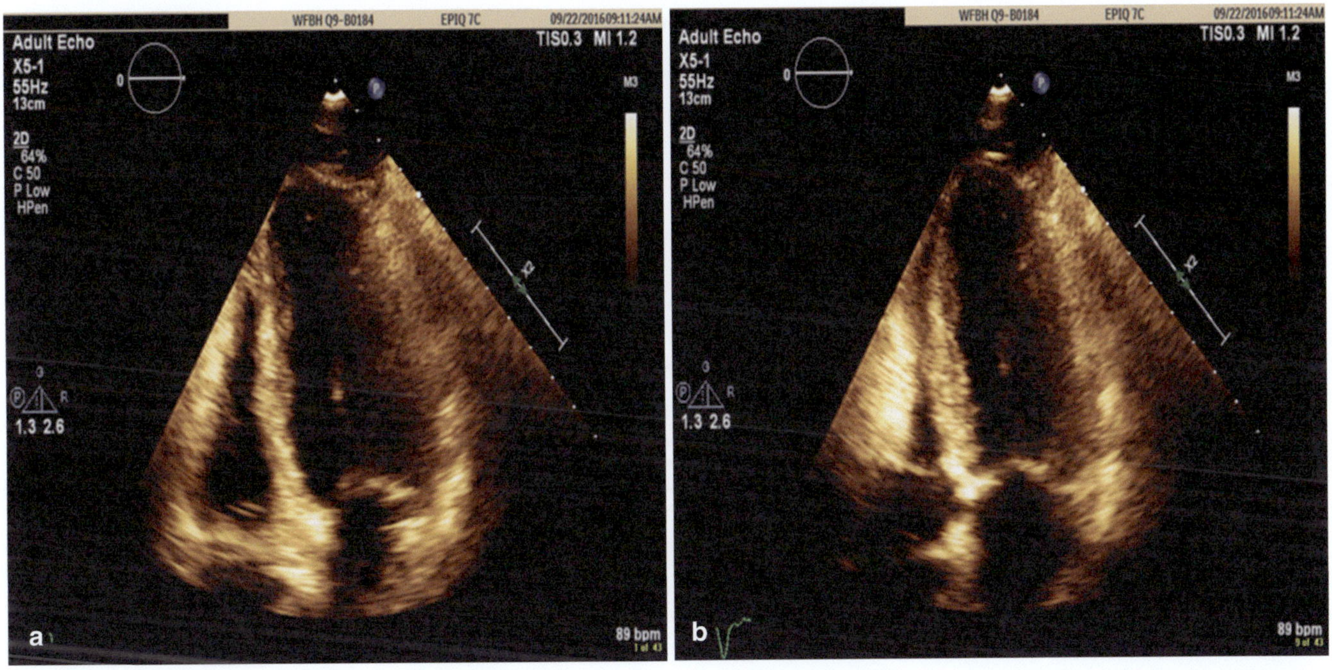

Fig. 4.10 (**a**) (Diastolic frame) and (**b**) (Systolic frame): Apical 4 chamber view of the heart shows show normal wall thickening and reduction of intra-cavity space only at the basilar level

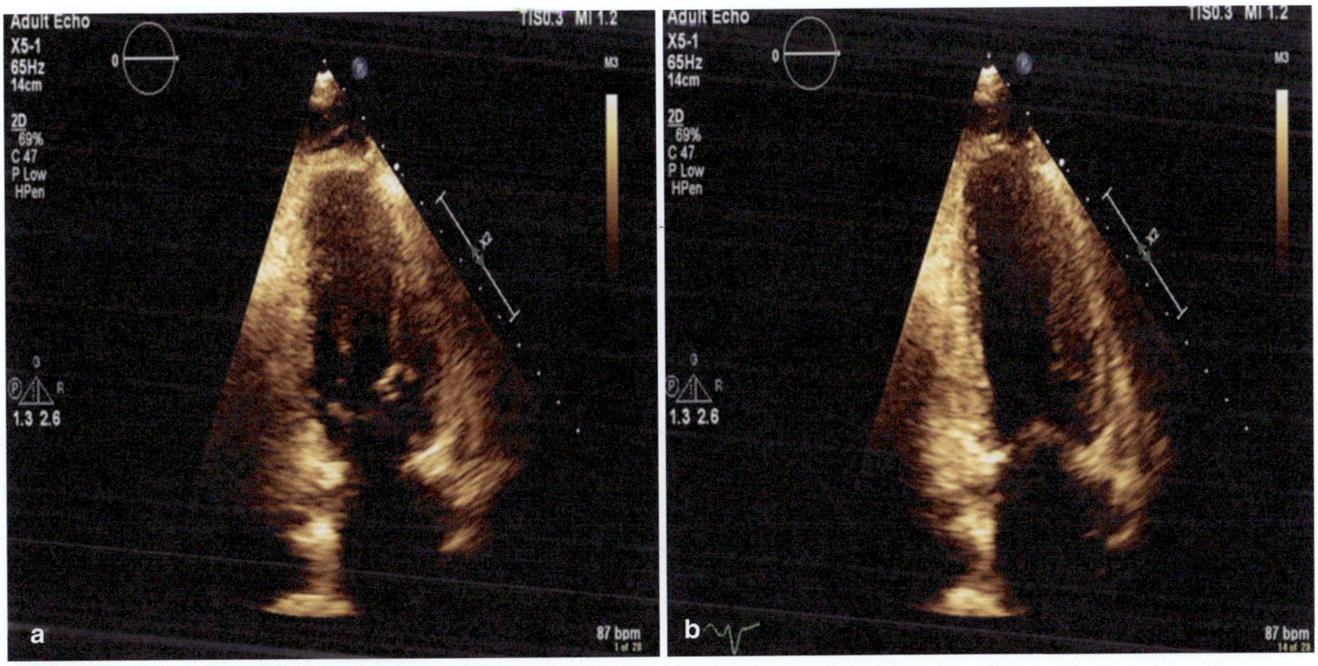

Fig. 4.11 (**a**) (Diastolic frame) and (**b**) (Systolic frame): Apical 2 chamber view of the heart shows normal wall thickening and reduction of intra-cavity space, only at the basilar level

as a differential when patients have an abrupt presentation similar to the one outlined above.

Munoz et al. have identified common stressors, i.e. surgery, radiation, chemotherapy, acute illness and emotional stressors as triggers for stress cardiomyopathy in cancer patient. Multiple studies have identified patients with malignancy as a vulnerable population for stress cardiomyopathy [5–7].

Follow up imaging

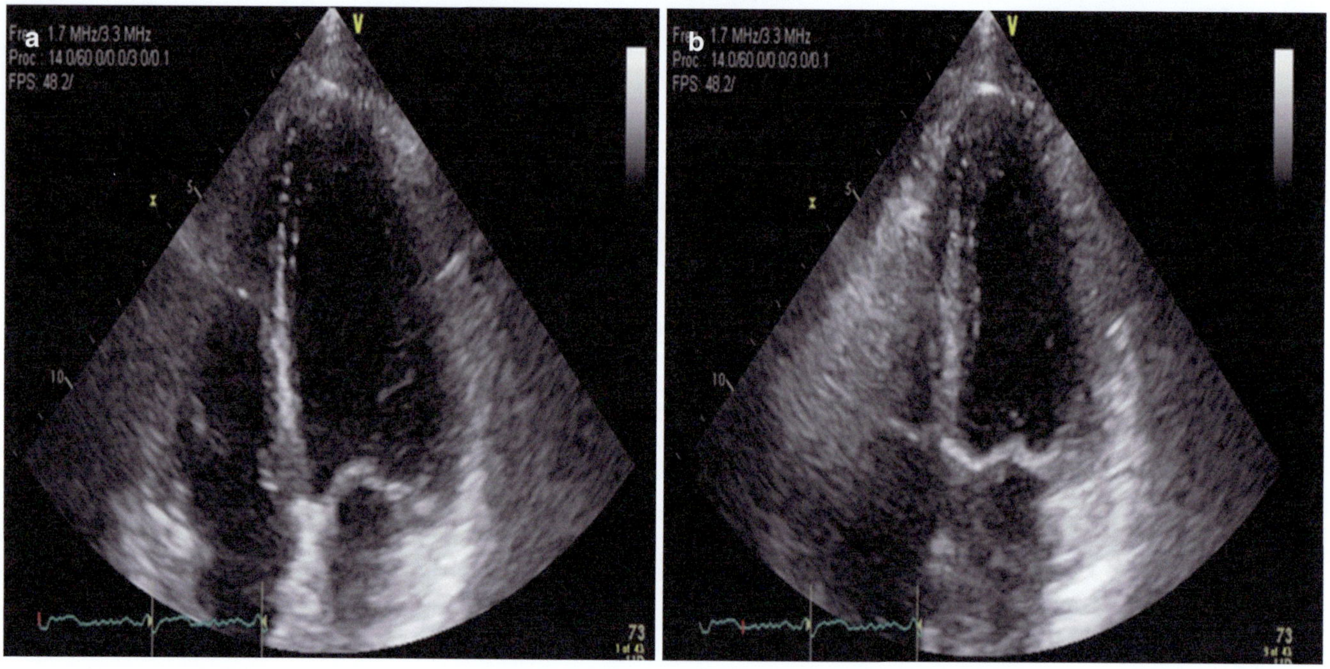

Fig. 4.12 (**a**) (Diastolic) and (**b**) (Systolic frame): Apical 4 chamber view of the heart shows normal wall thickening

Follow up imaging

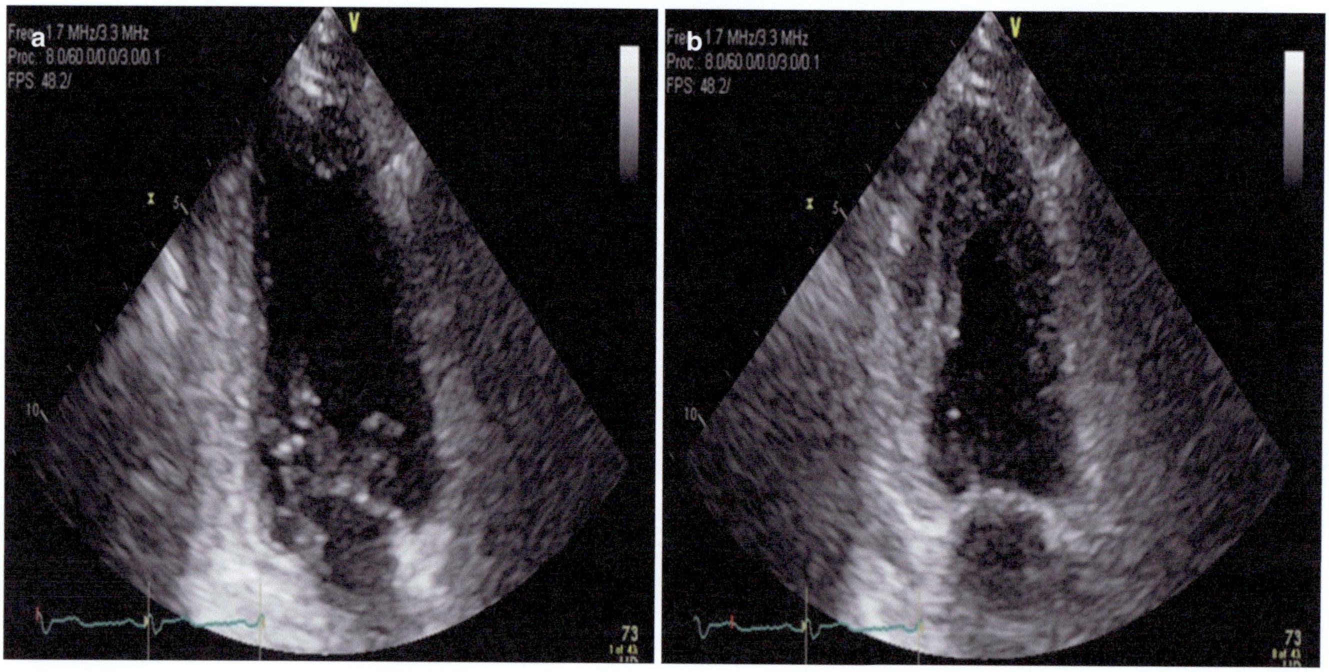

Fig. 4.13 (**a**) (Diastolic frame) and (**b**) (Systolic frame): Apical 2 chamber view of the heart showing normal wall thickening

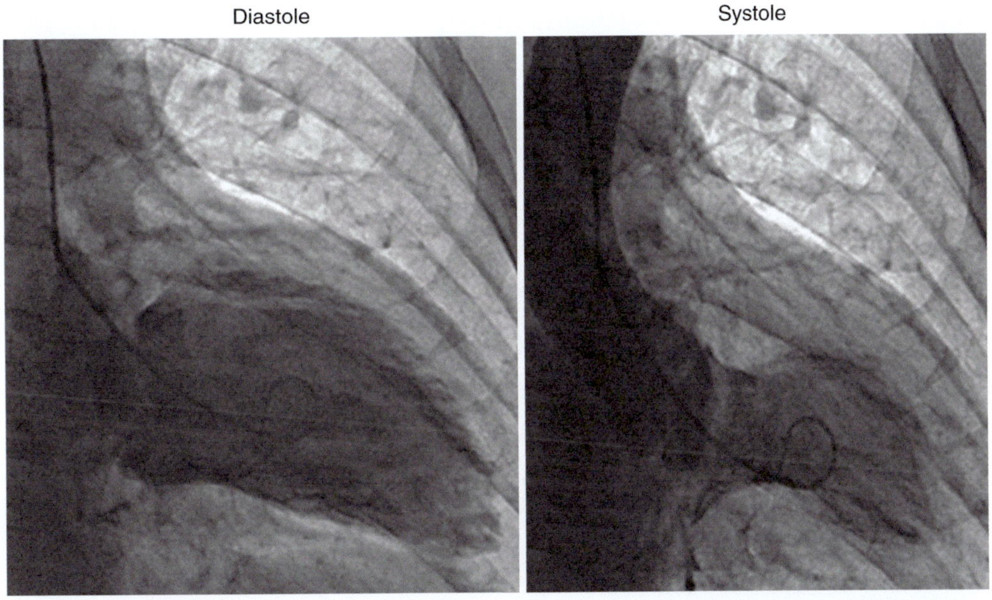

Fig. 4.14 LV gram from another patient with Takotsubo cardiomyopathy showing apical ballooning (Image courtesy of Dr. C. Iliescu)

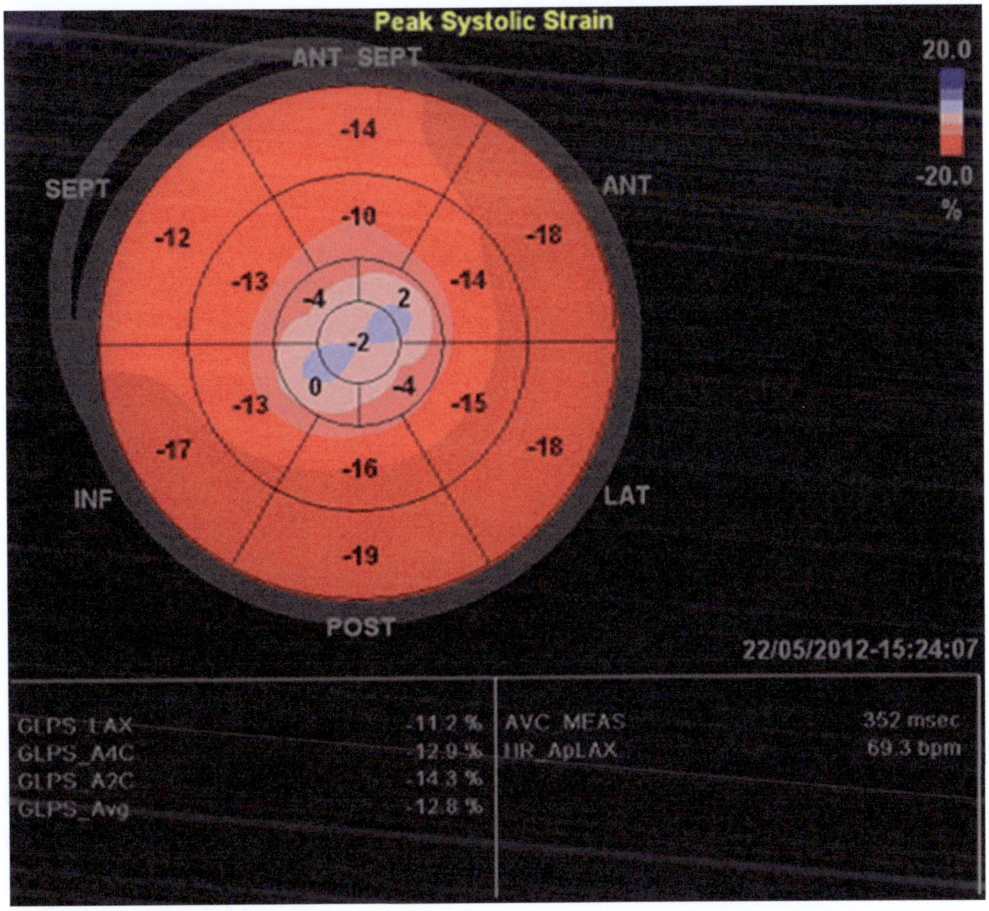

Fig. 4.15 Global longitudinal strain polar map: Predominant apical segmental abnormality polar map pattern in a patient with classic apical ballooning syndrome variant of stress cardiomyopathy. Note the marked difference isolated to the five apical segments on the polar map LV representation, atypical for a specific coronary distribution. (Image courtesy of Dr. J. Banchs)

Case 5: Other Causes of Cardiomyopathy in Patients with Cancer

While evaluating the etiology of heart failure, CMR can be helpful to identify amyloidosis, hypertrophic cardiomyopathy or iron overload. For example in amyloidosis, the basal slices show diffuse myocardial scar with preservation of the apex, as shown in Fig. 4.16. In addition the presence of transmural myocardial scar and right ventricular scar as well helps differentiate the types of amyloidosis (Transthyretin related amyloidosis) from light chain amyloidosis [8]. CMR can also be used to identify hypertrophic cardiomyopathy especially the phenotypic variants, i.e. Apical variant in addition to the asymmetric septal hypertrophy as outlined in this review by Maron et al. [9].

Basal slices are represented in A and B while the apical slice is shown in C. Basal slices have diffuse myocardial fibrosis in a near transmural pattern, in contrast to the apical slices which have no fibrosis. This correlates with the preservation of apical strain, with severe reduction of basal strain using echocardiography (Fig. 4.17).

Figure 4.18 shows the typical ECG and echocardiogram findings in a patient with biopsy proven cardiac amyloidosis.

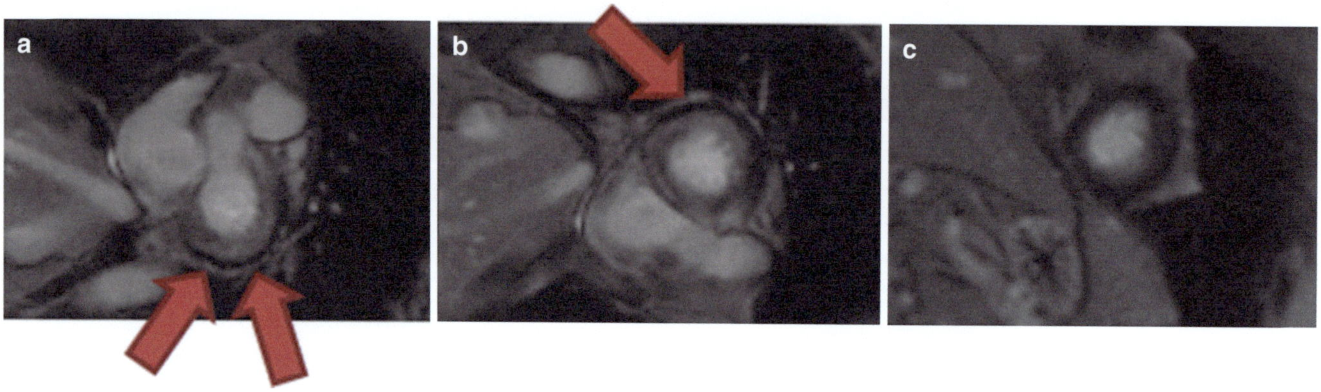

Fig. 4.16 CMR showing cardiac amyloidosis. Basal slices are represented in (**a**) and (**b**) while the apical slice is shown in (**c**). Basal slices have diffuse myocardial fibrosis in a near transmural pattern, in contrast to the apical slices which have no fibrosis

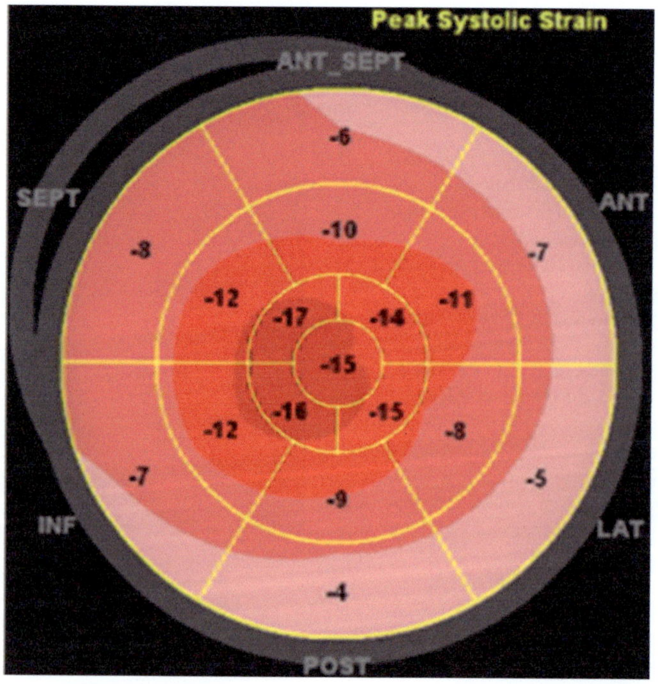

Fig. 4.17 Echocardiogram: Global longitudinal strain polar map, in a patient with cardiac amyloidosis, showing preservation of apical strain with severe reduction of basal strain (Image courtesy of Dr. S.W. Yusuf)

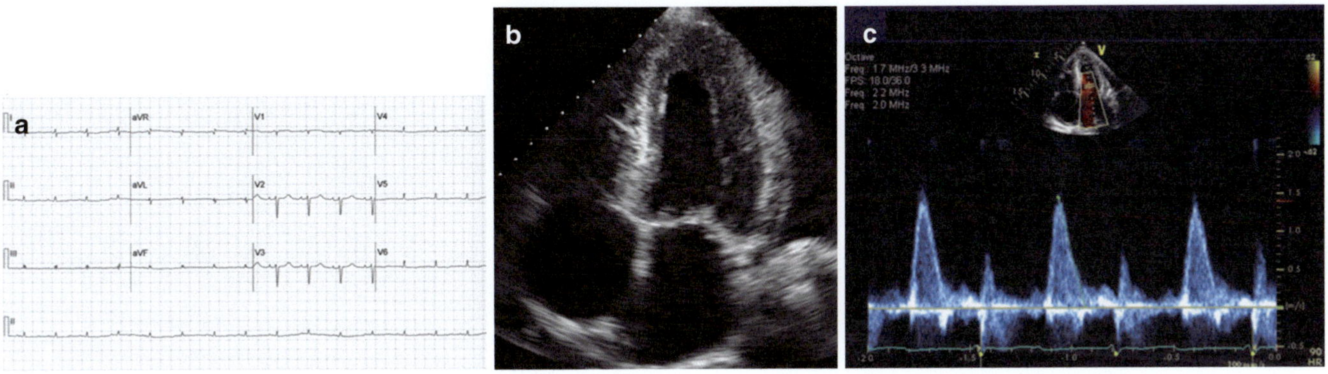

Fig. 4.18 Cardiac amyloidosis. (**a**) A 12 lead ECG showing low voltage complexes. (**b**) Echocardiogram: Apical 4 chamber view showing ventricular hypertrophy and atrial dilatation. (**c**) Mitral inflow showing restrictive pattern (Images courtesy of Dr. S.W. Yusuf)

References

1. Thavendiranathan P, Walls M, Giri S, Verhaert D, Rajagopalan S, Moore S, Simonetti OP, Raman SV. Improved detection of myocardial involvement in acute inflammatory cardiomyopathies using T2 mapping. Circ Cardiovasc Imaging. 2012;5:102–10.
2. Bohnen S, et al. Performance of T1 and T2 mapping cardiovascular magnetic resonance to detect active myocarditis in patients with recent-onset heart failure. Circ Cardiovasc Imaging. 2015;8:e003073. https://doi.org/10.1161/CIRCIMAGING.114.003073.
3. Esposito A, De Cobelli F, Ironi G et al. CMR in the assessment of cardiac masses. JACC Cardiovasc Imaging. 2014;7:1057–61.
4. Weinsaft JW, et al. Detection of left ventricular thrombus by delayed-enhancement cardiovascular magnetic resonance prevalence and markers in patients with systolic dysfunction. J Am Coll Cardiol. 2008;52:148–57.
5. Munoz E, et al. Takotsubo stress cardiomyopathy: "Good News" in cancer patients? J Am Coll Cardiol. 2016;68(10):1143–4.
6. El-Sayed AM, et al. Demographic and co-morbid predictors of stress (Takotsubo) cardiomyopathy. Am J Cardiol. 2012;110(9): 1368–72.
7. Tornvall P, et al. A case-control study of risk markers and mortality in Takotsubo stress cardiomyopathy. J Am Coll Cardiol. 2016;67(16):1931–6.
8. Dungu JN, et al. CMR-based differentiation of AL and ATTR cardiac amyloidosis. JACC Cardiovasc Imaging. 2014;7(2):133–42.
9. Maron MS, et al. Clinical utility of cardiovascular magnetic resonance in hypertrophic cardiomyopathy. J Cardiovasc Magn Reson. 2012;14:13.

Takotsubo Syndrome and Cancer

5

Joaquim Cevallos and Alexander Lyon

Abstract

Takotsubo Syndrome (TTS) is defined by transient ventricular dysfunction in the absence of culprit obstructive coronary artery disease. During acute presentation, patients present with typical ECG, echocardiographic and cardiac magnetic resonance imaging features. We present two cases of TTS in the context of cancer, with a wide range of complimentary tests, and then briefly discuss the pathophysiology and clinical presentation of TTS, highlighting the importance of appropriate management of TTS both during the acute phase and follow-up. The association between TTS and cancer is mentioned, with the possibility, in some cases, that TTS represents a paraneoplastic syndrome.

Keywords

Takotsubo syndrome • Stress cardiomyopathy • Heart failure • Prolonged QT • Metastatic cancer • Chemotherapy

Clinical Cases

Case 1

A 75 year old lady was admitted to her oncology unit after feeling generally unwell over the previous month, with increasing generalised pain, appetite suppression and dehydration. She had background of metastatic thyroid cancer, for which she had recently been started on multiple VEGFR kinase inhibitor Lenvatinib. She also had previous history of hypertension, which was treated with Propranolol and Amlodipine. Her blood pressure had been more difficult to control since initiation of Lenvatinib. Her cardiovascular assessment prior to treatment confirmed normal left ventricular ejection fraction (LVEF) with mild left ventricular hypertrophy with no regional wall motion abnormalities.

During her admission, most of her medications were discontinued, including her Lenvatinib and Propranolol. The patient became increasingly anxious as a result of her health condition and withdrawal of her targeted molecular cancer therapy. Four days following admission she awoke in the middle of the night with central chest pain. She remained haemodynamically stable and her initial ECG showed unspecific ST changes in the precordial leads with flattening T waves. As the patient remained pain-free and there was no definite ST elevation, an urgent angiogram was withheld. The next morning blood tests confirmed her Troponin I peaked at 158 ng/L (normal range < 20) with a BNP of 2202 ng/L (normal range < 20). Evolving ECGs showed isoelectric J point with widespread T wave inversion and prolonged QTc (Fig. 5.1). She was then transferred to our cardiac unit.

Her resting transthoracic echocardiogram showed apical akinesia (Fig. 5.2). This, in conjunction with a modest Troponin

J. Cevallos
Cardio-Oncology Service, Royal Brompton Hospital, London, UK

A. Lyon (✉)
Cardio-Oncology Service, Royal Brompton Hospital, London, UK

Imperial College, London, UK
e-mail: a.lyon@rbht.nhs.uk

S.W. Yusuf, J. Banchs (eds.), *Cancer and Cardiovascular Disease*, https://doi.org/10.1007/978-3-319-62088-6_5

Fig. 5.1 Successive ECG during presentation of TTS. (**a**) ST elevation in V2-V3 with minimal (<1mm) ST depression in I, aVL, V5 and V6. (**b**) Evolving changes with ST elevation in V2-3 and evolving T wave inversion. (**c**) Widespread deep T wave inversion in precordial leads with QTc 560 ms

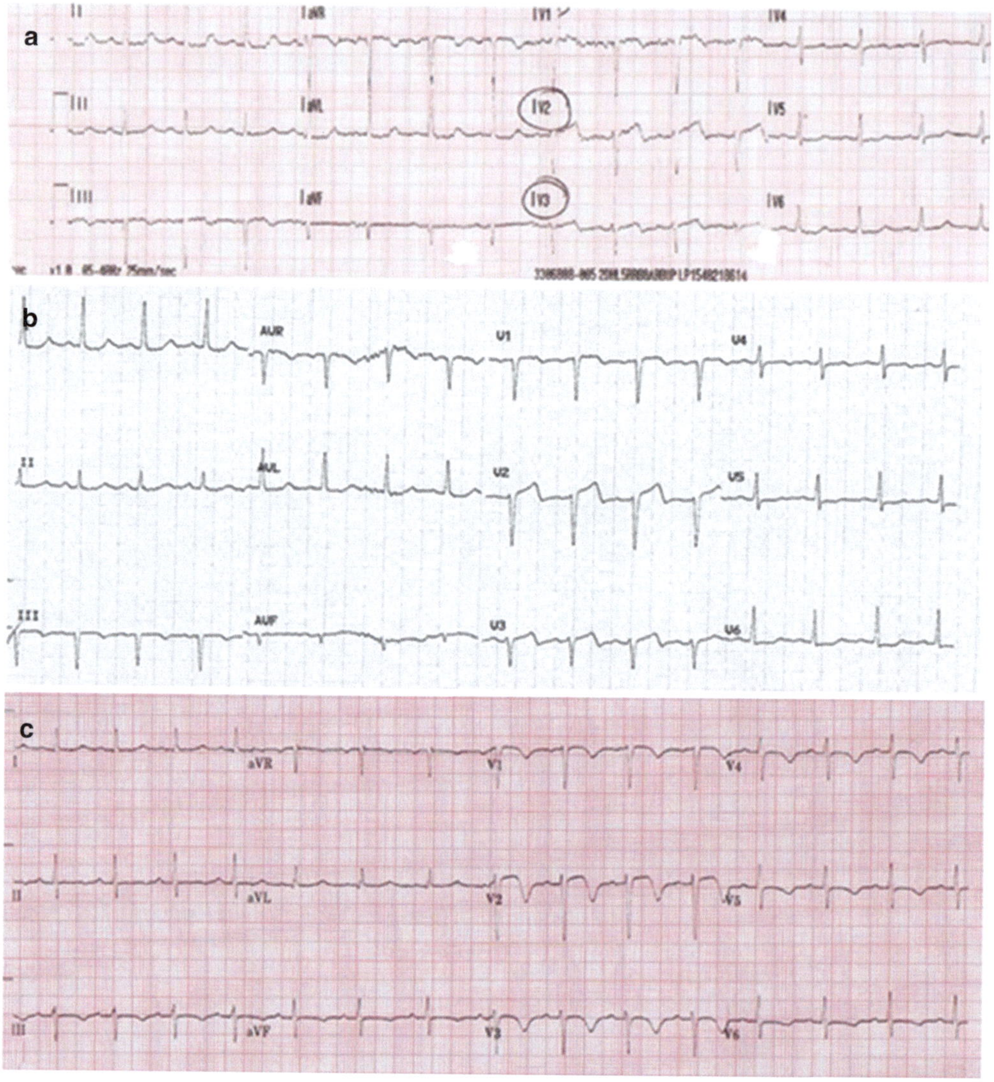

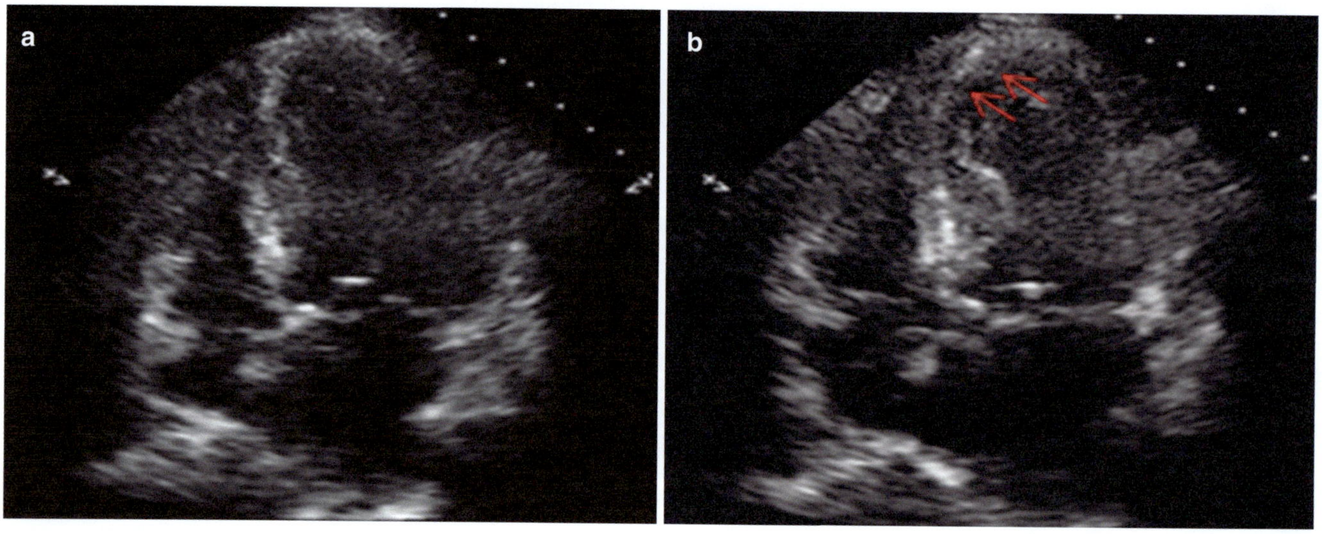

Fig. 5.2 Echocardiographic images during the acute phase of TTS. (**a**) Apical 4-chamber view at the end of diastole showing normal cavity size and myocardial thickness. (**b**) Apical 4-chamber view at the end of systole showing good contraction of basal segments with septo-apical dyskinesia (*arrows*).

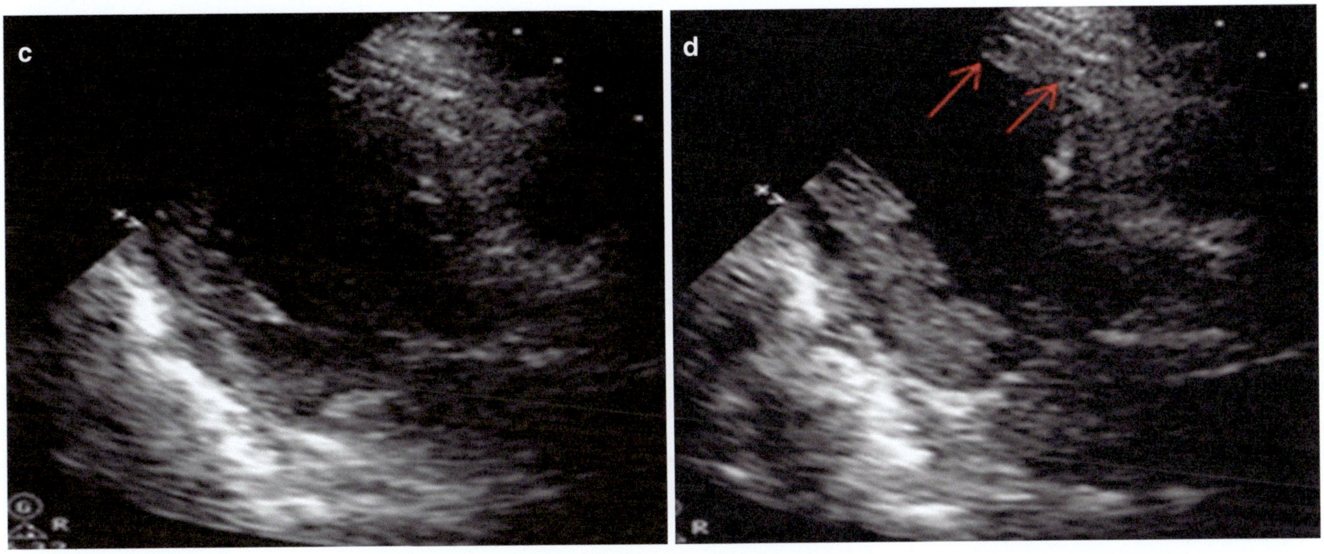

Fig. 5.2 (continued) (**c**) Modified parasternal long axis at end diastole. (**d**) Modified parasternal long axis showing dyskinetic apex (*arrows*)

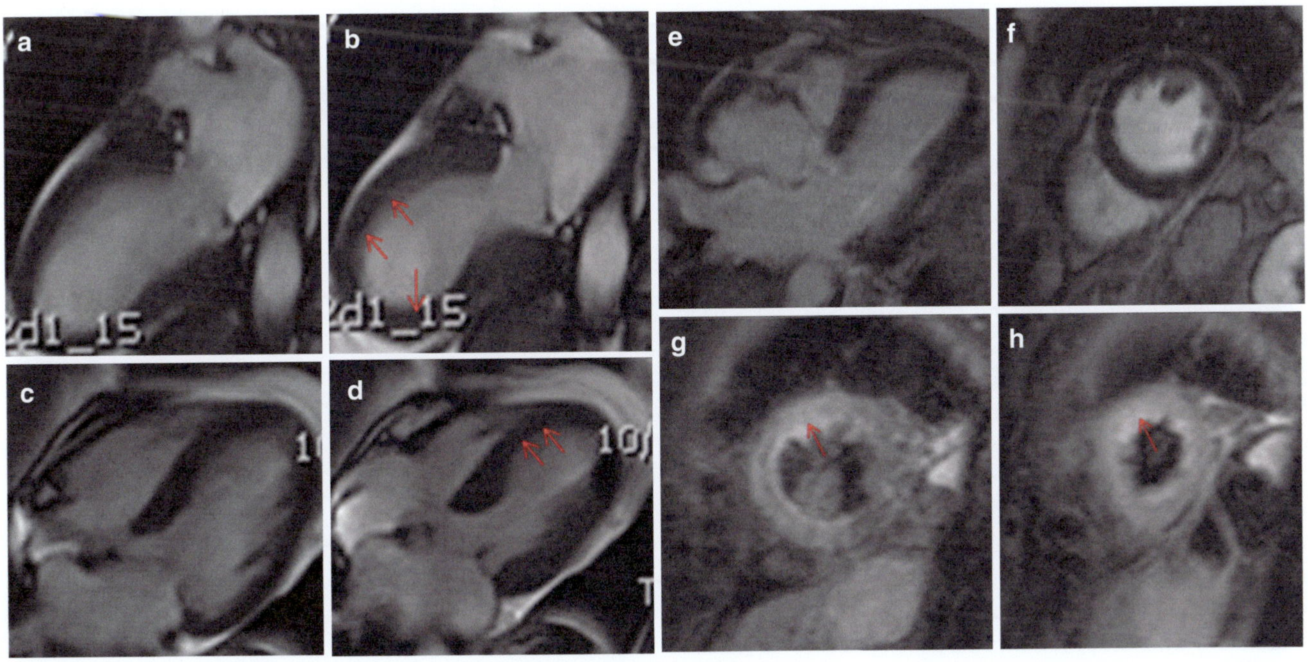

Fig. 5.3 CMR images with LGE and STIR. (**a**) Two-chamber view at end-diastole showing normal cavity size and wall thickness. (**b**) Two-chamber view at end-systole with apical dyskinesia (see *red arrows*). (**c**) Four-chamber view at end-diastole. (**d**) Four-chamber view at end-systole with septo-apical dyskinesia (see *red arrows*). (**e**) Four-chamber LGE. No evidence of uptake ruling out scarring or fibrosis. (**f**) Short axis LGE at mid-ventricular level. No evidence of LGE. (**g**) STIR image at mid-ventricular level. There is an area of oedema in the antero-septum (*red arrow*). (**h**) STIR image at the apex shows extension of oedema to the antero-apical segment (*red arrow*)

rise and substantial ECG changes and BNP elevation raised the suspicion of Takotsubo syndrome (TTS). A Cardiac Magnetic Resonance (CMR) scan was performed, which confirmed the diagnosis: apical akinesia in the absence of myocardial infarction on late gadolinium enhancement (LGE). Furthermore, the Short TI Inversion Recovery (STIR) sequences confirmed the presence of oedema/inflammation in the apical myocardium, as typically observed in TTS patients (Fig. 5.3). An invasive angiogram was deemed unnecessary and a CT coronary angiogram (CT-A) ruled out significant coronary disease (Fig. 5.4).

The patient was monitored in a level 2 setting under ECG monitoring and treated with low dose of Carvedilol. Her QTc remained prolonged (532 ms) with partial improvement with intravenous magnesium supplementation. She recovered over the next 4 days, and was discharged back home and cancer treatment was switched to Vandetanib. Unfortunately,

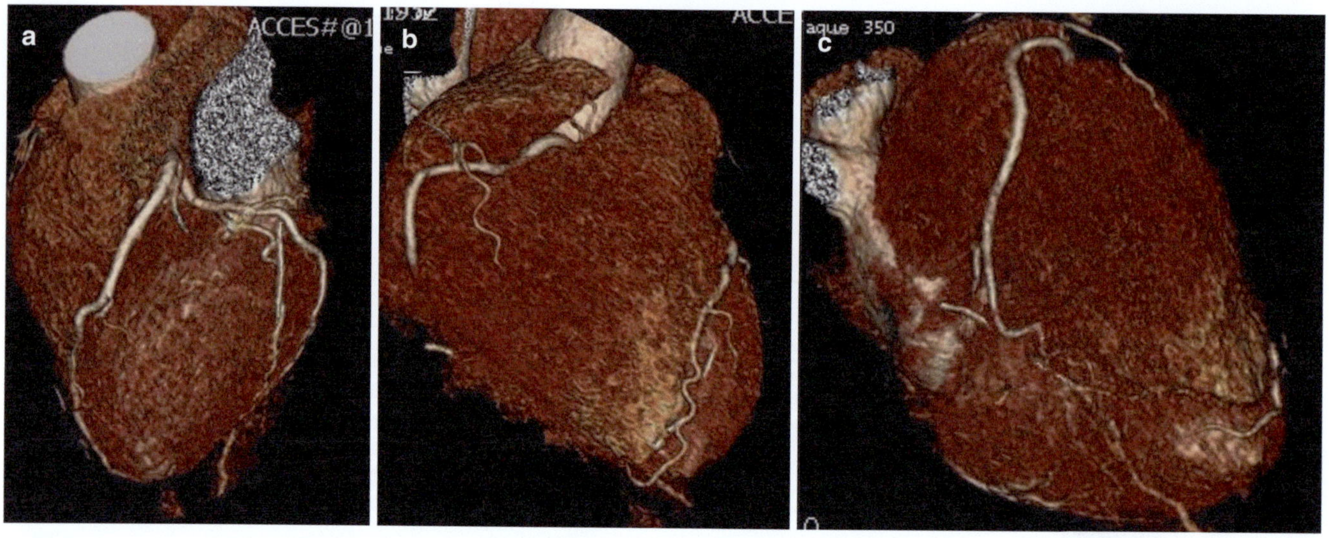

Fig. 5.4 CT-A showing absence of significant coronary disease. (**a**) Unobstructed left main (LM), Left Anterior Descending (LAD) and Circumflex coronary arteries. (**b**) Proximal Right Coronary Artery (RCA) with no evidence of atheroma. (**c**) Distal RCA and posterior descendant artery (PDA) with no significant disease

she did not tolerate chemotherapy and died 2 months later as a result of her metastatic malignancy.

Case 2

A 62 year old lady presented in the accident and emergency (A&E) Department with central chest pain. She had a background of hypertension and a previous hysterectomy with bilateral oophorectomy at the age of 45. She was on no regular medication. She had been under increasing stresses in the previous months due to personal issues including illness in a family member and death of her family dog. Her ECG showed acute ST changes (Fig. 5.5) which, in conjunction with persistent chest pain in spite of standard management, prompted an urgent coronary angiogram (Fig. 5.6). There were no flow-limiting lesions, albeit a significant lesion in the origin of the first diagonal. During the procedure, the patient ended pain free. As a consequence, she was managed medically with carvedilol, enalapril, aspirin and statins, with symptomatic relief.

An echocardiogram was performed (Fig. 5.7), showing apical and mid-ventricular circumferential hypokinesia with hyperdynamic basal segments. There was no significant left ventricular outflow tract obstruction. The CMR (Fig. 5.8) showed mid-ventricular and apical wall motion abnormalities, with no evidence of myocardial infarction or fibrosis. Active and extensive oedema of the hypokinetic segments was present on the STIR images. The patient remained monitored while her QTc remained extremely prolonged (> 500 ms), and she recovered over 6 days.

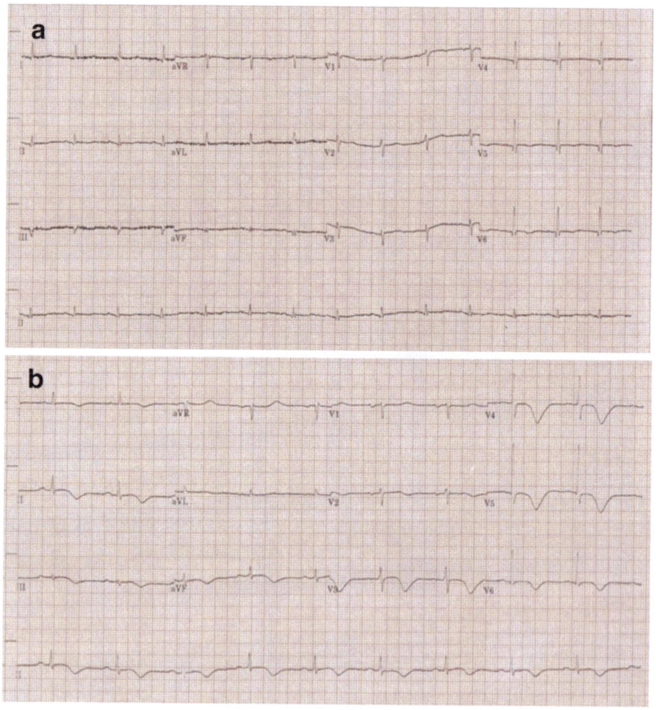

Fig. 5.5 Serial ECGs during acute phase of TTS. (**a**) Flattening T wave in the anterior leads with inversion in V4-V6. (**b**) Widespread T wave inversion with associated QTc prolongation (540 ms)

Following discharge, the patient was still reporting anginal symptoms, mainly on exertion but also in the context of anxiety. A physiological stress echocardiogram was performed (Fig. 5.9), which confirmed stress-inducible apical akinesia. For completion, a cardiac Iodine-123 meta-iodobenzyl-guanidine (mIBG) scan was requested to assess for sympathetic myocardial innervation (Fig. 5.10). It confirmed a reduction in the noradrenaline uptake and functional innervation of the apical segments, in keeping with a recent episode of TTS.

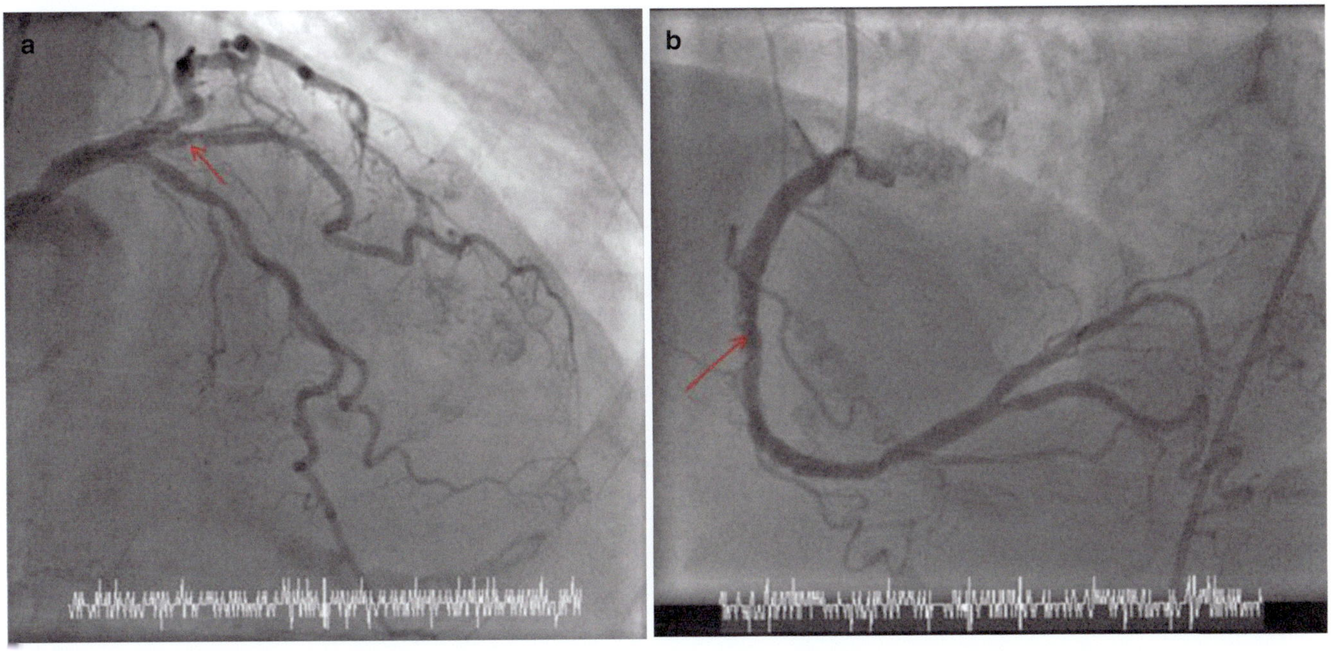

Fig. 5.6 Coronary angiography during acute presentation—significant but non-limiting flow lesions: (**a**) Unobstructed LM, LAD and Circumflex coronary arteries. There is a significant lesion in the first Diagonal branch (*red arrow*). (**b**) Moderate lesion in the mid RCA (see *red arrow*)

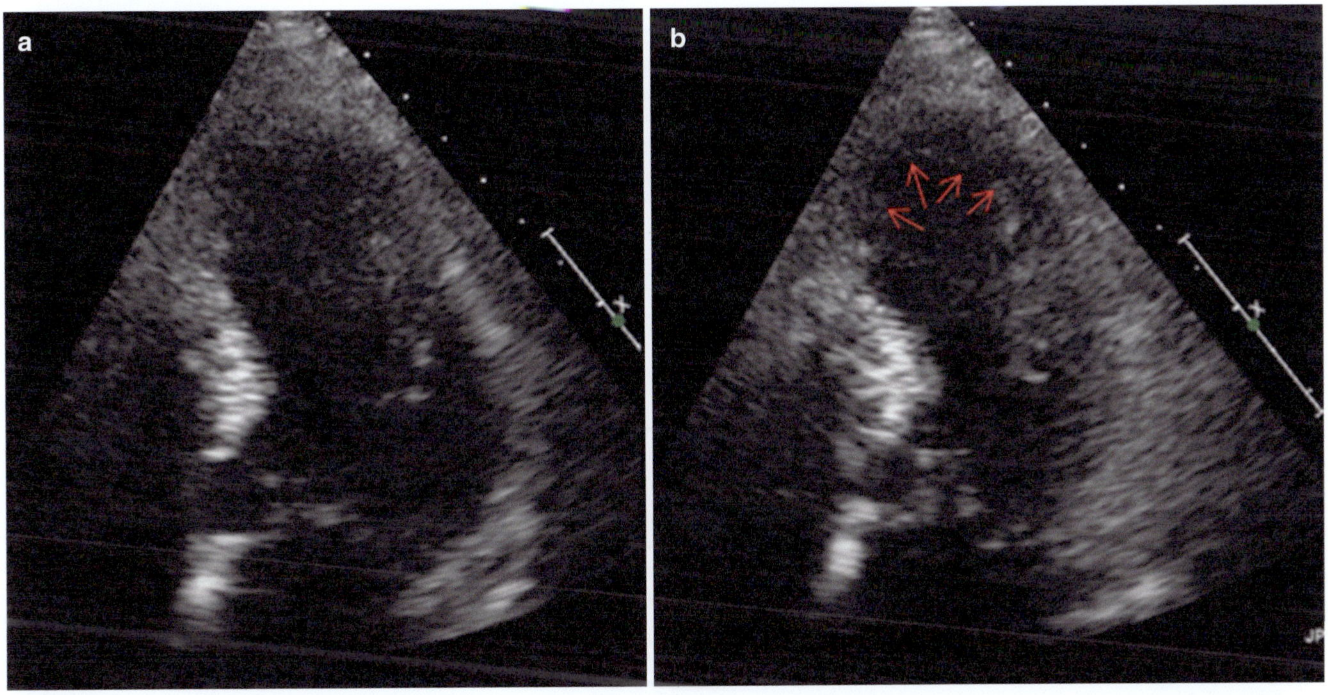

Fig. 5.7 Four-chamber apical views on transthoracic Echo. (**a**) End-diastole. (**b**) End-systole. Note hyperdynamic bases and apical *ballooning* (*red arrows*)

The patient was followed up in our heart failure service, with a program of cardiac rehabilitation and psychological input. She eventually managed to control her symptoms. Two years after the episode, she was diagnosed of a right breast cancer.

Discussion

Takotsubo syndrome (TTS) is defined by chest pain in the presence of transient regional wall motion abnormalities of left, right or both ventricles, which frequently extend beyond a single coronary distribution, in the absence of culprit coronary artery disease or other forms of cardiomyopathy [1]. The acute event is usually preceded by a stressful trigger, either emotional or physical. Contributing factors, although not diagnostic, are post-menopausal women (90% of cases), acute cerebrovascular accidents, drug abuse, mood disorders, malignancy, chronic liver disease and sepsis [2].

Electrocardiographic abnormalities comprise new and reversible ST-segment elevation or depression, acute left bundle branch block, T wave inversion (typically deep and widespread) and QTc prolongation, which is a risk factor for cardiac arrest and warrants ECG-monitoring in the acute

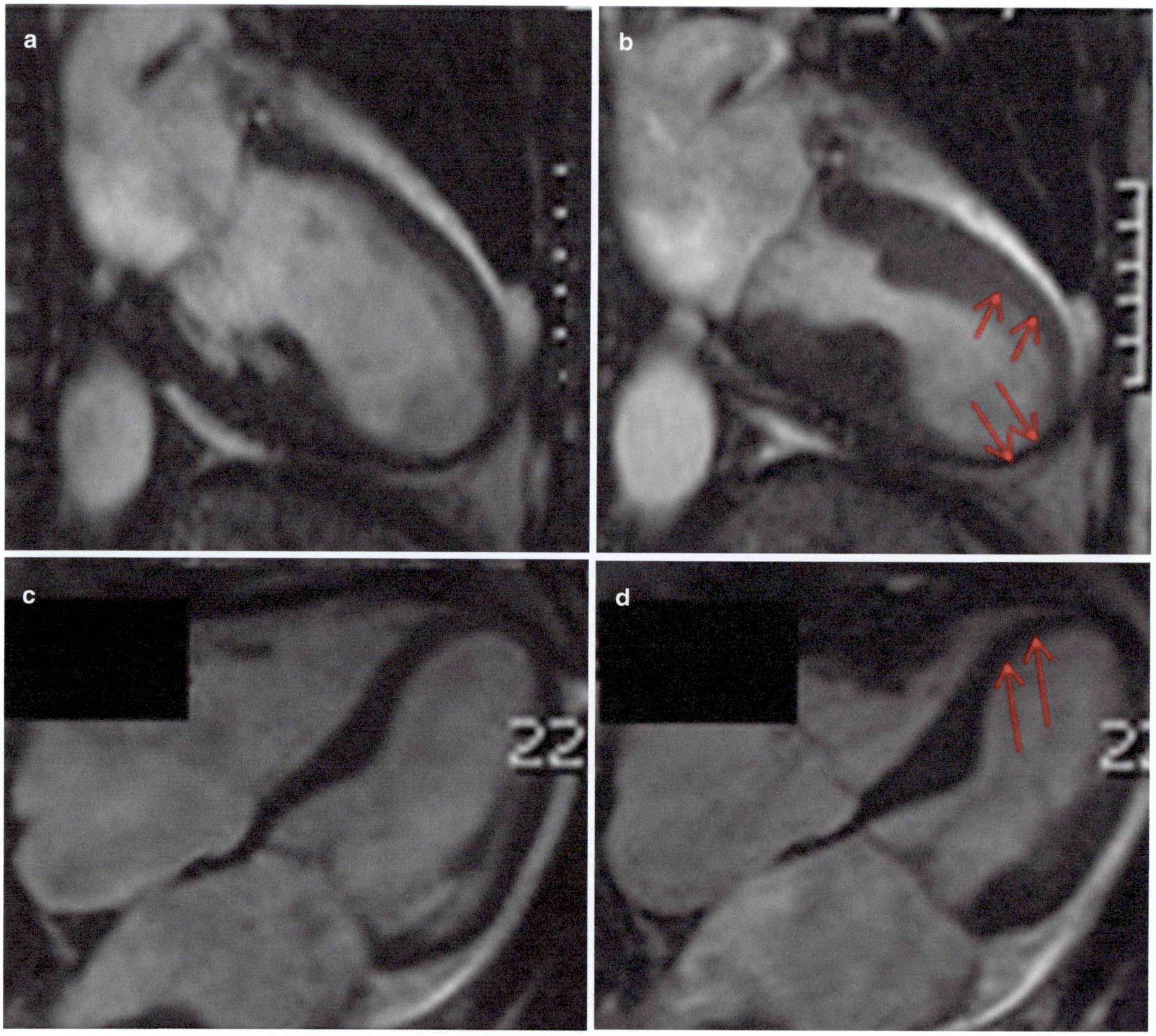

Fig. 5.8 CMR typical of Takotsubo syndrome. (**a**) Two-chamber (end-diastole). (**b**) Two-chamber (end-systole). Distinct apical dyskinesia (see *arrows*). (**c**) Four-chamber (end-diastole). (**d**) Four-chamber (end-systole). Distinct septo-apical dyskinesia (see *arrows*).

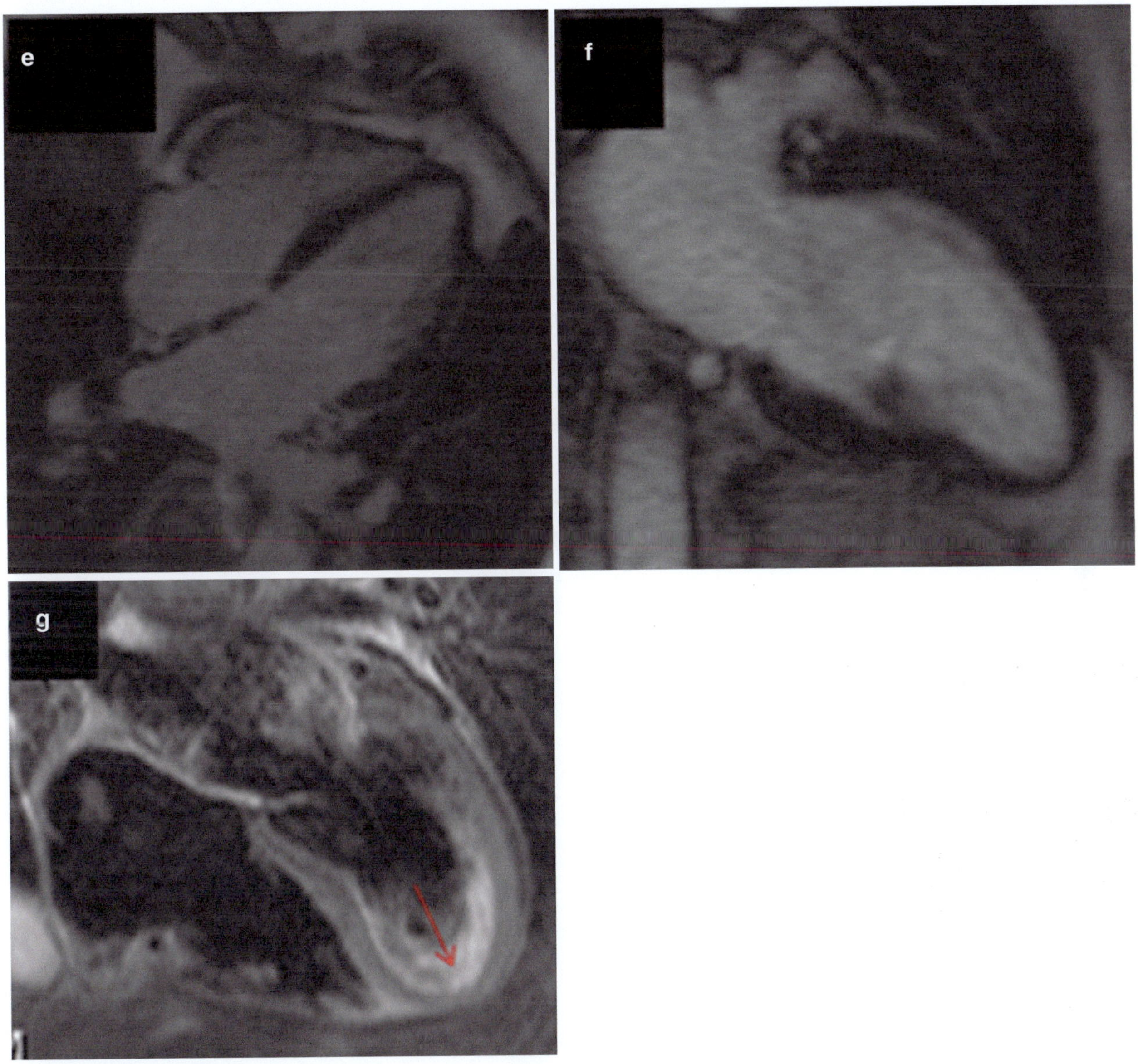

Fig. 5.8 (continued) (**e**) Absence of LGE in the 4-chamber view. (**f**) Absence of LGE in the 2-chamber view. (**g**) Extensive apical oedema in the STIR images (see *arrow*)

phase. The degree of elevation of natriuretic peptides (BNP or NT-proBNP) is disproportionately high as compared to a mild cardiac troponin rise, given the degree of myocardial dysfunction.

Based on cardiac imaging, there have been various anatomical variants of TTS, the most common being apical (80%), midventricular variant (10–15% of cases) and inverted or basal variant (5%). CMR will add information about tissue characterisation. Typically, there will be signs of acute oedema/inflammation on the STIR images in the absence of myocardial infarction on LGE.

The pathophysiology of TTS is complex and only partially understood [3, 4]. Based on animal models and secondary forms of TTS (phaeochromocytoma, subarachnoid haemorrhage), catecholamines appear to play an important role and frequently, although not always, there is a "sympathetic storm" following an acute stressor. This may lead to a form of catecholamine-induced cardiotoxicity. Hypotheses include stimulus trafficking of the β2-Adrenergic Receptor (β2-AR) in response to high levels of epinephrine, with a switch to the cardioprotective, but negatively inotropic G_i secondary messenger pathway. This pathway has cardioinhibitory and

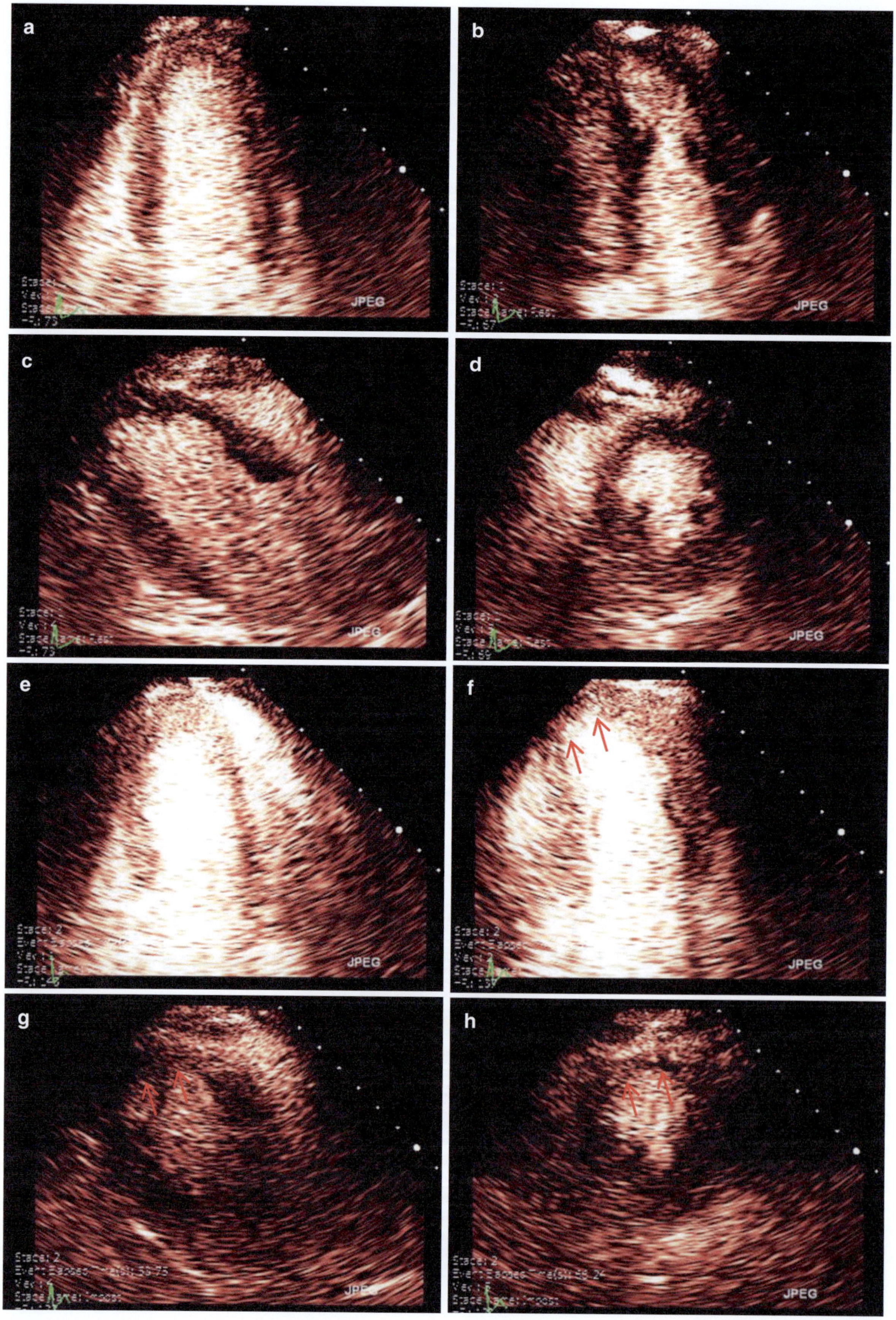

Fig. 5.9 Physiologic stress echocardiography with images at rest (**a–d**) and post-exercise (**e–h**) showing inducible septo-apical and antero-apical akinesia (*red arrows*). (**a**) Apical 4 Chamber (end-diastole). (**b**) Apical 4 Chamber (end-systole). (**c**) Parasternal long axis (end-systole). (**d**) Parasternal short axis at the level of papillary muscles (end-systole). (**e**) Stress Apical 4 Chamber (end-diastole). (**f**) Stress Apical 4 Chamber (end-systole). (**g**) Stress Parasternal long axis (end-systole). (**h**) Stress Parasternal short axis at the level of papillary muscles (end-systole)

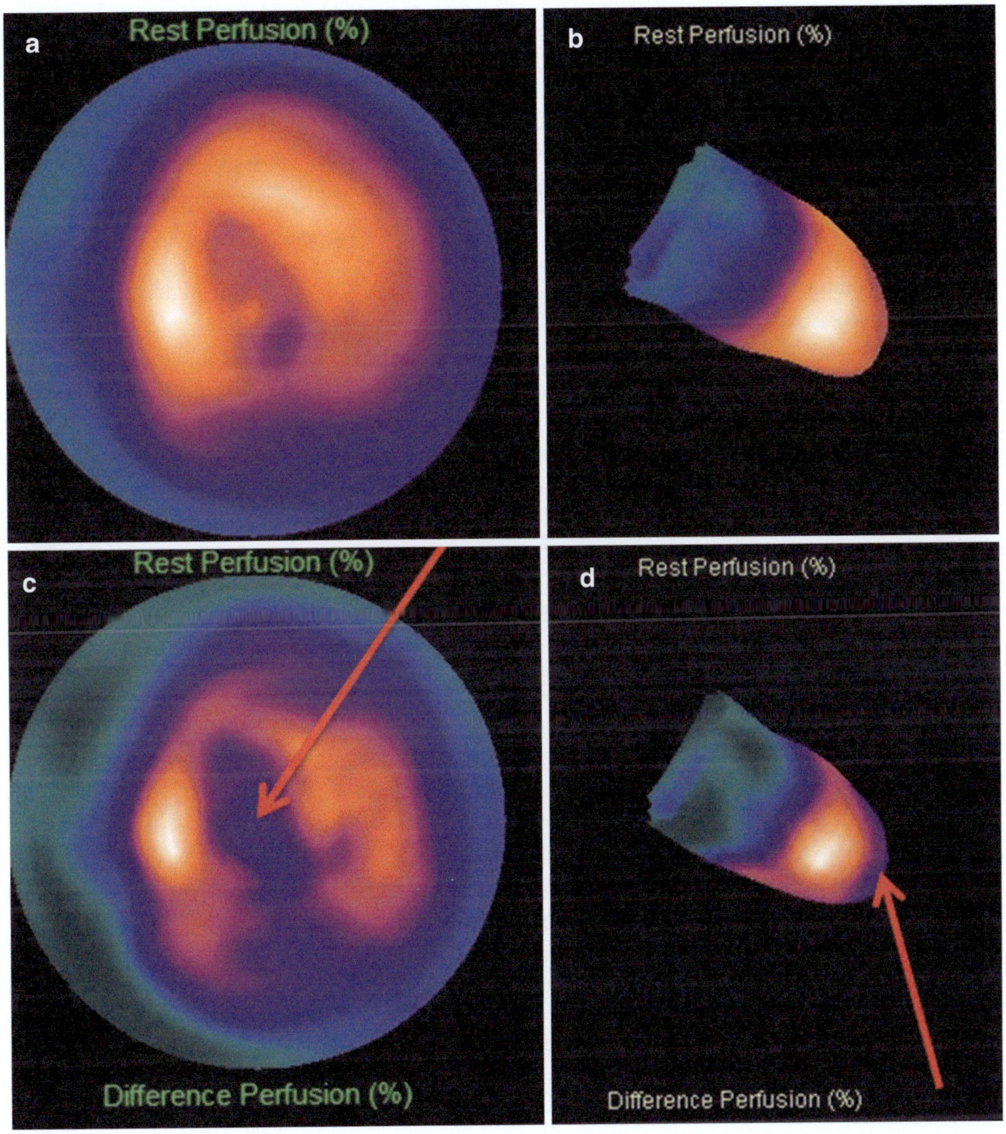

Fig. 5.10 Bull's eye (**a**, **c**) and 3D reconstruction (**b**, **d**) of left ventricular mIBG scan showing distinct apical defect (*red arrows*)

anti-apoptotic properties. Other features include increased afterload and possible diffuse coronary spasm, which altogether result in ventricular systolic dysfunction. Wall motion abnormalities are explained by regional differences in the density of β-adrenoceptors: these are higher in the apex, making this region more susceptible to circulating catecholamine levels; conversely, basal segments have higher rates of sympathetic innervation, leading to increased contractility. These findings are supported by mIBG scan findings following acute presentation, which can show reduced sympathetic innervation in the previously dysfunctional myocardial segments.

Consensus supports the definition of primary and secondary TTS [1], depending on whether TTS appears isolated (usually in the context of an emotional stressor) or triggered by another serious medical condition (phaeochromocytoma, thyrotoxicosis, neurosurgical emergencies, sepsis, cancer).

TTS is not as benign as previously reported. In the acute phase there are a variety of complications (ventricular arrhythmias, heart failure or cardiogenic shock) that require aggressive intervention, with ~50% cases having acute complications, and an inhospital mortality of ~5% across different published cohorts. Furthermore, during follow-up, survival is similar to STEMI and worse than matched population, specifically in the secondary TTS, due to additional comorbidities [5–7].

TTS in cancer patients is becoming increasingly frequent and warrants specific management [8]. This group of patients are frequently under increased levels of emotional stress that predispose to an acute event. The presence of cancer, frequently metastatic, may also be a trigger of secondary TTS via factors hitherto unknown, but may include paracrine factors. Furthermore, many cancer treatments may predispose to developing TTS including 5-Fluorouracil, Tyrosine kinase inhibitors, Anthracyclines, HER-2 inhibitors, ablative or surgical procedures [9].

As presented in our first case, these patients are frail and many times need to discontinue their cardiac medication (betablockers in this case), which could theoretically be another potential trigger. In this clinical context, electrolytic disturbances are not uncommon and may also lead to further electrical instability. All the above may lead to increased mortality in this subgroup of patients [6–8], with non-cardiac causes being the most frequent cause of death. Finally, as described in case 2, there is a small but growing number of patients who present with a new cancer diagnosis following an episode of TTS [7, 8]. This raises the possibility that, for some patients, TTS may be a form of paraneoplastic syndrome, which highlights the importance of long term follow-up in TTS patients, particularly in those without an identifiable acute triggering event.

Key Points

- TTS is defined by chest pain in the presence of transient regional wall motion abnormalities of left, right or both ventricles, in the absence of matching coronary disease.
- ECG abnormalities comprise ST-segment elevation or depression, acute left bundle branch block, T wave inversion and QTc prolongation. The latter is a risk factor for cardiac arrest and warrants ECG-monitoring in the acute phase.
- Given the degree of myocardial dysfunction, the troponin rise is modest, as opposed to a substantial elevation of natriuretic peptides.
- Based on cardiac imaging, there are mainly three anatomical variants of TTS: apical, midwall variant and inverted or basal variant.
- CMR will typically show absence of infarction on LGE but active oedema/inflammation on the STIR images.
- The pathophysiology of TTS is complex and only partially understood. One of the most accepted theories describes TTS as a form of catecholamine-induced cardiotoxicity.
- The hypothesis of stimulus trafficking of the β2-AR in response to high levels of epinephrine would explain regional wall motion abnormalities.
- TTS is defined as primary (whenever an emotional stress is identified) or secondary (triggered by another serious medical condition).
- TTS is not as benign as previously reported: in the acute phase there are a variety of cardiac complications (ventricular arrhythmias, heart failure or cardiogenic shock) that lead to an in hospital mortality of ~5% across different published cohorts.
- During follow-up, TTS survival is also worse than matching cohorts, mainly in the secondary TTS group.
- Cancer can predispose to TTS through various different mechanisms.
- TTS may be a paraneoplastic syndrome in patients with no primary stressor identified, which highlights the importance of follow-up in these subgroup of patients.

References

1. Lyon AR, et al. Current state of knowledge on Takotsubo syndrome: a position statement from the task force on Takotsubo syndrome of the Heart Failure Association of the European Society of Cardiology. Eur J Heart Fail. 2016;18:8–27.
2. El-Sayed AM, et al. Demographic and co-morbid predictors of stress (Takotsubo) cardiomyopathy. Am J Cardiol. 2012;110:1368–72.
3. Akashi YJ, et al. Epidemiology and pathophysiology of Takotsubo syndrome. Nat Rev Cardiol. 2015;12(7):387–97.
4. Lyon AR, et al. Stress (Takotsubo) cardiomyopathy—a novel pathophysiological hypothesis to explain catecholamine-induced acute myocardial stunning. Nat Clin Pract Cardiovasc Med. 2008;5(1):22–9.
5. Singh K, et al. Meta-analysis of clinical correlates of acute mortality in Takotsubo cardiomyopathy. Am J Cardiol. 2014;113:1420–8.
6. Isogai T, et al. Out-of-hospital versus in-hospital Takotsubo cardiomyopathy: analysis of 3719 patients in the Diagnosis Procedure Combination database in Japan. Int J Cardiol. 2014;176:413–7.
7. Morley-Smith AC, et al. Challenges of chronic cardiac problems in survivors of Takotsubo Syndrome. Heart Fail Clin. 2016;12(4):551–7.
8. Burgdof C, et al. Long-term prognosis of the transient left ventricular dysfunction syndrome (Tako-Tsubo cardiomyopathy): focus on malignancies. Eur J Heart Fail. 2008;10(10):1015–9.
9. Best L, et al. Microwave ablation of pulmonary metastases associated with perioperative Takotsubo cardiomyopathy. J Vasc Interv Radiol. 2014;25(7):1139–41.

6 Mechanism and Prevention of Cardiomyopathy Due to Chemotherapy

Rohit Moudgil and Edward T.H. Yeh

Abstract

The emergence of new oncological therapies has seen a great success in attenuating cancer and its metastases. However, the undesirable side-effect of cardiotoxicity has prevented utilization of anticancer therapies to its full potential. This chapter will elucidate some of the mechanisms behind the chemotherapy induced cardiomyopathy and will highlight the potential preventative and therapeutic measures to curb the cardiotoxic effect of anticancer agents. The aim of this chapter is to arm our clinicians with necessary knowledge and guidance as to how to treat chemotherapy related cardiomyopathy in our oncological patients.

Keywords

Chemotherapy • Cardiomyopathy

Introduction

The first "consensus" clinical description of cardiomyopathy was formulated by the cardiac review and evaluation committee supervising trastuzumab clinical trials, which defined drug-associated cardiotoxicity as one or more of the following: (1) cardiomyopathy characterized by a decrease in left ventricular ejection fraction (LVEF) due to regional or global wall motion abnormalities; (2) symptoms associated with congestive heart failure (CHF); (3) signs associated with CHF, such as S3 gallop, tachycardia, or both; (4) decline in initial LVEF of at least 5% to less than 55% with signs and symptoms of heart failure or asymptomatic decrease in LVEF of at least 10% to less than 55% [1]. This description has a limited scope as it does not encompass all the cardiotoxic effects secondary to chemotherapy (which was the original intention), albeit it does serves well as a definition for cardiomyopathy.

Chemotherapy-related cardiomyopathy has traditionally has been divided into two subtypes (Table 6.1). Anthracyclines belongs to chemotherapy-related cardiac dysfunction type I, characterized by irreversible, dose-dependent myocardial injury [2]. In contrast, type II chemotherapy-related cardiac dysfunction has been primarily seen with targeted therapies such as those directed against the human epidermal growth factor receptor-2 (HER2), e.g. trastuzumab [3]. Unlike type I cardiac dysfunction, the concept for type II involves cardiac dysfunction that shows no dose-dependent response, results in no ultrastructural changes and poses a favorable prognosis owing to its reversibility. However, the classification lacks well defined scientific data and is misguided as anthracyclines can lead to reversible effects and in rare instances the trastusumab related cardiomyopathy is also irreversible. Anthracycline administration can result in acute morbidity occurs during or shortly after the drug infusion and includes arrhythmias (supraventricular tachycardia, ventricular ectopy) accompanied, in some patients, by heart failure and pericarditis-myocarditis syndrome [4, 5]. The subacute cardiac toxicity occurs within few weeks, clini-

R. Moudgil, M.D., Ph.D. (✉)
Department of Cardiology, The University of Texas MD Anderson Cancer Center, Houston, TX 77030, USA
e-mail: rmoudgil@mdanderson.org

E.T.H. Yeh, M.D.
Professor of Medicine, Department of Cardiovascular Medicine, University of Missouri, Hospital Drive, Columbia, MO 65212, USA

S.W. Yusuf, J. Banchs (eds.), *Cancer and Cardiovascular Disease*, https://doi.org/10.1007/978-3-319-62088-6_6

Table 6.1 Chemotherapy-induced cardiac dysfunction

Characteristic of the agents	Doxorubicin	Trastuzumab
Clinical course, response to cancer related cardiac dysfunction (CRCD) therapy	May stabilize, but underlying damage appears to be permanent and irreversible; recurrence in months or years may be related to sequential cardiac stress	High likelihood of recovery (to or near baseline cardiac status) in 2–4 months (reversible)
Dose effects	Cumulative, dose related	Not dose related
Mechanism	Topoisomerase II Beta	Blocked ErbB2 signaling
Ultrastructure	Vacuoles; myofibrillar disarray and dropout; necrosis (changes resolve over time)	No apparent ultra structural abnormalities
Noninvasive cardiac testing	Decreased ejection fraction by ultrasound or nuclear determination: global decrease in wall motion	Decreased ejection fraction by ultrasound or nuclear determination: global decrease in wall motion
Effect of rechallenge	High probability of recurrent dysfunction that is progressive, may result in intractable heart failure and death	Increasing evidence for the relative safety of rechallenge; additional data needed
Effect of late sequential stress	High likelihood of sequential stress related cardiac dysfunction	Low likelihood of sequential stress-related cardiac dysfunction

Modified from Ewer MS, Lippman SM. Type II chemotherapy-related cardiac dysfunction: time to recognize a new entity. J Clin Oncol. 2005;23:2900–2902

cally resembles myocarditis with edema and thickening of the left ventricular walls, and is associated with diastolic dysfunction and increased mortality [6]. In contrast to the late anthracycline mediated cardiotoxicity, improvement in left ventricular function has been noted to occur in these subacute patients [4, 7, 8].

Figure 6.1 Illustrates the case of improvement in LVEF in a patient with cardiomyopathy, secondary to adriamycin based chemotherapy. The case presented is of a 19-year-old gentleman with osteosarcoma of the L5 and S1 vertebrae for which he underwent surgery and anthracycline based chemotherapy, with a total cumulative dose of Adriamycin of 540 mg/m^2, completed in Dec 2003. Soon afterwards, he was admitted with symptoms and signs of cardiac dysfunction and an echocardiogram in Jan 04, showed an LVEF of 20%, with a thrombus in his left ventricle. He was started on low molecular heparin for the thrombus and ACE-I, beta-blockers and spironolactone for his cardiomyopathy. Over the next few months, his LV function recovered and remained normal on subsequent follow ups (last follow up at our institution was in March 2007), as he continued to take his cardiac medications

Alternatively trastuzumab, can also show irreversible cardiac dysfunction, although the incidence is very low [9]. Recent PHARE trials showed that their seems to be a time dependent increase in cardiotoxicity among patients treated with trastuzumab and a small portion of patients among the treated cohort had irreversible cardiac dysfunction at the end of 2 year [9]. Therefore, it is time to revisit the classification

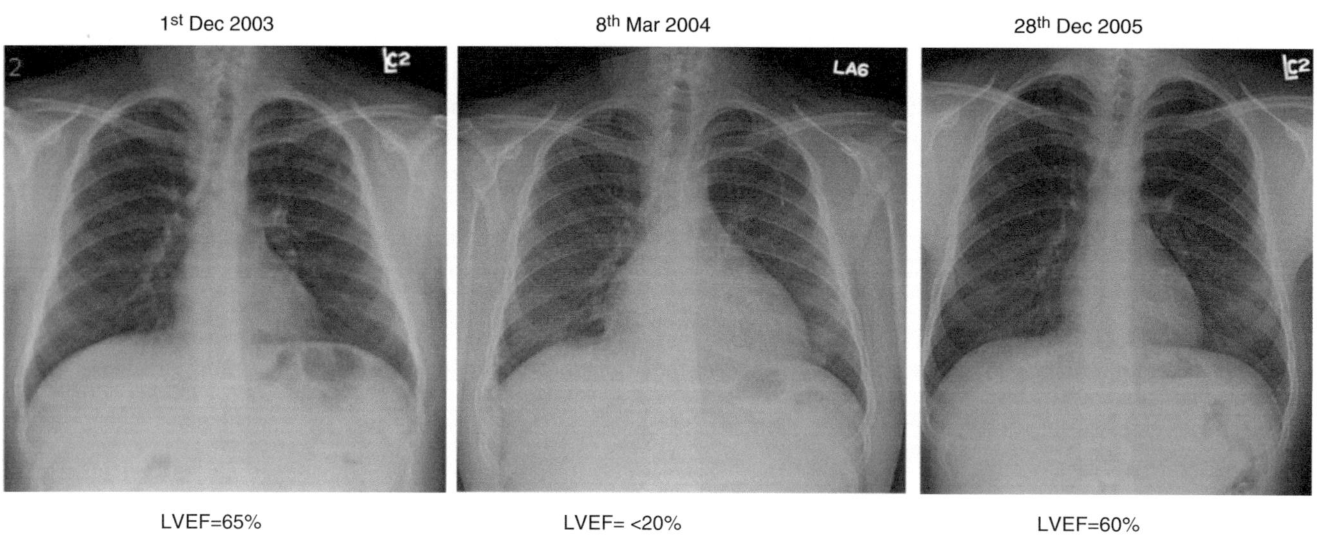

Fig. 6.1 A 19-yead-old gentleman with osteosarcoma of the L5 and S1 vertebrae. He underwent surgery and chemotherapy, with a total cumulative dose of Adriamycin of 540 mg/m^2, completed in Dec 2003. He was admitted with symptoms and signs of cardiac dysfunction and an echocardiogram in Jan 04, showed an LV ejection fraction of 20%, with a thrombus in his left ventricle. He was started on low molecular heparin for the thrombus and ACE-I, beta-blockers and spironolactone for his cardiomyopathy. Over the next few month his LV function recovered and remained normal on subsequent follow ups (last follow up at our institution was in March 2007), as he continued to take his cardiac medications. The chest X ray done when the LVEF was 20% shows cardiomegaly, with normal heart size prior to chemotherapy and subsequently on normalization of LVEF. (Image courtesy of Dr. S.W. Yusuf)

as recent studies have created a grey area in this dichotomous subtype.

Case Presentation #1

A 47 year old female was diagnosed with intra-ductal carcinoma of the breast. As a part of therapeutic regimen she underwent neo-adjuvant chemotherapy with doxorubicin (300 mg/m^2). An baseline echocardiogram was done which showed an LVEF of 63%. Subsequently, she received the chemotherapy and 6 months later, as part of cardiac surveillance, she underwent an echocardiogram which showed an LVEF of 53%. Therefore, the question arises as to what is/are the molecular mechanism(s) underlying this objective deterioration and what therapeutic strategies can be used, if any, in this asymptomatic patient.

Anthracyclines

Clinical Perspective

In a retrospective analysis of over 4000 patients treated with doxorubicin (DOX), von Hoff and colleagues [10] found that 2.2% of the patients developed clinical signs and symptoms of CHF. Since the study identified CHF based on clinical assessment, incorporation of subclinical left ventricular dysfunction would result in higher incidence of the cardiovascular disease in DOX treated patients; as acknowledged by the authors themselves [10]. This study went on to conclude that the prevalence of heart failure markedly increased with a cumulative dose of 550 mg/m^2 of DOX [10], which is now recognized as one of the greatest determinants in the development of anthracycline mediated heart failure [11].

Subsequently, the cardiotoxicity in DOX treated patients was prospectively assessed in three clinical trials (two in breast and one in non-small cell lung cancer) conducted between 1988 and 1992. The cumulative findings highlighted that it seemed to have dose-dependent damage (CHF was 5% at a cumulative dose of 400 mg/m^2, 16% at a dose of 500 mg/m^2 and 26% at a dose of 550 mg/m^2) [11]. This was also true in pediatric population who had a lifetime increased risk of cardiac dysfunction with increased anthracycline dose (Fig. 6.2). Histo-pathologically, changes can be seen in endomyocardial biopsy specimens from patients who have received as little as 240 mg/m^2 of DOX [12]. Moreover, subclinical events occurred in about 30% of the patients, even at doses of 180–240 mg/m^2 [13], although they were observed 13 years after the treatment was received. Even doses as low as 100 mg/m^2 have been associated with reduced cardiac function [12, 14]. These findings suggest that there is no safe dose of anthracyclines. Conversely, early studies suggested that some patients had no significant cardiac complications despite achievement of the doses as high as 1000 mg/m^2 [10]. Therefore, individual susceptibility to cardiomyopathy may vary. However, the current consensus is that DOX causes cardiomyopathy.

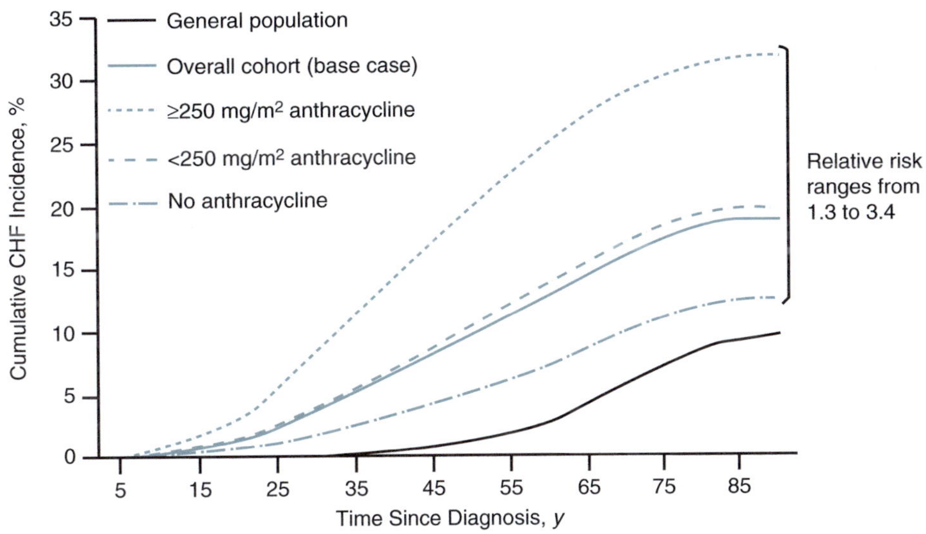

Fig. 6.2 Life-time incidence of HF in pediatric cancer survivors stratified by cumulative anthracycline dose. (Yeh JM, Nohria A, Diller L. Routine echocardiography screening for asymptomatic left ventricular dysfunction in childhood cancer survivors: a model-based estimation of the clinical and economic effects. Ann Intern Med 2014;160:661–71; with permission)

Pathophysiological Mechanisms

Anthracycline mediated cardiomyopathy has been studied extensively. Among the pathways implicated in anthracycline mediated toxicity involves production of reactive oxygen species, formation of iron complexes resulting in intracellular damage. However, new evidence highlights the role of topoisomerase II beta (Top II B) as a direct target of DOX that provides a unifying mechanism encompassing most of the implicated pathways in DOX mediated cardiomyopathy.

It has been well-studied that one of the mechanisms of DOX induced tumor-cytotoxic effect is mediated by topoisomerase II alpha inhibition [15]. However, the heart only expresses Top II B. Recent research looking at the effects of DOX in Top II B has identified that by virtue of forming a ternary complex (DNA/DOX/Top II B) double stranded breaks were generated, reactive oxygen species and mitochondrial damage ensued, thus disrupting myofibrillar apparatus culminating into cardiac dysfunction. The end result was an increase in end systolic and end-diastolic volumes with decrease in ejection fraction [16] (Fig. 6.3). Other studies also identified the activation of the p53 pathway to DNA-damage and the consequent apoptosis and mitochondrial dysfunction in cultured cardiomyocytes treated with DOX [17, 18].

The corroborating evidence of Top II B mechanism is provided by the use of dexrazoxane (DEX). In vivo, DEX has shown significant cardio-protection against DOX in various preclinical models such as mouse, rat, hamster, rabbit, and dog [19–22]. In addition, the cardioprotective effects were evident in both acute and chronic models of DOX-induced cardiomyopathy [23, 24]. These findings were extended to human subjects in various clinical trials also [21, 25–28]. It appears that DEX can block ATP hydrolysis and inhibit the reopening of the ATPase domain, thereby trapping the topoisomerase complex on DNA and blocking enzyme turnover [29]which may be its predominant mechanism. Therefore, DEX inhibits DOX's activity on TOP II B catalytic site, thereby providing cardio-protection. In essence, DOX/DNA/Top II B ternary complex may be the prime mediator of anthracycline mediated cardiomyopathy.

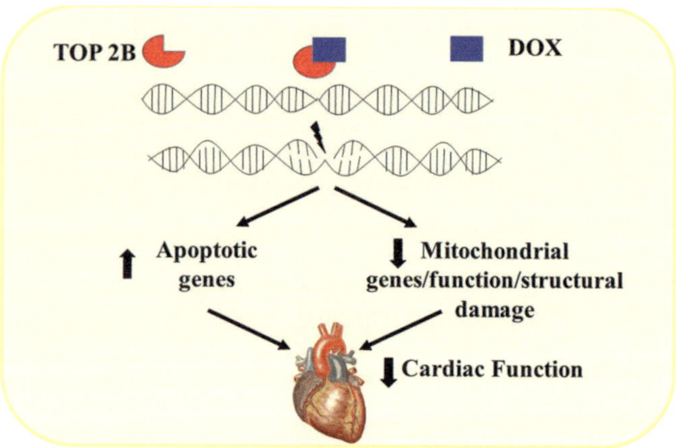

Fig. 6.3 Schematic representation of DOX/DNA/Top II Beta ternary Complex. Activation of the ternary complex results in upregulation of apoptotic signaling pathway. Furthermore, there is a downregulation of mitochondrial function. Both pathways culminates into decreased overall cardiac function resulting in congestive heart failure

Current Therapies to Prevent Anthracycline Mediated Cardiomyopathies

Primary Prevention

Continuous Infusion

Replacing bolus administration with slow infusions does not significantly affect anthracycline area under the curve (AUC) but diminishes anthracycline Cmax and anthracycline accumulation in the heart [30]. A Cochrane review [31] identified seven randomized clinical trials (RCTs) and showed a significantly lower rate of clinical heart failure with an infusion duration of 6 h or longer as compared to a shorter infusion duration (relative risk (RR) = 0.27; 95% confidence interval (CI) 0.09 to 0.81; 5 studies; 557 patients). As far as the peak dose is concerned, neither less than 60 mg/m^2 DOX versus 60 mg/m^2 or more (two RCTs), liposomal DOX at 25 mg/m^2 versus 50 mg/m^2 (one RCT), and epirubicin peak dose of 83 mg/m^2 versus 110 mg/m^2 (one RCT) showed promise for a lower incidence of clinical HF [31]. Thus, increased duration of anthracycline infusion to 6 h or longer reduce the risk of clinical heart failure and subclinical cardiac damage to some extent [71]. However, the review was only performed in adult population inflicted with solid tumors.

In pediatric populations, the results of infusion of anthracycline have been disappointing. A randomized trial in children with high-risk ALL found that continuous infusion offered no additional cardiac protection over bolus administration in a median follow-up of 8 years post-diagnosis [32]. A follow-up at 10 years also revealed no incremental therapeutic efficacy for infusion [32]. This is further supported by other studies, which also looked at cardiovascular outcomes in patients 5–7 years after treatment [33, 34]. However, despite a lack of evidence for cardioprotection, anthracycline administration by continuous infusion is still incorporated into pediatric treatment protocols for cardioprotection [32].

PEGylated Liposomal DOX

PEGylated liposomal DOX comprises an aqueous core of DOX hydrochloride encapsulated in liposomes with a protective hydrophilic outer coating of surface-bound methoxypolyethylene glycol [35, 36]. Delivery of DOX in a PEGylated liposomal form decreases the circulating concentrations of free DOX and result in selective uptake of the agent in tumor cells.

In three randomized [37–39], open-label, multi-center trials, monotherapy conducted with PEGylated liposomal DOX showed that it is as effective as DOX or capecitabine in the first-line treatment of metastatic breast cancer, and as effective as vinorelbine or combination mitomycin plus vinblastine in taxane-refractory metastatic breast cancer.

PEGylated liposomal DOX exhibited a favorable cardiac safety profile compared with conventional DOX and other available chemotherapy agents. The most common treatment-related adverse events included myelosuppression, palmar-plantar erythrodysesthesia and stomatitis, although these are manageable with appropriate supportive measures [40]. Thus, PEGylated liposomal DOX is a useful option in the treatment of various malignancies, including metastatic breast cancer, ovarian cancer, multiple myeloma and AIDS-related Kaposi's sarcoma [41]. However, the cost associated with administering the drug has prevented its widespread adoption as a conventional anthracycline therapy [42].

Dexrazoxane

DEX (ICRF-187, ADR-529) and the corresponding racemic mixture—razoxane (ICRF-159, ADR-159)—belong to the bisdioxopiperazine agents originally developed by Creighton et al. [43], as a potential anticancer agent. While it was being developed as anti-cancer agent, using H9c2 myoblasts and fibroblasts from TOP II B knockout mice, Lyu et al. [44] have suggested that the parent compound DEX may be protective through inhibition of anthracycline-induced and TOP II B-mediated DNA damage, thus opening a window of DEX as a protective agent for anthracycline induced cardio-toxicity.

More evidence of support emerged when DEX was shown to be cardioprotective in DOX treated populations. The salient effects of DEX against anthracycline-induced cardiotoxicity have been unanimously demonstrated in numerous clinical trials and in both adults and children [27, 28, 45–50]. Importantly, significant cardioprotection has been achieved in various chemotherapy regimens, using different DEX-to-anthracycline ratios and different subtypes of anthracycline in clinical use. Cardioprotective potential of DEX has been evaluated by clinical examination (incidence of cardiac events and symptoms of CHF), using cardiac function examinations (echocardiography or radionuclide ventriculography), by analysis of biochemical markers (e.g., plasma concentrations of cardiac troponins) and/or endomyocardial biopsy [27, 28, 45, 46, 48, 50]. Today, DEX had passed all the stages of preclinical and clinical research and has been finally approved in Europe and the United States for cardioprotection in patients treated with anthracyclines (Cardioxane and Zinecard) with several generic preparations recently available (Procard and Cardynax). More recently, DEX has been also approved for treatment of accidental extravasation of anthracyclines (Savene). Thus, DEX role as protective agent against anthracycline induced cardio-toxicity has been firmly established.

Significant, although not well evidenced, suspicion on potential interference of DEX with anticancer effects of anthracycline has arisen from one of the phase III trials [28]. In this trial ($n = 293$), a significant difference in objective response has been reported (47% vs. 61%, respectively, $p = 0.019$). While high response in the placebo group was quite unusual, no other endpoints (including survival or time to progression) were affected in either of these studies, DEX nevertheless became scrutinized for potential negative effects on tumor response [28, 49]. Careful meta-analyses of all available randomized clinical trial data have, however, found no evidence for this hypothesis [47, 51]. Still, the American Society of Clinical Oncology, Chemotherapy and Radiotherapy Expert Panel remain cautious and recommend using DEX only in very limited conditions (e.g., patients who have received more than 300 mg/m^2 for metastatic breast cancer and who may benefit from continued DOX treatment) [52]. The time has come to revisit this cautionary note.

Secondary Prevention

Beta-Blocker

Beta Blockers have been at the cornerstone of treating various cardiovascular disease. Initial investigations, with small sample size demonstrated the beneficial effects of beta-blockers for anthracycline cardiotoxicity [53–55]. In a small, randomized placebo-controlled study, patients treated with carvedilol at anthracycline initiation had preserved systolic and diastolic function at 6 months [53]. Recent data from the OVERCOME (preventiOn of left Ventricular dysfunction with Enalapril and caRvediolol in patients submitted to intensive ChemOtherapy for the treatment of Malignant hEmopathies) trial have also shown that beta-blocker therapy, in combination with angiotensin converting enzyme (ACE) inhibitor therapy, may be beneficial in preventing anthracycline-induced cardiotoxicity, with treated patients demonstrating less significant changes in LVEF and a lower incidence of death or HF compared with placebo [56]. Table 6.2 provides a summary of some of the clinical trials.

PRADA (PRevention of cArdiac Dysfunction during Adjuvant breast cancer therapy) trial was designed as largest clinical trial to look at the chemotherapy mediated cardio-toxicity. It was a randomized, placebo-controlled, 2 × 2 factorial, double-blind trial to assess whether left ventricular dysfunction and/or injury is preventable, completely or partly, by the concomitant administration of the angiotensin receptor blocker (ARB), candesartan, and the beta

Table 6.2 Cardio-protective therapies in chemotherapy mediated cardiac dysfunction

Therapies and authors	Population and treatment	Total number of patients	Therapy	Duration of follow-up	Findings
Beta-blockers					
Kalay et al. [53]	Anthracylines in breast, lymphoma etc.	50	Carvedilol 12.5 mg once daily vs. placebo	6 months	Preserved ejection fraction in carvedilo l 68.9 vs. 52.3 (P < 0.001)
Seicean et al. [54]	Anthracycline and Trastuzumab	318	Continuous BB (n = 106) vs. not on continuous BB (n = 212)	3.2 years	Lower incidence of new onset heart failure (HF). HF events 5 vs. 27 (P = 0.008) in continuous BB vs. no BB group
Kaya et al. [55]	Breast cancer and planned chemotherapy	45	Nebivolol 5 mg daily vs. placebo	Echocardiogram and NT pro-BNP at baseline and 6 months of chemo	Preservation of LVEF, end-systolic and end-diastolic volume in nebivolol (P = 0.01) Reduced NT BNP in treatment group
Angiotensin converting enzyme inhibitor/angiotensin receptor antagonist					
Cardinale et al. [59]	High dose chemo for AML, relapsed, or refractory Hodgkins lymphoma, Ewing's sarcoma	114	Enalapril 20 mg daily vs. none	1 month after last high-dose chemo, continued 1 year	Absolute decrease in LVEF > 10% to decline below normal value (LVEF, 50%) (43% vs. 0%) (P < 0.001)
Cadeddu et al. [65]	Epirubicin in solid tumors	49	Telmisartan 40 mg daily vs. placebo	Echo, TD, strain/strain rate (SR) and plasma levels of inflammatory and oxidative stress markers at baseline and at 7 days after every new epirubicin	Impairment in strain rate peak epi dose of 200 mg/m^2 (no significant difference between groups) but at 300 and 400 mg/m^2 SR normalized only in telmisartan group (P < 0.001) Significant increase in ROS and interleukin-6 in placebo
Nakamae et al. [66]	CHOP in Non-Hodgkin's lymphoma	40	Valsartan 80 mg daily vs. none	Neurohormonal, echo, and ECG Parameters measured before, days 3, 5, 7 and after initiation of CHOP 7 days	Valsartan significantly prevented increases in LVEDd, QTc dispersion and BNP elevation (P < 0.05) with no significant change in BP or HR
Spironolactone					
Akpek et al. [68]	Anthracycline for breast cancer	83	25 mg/day vs. placebo	LVEF, CKMB, troponin, oxidative stress index and diastolic parameters	LVEF decrease from 67.0 ± 6.1 to 65.7 ± 7.4 (*P* = 0.094) in the spironolactone group, and from 67.7 ± 6.3 to 53.6 ± 6.8 in the control group (*P* < 0.001) The diastolic functional grade was protected in treatment group (*P* < 0.001). CKMB, troponins and oxidative stress index was lower in treatment group

blocker, metoprolol, during postoperative chemotherapy and radiotherapy [57]. The important finding in PRADA was that unlike the angiotensin receptor blocker candesartan, metoprolol, a beta blocker, didn't prevent the early drop in LVEF commonly seen in breast cancer patients treated with anthracyclines and trastuzumab, even though both classes of heart medications are at the hub of treating ischemic and hypertensive cardiomyopathy [58]. These findings may be due to some of the study limitations. Foremost concern was the small number of participants in the study, even though it is the largest clinical trial in chemotherapy mediated cardiotoxicity. Another limitation is that this was an extremely low-cardiovascular-risk patient cohort: the baseline prevalence of diabetes was less than 4% per group, and fewer than 7% of patients had hypertension. Therefore, the incidence of moderate and severe heart failure was extremely low and thereby hard to extrapolate to our symptomatic population. Furthermore, the incidence of cardiomyopathy following breast cancer therapy is known to increase over time, the short duration of follow-up in the study was also concerning from beta-blocker perspective.

Angiotensin Converting Enzyme Inhibitors (ACEI) and Angiotensin 2 Receptor Blockers (ARB)

Role of enalapril was studied in 114 patients with a baseline normal LVEF but an elevated troponin I level within 72 h after high-dose anthracycline administration. These patients were then randomized to enalapril or placebo after completion of chemotherapy and followed for 12 months [59]. Roughly, half of the control cohort (43%) and none of the ACE inhibitor–treated patients met the primary end point (decrease in LVEF of >10%). Additionally, there were 30 cardiac events in the control patients and only 1 cardiac event in ACE inhibitor–treated patients [59]. Thus, early administration of enalapril proved to be cardio-protective [59]. A prospective study examined the effects of angiotensin-converting enzyme (ACE) inhibitors in breast cancer patients treated with epirubicin. Patients receiving ACE inhibitors had an increase in their LVEF, suggesting that ACE inhibitors should be part of the treatment of LV dysfunction in cancer patients [60]. These studies were at the footsteps of OVERCOME trial which showed beneficial effects with ACEI [56].

Conversely, in younger population, a trial in 18 doxorubicin-treated long-term childhood cancer survivors reported improved LV function with enalapril treatment, but this improvement was lost 10 years after treatment, suggesting that the effects of ACE inhibitors are transient [61]. In 2004, Silber et al. [62] reported the results of a randomized, double-blind, controlled clinical trial comparing enalapril to placebo in 135 long-term survivors of pediatric cancer who had at least 1 cardiac abnormality identified at any time after anthracycline exposure. There was no difference in the rate of change in maximal cardiac index per year between enalapril and placebo groups (0.30 L/min/m^2 vs. 0.18 L/min/m^2; $P = 0.55$).

One possible explanation is that ACE inhibitors do not provide long-term protection in children because of the restrictive nature of anthracycline-induced cardiomyopathy [63]. In addition to the lack of evidence of a long-term benefit in children compliance may be an issue with this cohort. In pediatric cancer population who are undergoing chemotherapy, adverse effects of ACE-inhibitor therapy are well known, including hypotension, dizziness, fatigue, and chronic neurohormonal suppression [64]. This may lead to compliance issues. Thus, ACEI's effects may limited in pediatric cancer population over the long-term.

ARBs have also been studied as cardioprotective agents in patients receiving anthracycline therapy [65]. Valsartan was found to have a protective effect against acute cardiotoxicity in a small study of patients who received doxorubicin for Hodgkin's lymphoma [66]. In a randomized control trial, patients who received telmisartan with epirubicin also showed preserved systolic function by LVEF and strain rate [67]. Overall, ARB seems to have the same efficacy of cardio-protection as the ACEI.

Spironolactone

While the studies in beta-blocker and ACEI are limited, role of spironolactone was identified in one study. Eighty-three female patients who were diagnosed with breast cancer were randomized into spironolactone and control groups [68]. A dose of 25 mg/day spironolactone was administered to the patients in the spironolactone group. There were 43 patients (mean age 50 ± 11 years) in the spironolactone group and 40 patients (mean age 51 ± 10 years) in the control group. LVEF decreased from 67.0 ± 6.1 to 65.7 ± 7.4 ($P = 0.094$) in the spironolactone group, and from 67.7 ± 6.3 to 53.6 ± 6.8 in the control group ($P < 0.001$) [68]. When the general linear model was applied, the interaction of LVEF decrease between groups was significantly lower in the spironolactone group than in the control group ($P < 0.001$) [68]. The diastolic functional grade of subjects in the spironolactone group was protected ($P = 0.096$), whereas it deteriorated in the control group ($P < 0.001$) [68]. Thus, the study showed that spironolactone may have a role to play in cardioprotection against chemotherapy mediated cardio-toxicity. Future clinical trial NCT01708798 is being conducted where the potential ability of the aldosterone antagonist, eplerenone, to prevent doxorubicin-induced cardiotoxicity, will be explored in a randomized controlled trial in the breast cancer patients.

Statins

Clinical data regarding statin therapy for anthracycline-induced cardiotoxicity in humans is sparse. In a retrospective observational study of 201 breast cancer patients treated with anthracyclines, concomitant statin use for other indications in

64 patients was associated with a reduced risk of HF hospitalization compared with propensity-matched controls (hazard ratio 0.3, 95% CI 0.1–0.9, P < 0.03) [69]. In a small trial, 40 patients receiving anthracycline containing chemotherapy regimens were randomized to receive atorvastatin or no intervention. The control group showed statistically significant worsening of LVEF and change in LV dimensions as compared with the atorvastatin group. The incidence of LVEF of less than 50% was lower (although not statistically significant) in patients on atorvastatin as compared with those in the control group (5 versus 25%, P < 0.18) [70]. A summary of cardio-protective therapy in provided in Table 6.2.

Despite a wide array of heart failure medication at hand, prompt administration is at the cornerstone of curbing anthracycline mediated cardiomyopathy. In a study comprising of 201 patients with a left ventricular ejection fraction (LVEF) ≤45% due to anthracycline mediated cardiomyopathy Beta blocker (carvediolol) and ACEI (enalapril) was administered when decrease in LVEF was noted. LVEF was measured at enrollment, every month for the first 3 months, every 3 months during the first 2 following years, and every 6 months afterward (mean follow-up 36 ± 27 months). Patients were considered responders, partial responders, or non-responders according to complete, partial, or no recovery in LVEF, respectively. The study showed roughly half of the patient population responded to therapy (Fig. 6.4). In this study, responders showed a lower rate of cumulative cardiac events than partial and non-responders (5%, 31% and 29% respectively; p< 0.001) [71]. Additionally, the proportion of non-responder increased with time duration between the anthracycline administration and implementation of heart failure medications [71] (Fig. 6.5). Therefore, prompt diagnosis and immediate therapeutic intervention should be at the hub of the cardiac clinical care provided to the oncological patients (Fig. 6.5) [71].

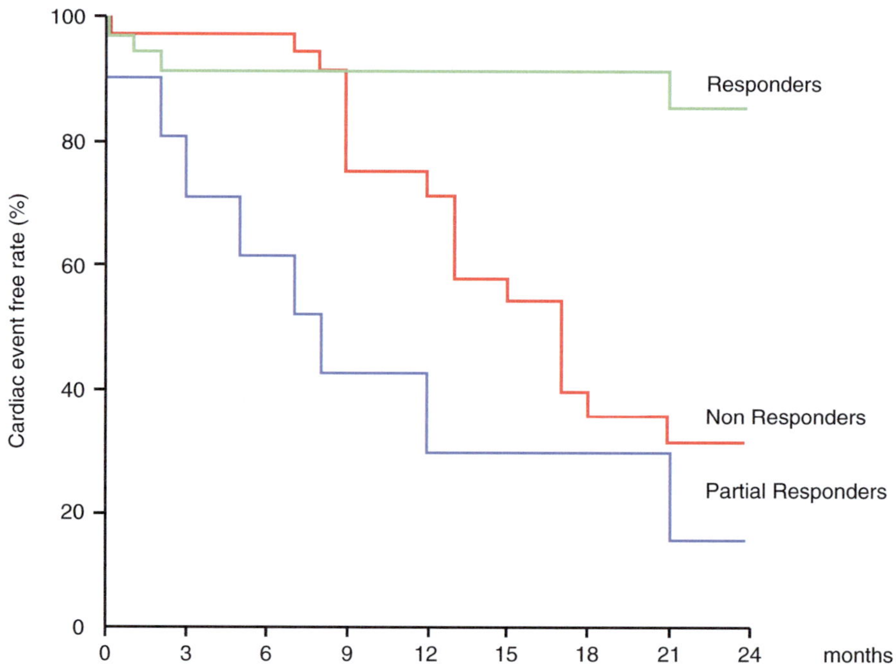

Fig. 6.4 Cumulative rate of cardiac events over 2 year study time. (Cardinale D et al. *J Am Coll Cardiol.* 2010;55:213-220. with permission)

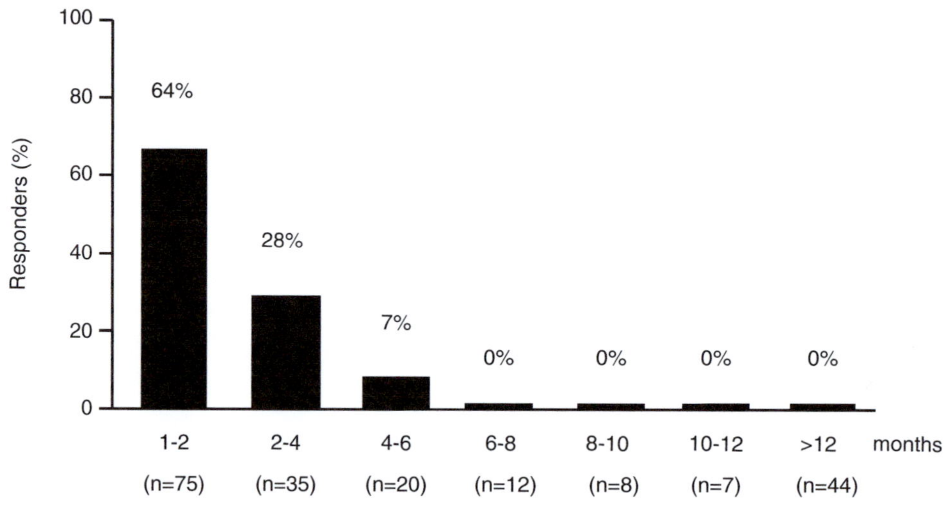

Fig. 6.5 Percentage of responders from the time of anthracycline administration to the time of the initiation of heart failure therapy. (Cardinale D et al. *J Am Coll Cardiol.* 2010;55:213–220. with permission)

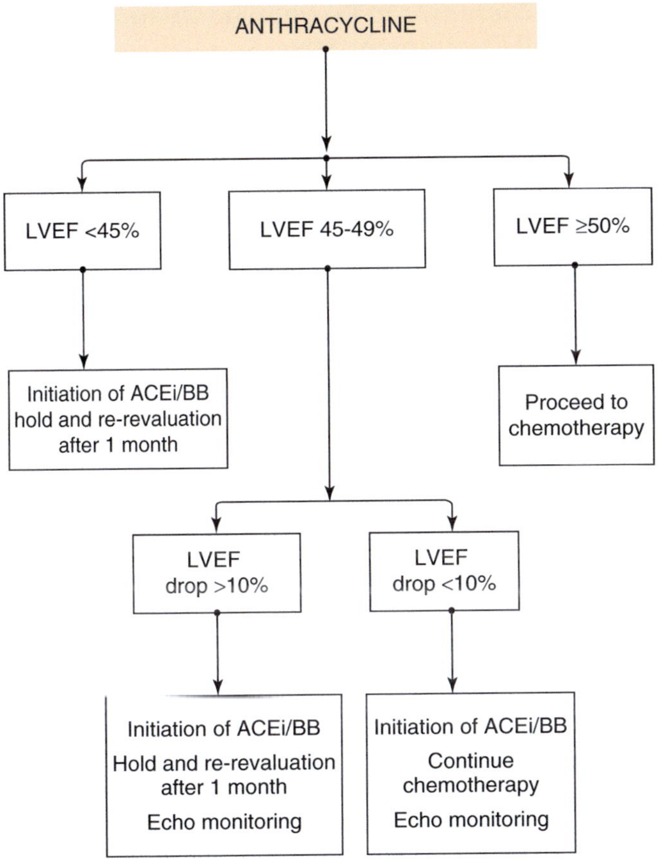

Fig. 6.6 Hassan, S. and Banchs, J. *Monitoring Cardiotoxicity with Left Ventricular Ejection Fraction*. **MD Anderson Practices in Onco-Cardiology** 2015

Revisiting the Case #1

A 47 year old female who was treated with doxorubicin for intra-ductal carcinoma of the breast had an asymptomatic decrease in her ejection fraction from 63 to 53%. In clinical practice we would hold anthracycline temporarily (after discussion with the oncologist) and initiate beta-blockers and ACEI with continuation of chemotherapy and close echocardiographic monitoring. Ideally, re-initiation of chemotherapy should be with slow continuous infusion over 6 h as it has been shown to be cardioprotective. A succinct experience based clinical practice has been outlined in our institutional booklet, M.D. Anderson Practices in Onco-Cardiology which is available online for free download (Fig. 6.6) [72].

Case Presentation #2

Fifty-two year old female with breast cancer was found to have Her 2 positive lymph nodes as she underwent mastectomy and lymph node biopsy. The pre-chemotherapeutic echocardiogram showed ejection of 57%. At 6-month follow-up she reported fatigue after using traztuzumab and echocardiogram showed ejection fraction of 47% by Simpson's method. Therefore, question remains as to what is the molecular mechanism in precipitating type II cardiomyopathy and what are the therapeutic strategies one can employ to curb the ejection fraction decrease. Most importantly, can we re-introduce traztuzumab to complete the course of chemotherapy despite this decrease in ejection fraction?

HER-2/ERB-2 Targeted Therapies

Clinical Perspective

Trastuzumab is a monoclonal antibody against the human epidermal growth factor receptor tyrosine kinase (HER2-ErbB2), which is a member of a cell-receptor family that regulates cell growth and intracellular repair [73]. Overexpression of human epidermal growth factor receptor-2 (HER2) receptor occurs in approximately 25% of breast cancers and confers increased proliferative and metastatic potential. Trastuzumab has been used in human epidermal growth factor receptor-2 positive (HER2+ve) breast cancers with significant reductions in recurrence rates and overall mortality. In agreement, a pivotal study in the metastatic setting demonstrated a 33% reduction in mortality at 1 year and an increase in median survival by 5 months [74].

The cardiac side effect of trastuzumab was first noticed following the trials leading to its approval by the Food and Drug Administration in 1998 [1]. In these trials, trastuzumab was administered on top of the standard therapy, which consisted of either paclitaxel or doxorubicin and cyclophosphamide. Post-hoc analyses revealed an incidence of "cardiotoxicity" of up to 11% in patients receiving trastuzumab on top of paclitaxel compared with only 1–4% in those who received paclitaxel alone [74]. There was an even greater incidence of cardiotoxicity in patients receiving the combination of trastuzumab and anthracyclines. Anthracyclines, such as doxorubicin [75], are themselves cardiotoxic, but addition of trastuzumab leads to a synergistic increased in incidence of cardiac symptoms from 13% (with doxorubicin alone) to 27% (when combined with trastuzumab). Moreover, severe chronic heart failure (New York Heart Association class III and IV) occurred in 16% of patients treated with this combination [1]. Subsequently, several large clinical trials confirmed the importance of trastuzumab in increasing disease-free survival from cancer, but also established trastuzumab's association with heart failure [76, 77]. The incidence of cardiomyopathy dropped to 13% when anthracyclines were not administered concurrently with trastuzumab; although these patients were previously treated with anthracycline. In the adjuvant trials, 1.7–4.1% of trastuzumab-treated patients developed CHF [76, 77] when anthracycline was not part of the therapeutic regimen. Thus, trastuzumab came with a black box warning of possibly inducing cardiomyopathy.

Trastuzumab-related cardiac damage includes various degrees of LV systolic dysfunction, occasionally leading to CHF. ECG changes are not seen [78]. Symptoms are usually mild or moderate and improve following medical management and termination of drug administration [79, 80]. The improvement is usually seen in about 6 weeks after trastuzumab withdrawal and can be earlier [81]. After symptomatic improvement, the re-institution of trastuzumab treatment is usually possible [79–81]. The reversibility of trastuzumab-induced cardiac toxicity may be explained by the fact that this compound does not cause cell death but only temporary dysfunction by inducing changes in the structure of contractile proteins [82]. In further agreement, the risk of cardiotoxicity is confined to the time of administration, as illustrated in randomized controlled trials. These are the characteristics of type II chemotherapy-related cardiac damage [3].

Pathophysiological Mechanisms

Early studies indicated that the murine Erb-B2 Receptor Tyrosine Kinase 2 (ERBB2), and its activating ligand, neuregulin-1 (Nrg1), play an integral role in the cardiac development. ErbB2 activation activates the ERK and PI3K/Akt pathways promoting cardiomyocyte survival [83]. Expression of the anti-apoptotic protein Bcl-XL in the hearts of mice with cardio-specific ERBB2 deletion partially prevented the heart chamber dilation and the impaired contractility seen in the adulthood and suggests that ERBB2 signaling is important for normal cardiomyocyte function per se [84].

Trastuzumab is a humanized monoclonal antibody to subdomain IV of ErbB2 [85]. This leads to disruption of ErbB2-ErbB3 complexes which are preferentially formed when ErbB2 is overexpressed in the absence of ligand-binding to ErbB3 [85]. The exact mechanisms of this disruption are still unclear. Disruption of these complexes inhibits PI3K signaling and Akt activation and explains the antiproliferative effects of trastuzumab in ErbB2-amplified tumor cells. Hence, trastuzumab inhibits only ligand-independent signaling [86]. On the other hand, pertuzumab is a humanized monoclonal antibody to subdomain II, the dimerization arm of ErbB2 [87]. Pertuzumab leads to inhibition of ligand-induced ErbB2 signaling, not of ligand-independent ErbB2 signaling, thus inhibiting the signal transduction mechanism only in the presence of a ligand [86]. Alternatively, lapatinib is a small molecule tyrosine kinase inhibitor of ErbB1 and ErbB2 [88]. Lapatinib blocks tyrosine kinase activity, independently of whether this activity has been triggered by a ligand or not, thus inhibiting both ligand-dependent and independent mechanism [86, 89, 90]. With this assertion then lapatinib should cause a similar, if not more, incidence of cardiomyopathy which is not the case clinically. Thus, precise mechanisms is not clearly delineated yet.

Current Therapies to Prevent Trastuzumab Mediated Cardiomyopathy

In a Cardiac Review and Evaluation Committee (CREC) analysis of 82 women with trastuzumab induced cardiomyopathy [3], Seventy-nine percent responded to conventional therapy including ACEIs, diuretics, cardiac glycosides and other inotropic agents. There was a significant difference in the recovery potential between patients with and without additional anthracycline therapy and those with and without cardiac troponin elevation, which was noted at baseline or with the first two cycles of trastuzumab, suggestive of an interactive phenomenon as further outlined below [3, 91] Withdrawal of trastuzumab resulted in complete recovery in ejection fraction in 84% of the patients within a mean time of 1.5 months [3]. Over 75% of patients in this cohort were re-introduced to trastuzumab and 88% of these showed no further change in cardiac parameters [3].

In 2009, the United Kingdom National Cancer Research Institute released recommendations for management of cardiac health in trastuzumab-treated patients with breast cancer. The readers are referred to this clinical resource for an effective management of trastuzumab-induced cardiomyopathy [92]. Furthermore, MD Anderson Practices in Onco-Cardiology also outlines how to treat heart failure in the context of chemotherapeutic agents and how to proceed with various treatments [72]. Readers are encouraged to use this free source of information for their clinical practice.

Preventative Strategies

Cardiovascular co-morbidities confers adverse outcomes in patients who are subjected to cardio-toxic chemotherapies. The disease and treatment burden has been shown to contribute to both weight gain [93] and decrease in physical activity [94, 95] thus potentially raising cardiovascular disease risk. In 5721 asymptomatic women who underwent baseline evaluation in the St. James Women Take Heart Project, exercise tolerance measured by metabolic equivalents on treadmill testing predicted a 17% increase in Framingham Risk Score-adjusted mortality with each unit decline in MET level [96]. This can be attenuated by exercise training in women as it improves cardiovascular function, especially in breast cancer patients [97, 98]. Furthermore, a Cochrane review in 2012 showed benefit of a regular exercise program on quality of life in cancer patients [99]. Taken together, these reports underscore the importance of cardiovascular fitness. Therefore, prevention and treatment should be centered-around these adverse risk factors.

It is recommended that all patients should have a baseline screening transthoracic echocardiography done prior to initiation of chemotherapy with agents known to cause cancer therapeutics-related cardiac dysfunction (CRTCD) (grade

IA from European Society for Medical Oncology (ESMO) guidelines) [100]. This recommendation identifies patients with pre-existing compromised cardiac function so that their treatment regimen may be modified. Other methodologies such as biomarkers and risk prediction models can be used to risk stratify the patients. However, use of biomarkers and risk prediction model has not been integrated in the standard of practice. ESMO guidelines recommend assessment of cardiac function at baseline and at 3, 6, and 9 months during treatment as well as at 12 and 18 months after initiation of treatment (grade IA) [100]. Thereafter, recommended monitoring with TTE is annual or biannual depending on the clinical indication [100]. A TTE should include assessment of LVEF, wall motion, diastolic dysfunction, and strain. American Society of Echocardiography (ASE) and European Association of Echocardiography (EAE) both recommend calculating LVEF using the modified biplane Simpson's technique in combination with the wall motion score index [1, 101, 102]. While these recommendations are largely based on studies stemming from anthracycline treatments, the data on trastuzumab is sparse. However, a comprehensive table outlining various monitoring strategies recommended by various medical institutions is outlined in Table 6.3 [103–105].

For secondary prevention, in women with early breast cancer, treatment with the cardiotoxic agent should be discontinued and non-cardiotoxic therapy substituted where possible. For women with metastatic HER-2 amplified breast cancer, temporarily discontinuing HER-2 targeted agents, treatment with blockers and ACEIs and then cautious re-introduction of the HER-2 targeted agent is often successful with continued indefinite use of the beta blocker and ACE inhibitor [106]. Furthermore, the general population experience, it is clear that individuals with an asymptomatic ejection fraction below 50% have a ~3.5-fold increase in all-cause mortality over the ensuing 9–10 years [107]. Therefore, as per ESMO guidelines, use of ACEI should be considered in asymptom-

Table 6.3 Guideline recommendations for detecting cardiac dysfunction

	Guidelines/position paper	Year	Recommendations
Plana et al. [103]	American Society of Echocardiography/European Association of Cardiovascular Imaging: Multimodality Imaging Evaluation	2014	Treatment with anthracycline → baseline LVEF assessment with 3D or 2D Echo, GLS, and troponin I measurement. If abnormal, cardiology consultation. If normal, follow-up at completion of therapy and 6 months later. If the dose if >240 mg/m^2, recommend LVEF, GLS and troponin prior to each additional 50 mg/m^2
Virani et al. [104]	Canadian Cardiovascular Society Guidelines for Evaluation and Management of Cardiovascular Complications of Cancer Therapy	2016	1. We recommend the same imaging modality and method be used to determine LVEF before, during, and after completion of cancer therapy (Suggestion, Low-Quality Evidence)
			2. We suggest that myocardial strain imaging be considered a method for early detection of subclinical LV dysfunction in patients treated with potentially cardiotoxic cancer therapy (Suggestion, Low-Quality Evidence)
			3. We suggest that serial use of cardiacbiomarkers (e.g., BNP, troponin) be considered for early detection of cardiotoxicity in cancer patients who receive cartiotoxictherapies implicated in the development of LV dysfunction (Weak Recommendation, Moderate Quality Evidence)
Zamorano et al. [105]	ESC Position Paper on cancer treatments and cardiovascular toxicity developed under the auspices of the ESC Committee for Practice Guidelines	2016	Echocardiography: -3D-based LVEF - 2D Simpson's LVEF–GLS
			• LVEF: >10 percentage points decrease to a value below the LLN suggests cardiotoxicity
			• GLS: >15% relative percentage reduction from baseline may suggest risk of cardiotoxicity
			Nuclear cardiac imaging (MUGA)
			• >10 percentage points decrease in LVEF with a value <50% identifies patients with cardiotoxicity
			Cardiac magnetic resonance
			• Typically used if other techniques are non-diagnostic or to confirm presence of LV dysfunction if LVEF is borderlines
			Cardiac biomarkers:- (Troponin I - High-sensitivity Troponin I - BNP - NT-proBNP)
			• A rise identifies patients receiving anthracyclines who may benefit form ACE-Is
			• Routine role of BNP and NT-proBNP in surveillance of high-risk patient needs further investigation

atic woman with LVEF of <50%. Furthermore, a combination of ACEI and beta-blockers are recommended for both symptomatic and asymptomatic patients with LVEF below 40% [100]. Additionally, algorithms have also been proposed by the ESMO Clinical Practice Guideline for when to hold or discontinue treatment with trastuzumab based on serial LVEF measures [100]. Therefore, decisions to modify or stop cancer therapy should be made by the treating team comprised of cardiologist, oncologist, other healthcare participants and patient himself/herself.

Revisiting the Case Presentation #2

A 52 year old female with pre-chemotherapeutic echocardiogram showing and LVEF of 57%, had fatigue at 6 months after the initiation of trastuzumab, with the echocardiogram showing an LVEF of 47% by Simpson's method. Therefore, the strategy would be to halt the administration of trastuzumab. Cardioprotective agents such as ACEI and beta-blockers can be started with close surveillance with echocardiogram. Once the target ejection fraction is achieved (≥54%), trastuzumab can be re-introduced. The process of recovery tends to be quick and possibility of relapse to cardiac dysfunction is minimal.

Conclusion

Cardiomyopathy is a well-recognized cardio-toxicity of many anticancer agents. Primary prevention is essential and therefore a proactive approach of identifying and treating underlying cardiac risk factors is of paramount importance. Additionally, a succinct, and an effective approach should be undertaken early in the course of the disease in patients suffering from chemotherapy related cardiomyopathy. It is also essential to delineate the type of cardiomyopathy as the therapeutic approach is not only different but the outcomes are diverse also. Hence all other possible etiologies (e.g. coronary artery disease, myocarditis) as contributing or sole cause should be excluded. Thus, we cannot paint all the cardiomyopathies/cardiotoxicity with the same brush, and there is a need still to advance our knowledge in this area to identify, understand and thereby attenuate, if not ameliorate, chemotherapy-induced cardiomyopathy.

References

1. Seidman A, Hudis C, Pierri MK, et al. Cardiac dysfunction in the trastuzumab clinical trials experience. J Clin Oncol. 2002;20:1215–21.
2. Theodoulou M, Seidman AD. Cardiac effects of adjuvant therapy for early breast cancer. Semin Oncol. 2003;30:730–9.
3. Ewer MS, Lippman SM. Type II chemotherapy-related cardiac dysfunction: time to recognize a new entity. J Clin Oncol. 2005;23:2900–2.
4. Hayek ER, Speakman E, Rehmus E. Acute doxorubicin cardiotoxicity. N Engl J Med. 2005;352:2456–7.
5. Bristow MR, Mason JW, Billingham ME, Daniels JR. Doxorubicin cardiomyopathy: evaluation by phonocardiography, endomyocardial biopsy, and cardiac catheterization. Ann Intern Med. 1978;88:168–75.
6. Lenihan DJ. Progression of heart failure from AHA/ACC stage A to stage B or even C: can we all agree we should try to prevent this from happening? J Am Coll Cardiol. 2012;60:2513–4.
7. Bristow MR, Thompson PD, Martin RP, Mason JW, Billingham ME, Harrison DC. Early anthracycline cardiotoxicity. Am J Med. 1978;65:823–32.
8. Dazzi H, Kaufmann K, Follath F. Anthracycline-induced acute cardiotoxicity in adults treated for leukaemia. Analysis of the clinico-pathological aspects of documented acute anthracycline-induced cardiotoxicity in patients treated for acute leukaemia at the University Hospital of Zurich, Switzerland, between 1990 and 1996. Ann Oncol. 2001;12:963–6.
9. Pivot X, Romieu G, Debled M, et al. 6 months versus 12 months of adjuvant trastuzumab for patients with HER2-positive early breast cancer (PHARE): a randomised phase 3 trial. Lancet Oncol. 2013;14:741–8.
10. Von Hoff DD, Layard MW, Basa P, et al. Risk factors for doxorubicin-induced congestive heart failure. Ann Intern Med. 1979;91:710–7.
11. Swain SM, Whaley FS, Ewer MS. Congestive heart failure in patients treated with doxorubicin: a retrospective analysis of three trials. Cancer. 2003;97:2869–79.
12. Nysom K, Holm K, Lipsitz SR, et al. Relationship between cumulative anthracycline dose and late cardiotoxicity in childhood acute lymphoblastic leukemia. J Clin Oncol. 1998;16:545–50.
13. Vandecruys E, Mondelaers V, De Wolf D, Benoit Y, Suys B. Late cardiotoxicity after low dose of anthracycline therapy for acute lymphoblastic leukemia in childhood. J Cancer Surviv. 2012;6:95–101.
14. van der Pal HJ, van Dalen EC, Hauptmann M, et al. Cardiac function in 5-year survivors of childhood cancer: a long-term follow-up study. Arch Intern Med. 2010;170:1247–55.
15. Bodley A, Liu LF, Israel M, et al. DNA topoisomerase II-mediated interaction of doxorubicin and daunorubicin congeners with DNA. Cancer Res. 1989;49:5969–78.
16. Zhang S, Liu X, Bawa-Khalfe T, et al. Identification of the molecular basis of doxorubicin-induced cardiotoxicity. Nat Med. 2012;18:1639–42.
17. L'Ecuyer T, Sanjeev S, Thomas R, et al. DNA damage is an early event in doxorubicin-induced cardiac myocyte death. Am J Physiol Heart Circ Physiol. 2006;291:H1273–80.
18. Liu J, Mao W, Ding B, Liang CS. ERKs/p53 signal transduction pathway is involved in doxorubicin-induced apoptosis in H9c2 cells and cardiomyocytes. Am J Physiol Heart Circ Physiol. 2008;295:H1956–65.
19. Hasinoff BB, Herman EH. Dexrazoxane: how it works in cardiac and tumor cells. Is it a prodrug or is it a drug? Cardiovasc Toxicol. 2007;7:140–4.
20. Herman EH, el-Hage A, Ferrans VJ. Protective effect of ICRF-187 on doxorubicin-induced cardiac and renal toxicity in spontaneously hypertensive (SHR) and normotensive (WKY) rats. Toxicol Appl Pharmacol. 1988;92:42–53.
21. Herman EH, Ferrans VJ. Preclinical animal models of cardiac protection from anthracycline-induced cardiotoxicity. Semin Oncol. 1998;25:15–21.
22. Herman EH, Zhang J, Chadwick DP, Ferrans VJ. Comparison of the protective effects of amifostine and dexrazoxane against the

toxicity of doxorubicin in spontaneously hypertensive rats. Cancer Chemother Pharmacol. 2000;45:329–34.
23. Herman EH, Ferrans VJ. Timing of treatment with ICRF-187 and its effect on chronic doxorubicin cardiotoxicity. Cancer Chemother Pharmacol. 1993;32:445–9.
24. Rao VA, Zhang J, Klein SR, et al. The iron chelator Dp44mT inhibits the proliferation of cancer cells but fails to protect from doxorubicin-induced cardiotoxicity in spontaneously hypertensive rats. Cancer Chemother Pharmacol. 2011;68:1125–34.
25. Imondi AR. Preclinical models of cardiac protection and testing for effects of dexrazoxane on doxorubicin antitumor effects. Semin Oncol. 1998;25:22–30.
26. Lipshultz SE, Colan SD, Gelber RD, Perez-Atayde AR, Sallan SE, Sanders SP. Late cardiac effects of doxorubicin therapy for acute lymphoblastic leukemia in childhood. N Engl J Med. 1991;324:808–15.
27. Marty M, Espie M, Llombart A, et al. Multicenter randomized phase III study of the cardioprotective effect of dexrazoxane (Cardioxane) in advanced/metastatic breast cancer patients treated with anthracycline-based chemotherapy. Ann Oncol. 2006;17:614–22.
28. Swain SM, Whaley FS, Gerber MC, et al. Cardioprotection with dexrazoxane for doxorubicin-containing therapy in advanced breast cancer. J Clin Oncol. 1997;15:1318–32.
29. Nitiss JL. Targeting DNA topoisomerase II in cancer chemotherapy. Nat Rev Cancer. 2009;9:338–50.
30. Minotti G, Menna P, Salvatorelli E, Cairo G, Gianni L. Anthracyclines: molecular advances and pharmacologic developments in antitumor activity and cardiotoxicity. Pharmacol Rev. 2004;56:185–229.
31. van Dalen EC, van der Pal HJ, Caron HN, Kremer LC. Different dosage schedules for reducing cardiotoxicity in cancer patients receiving anthracycline chemotherapy. Cochrane Database Syst Rev. 2009;(4):CD005008.
32. Lipshultz SE, Miller TL, Lipsitz SR, et al. Continuous versus bolus infusion of doxorubicin in children with ALL: long-term cardiac outcomes. Pediatrics. 2012;130:1003–11.
33. Gupta M, Steinherz PG, Cheung NK, Steinherz L. Late cardiotoxicity after bolus versus infusion anthracycline therapy for childhood cancers. Med Pediatr Oncol. 2003;40:343–7.
34. Levitt GA, Dorup I, Sorensen K, Sullivan I. Does anthracycline administration by infusion in children affect late cardiotoxicity? Br J Haematol. 2004;124:463–8.
35. Pignata S, Scambia G, Ferrandina G, et al. Carboplatin plus paclitaxel versus carboplatin plus pegylated liposomal doxorubicin as first-line treatment for patients with ovarian cancer: the MITO-2 randomized phase III trial. J Clin Oncol. 2011;29:3628–35.
36. Sharpe M, Easthope SE, Keating GM, Lamb HM. Polyethylene glycol-liposomal doxorubicin: a review of its use in the management of solid and haematological malignancies and AIDS-related Kaposi's sarcoma. Drugs. 2002;62:2089–126.
37. Al-Batran SE, Guntner M, Pauligk C, et al. Anthracycline rechallenge using pegylated liposomal doxorubicin in patients with metastatic breast cancer: a pooled analysis using individual data from four prospective trials. Br J Cancer. 2010;103:1518–23.
38. Keller AM, Mennel RG, Georgoulias VA, et al. Randomized phase III trial of pegylated liposomal doxorubicin versus vinorelbine or mitomycin C plus vinblastine in women with taxane-refractory advanced breast cancer. J Clin Oncol. 2004;22:3893–901.
39. O'Brien ME, Wigler N, Inbar M, et al. Reduced cardiotoxicity and comparable efficacy in a phase III trial of pegylated liposomal doxorubicin HCl (CAELYX/Doxil) versus conventional doxorubicin for first-line treatment of metastatic breast cancer. Ann Oncol. 2004;15:440–9.
40. Agency EM. Caelyx (doxorubicin hydrochloride in a pegylated liposomal formulation). 2011. http://www.ema.europa.eu/docs/en_GB/document_library/EPAR_-_Product_Information/human/000089/WC500020180.pdf
41. Duggan ST, Keating GM. Pegylated liposomal doxorubicin: a review of its use in metastatic breast cancer, ovarian cancer, multiple myeloma and AIDS-related Kaposi's sarcoma. Drugs. 2011;71:2531–58.
42. Smith DH, Adams JR, Johnston SR, Gordon A, Drummond MF, Bennett CL. A comparative economic analysis of pegylated liposomal doxorubicin versus topotecan in ovarian cancer in the USA and the UK. Ann Oncol. 2002;13:1590–7.
43. Creighton AM, Birnie GD. The effect of bisdioxopiperazines on the synthesis of deoxyribonucleic acid, ribonucleic acid and protein in growing mouse-embryo fibroblasts. Biochem J. 1969;114:58P.
44. Lyu YL, Kerrigan JE, Lin CP, et al. Topoisomerase IIbeta mediated DNA double-strand breaks: implications in doxorubicin cardiotoxicity and prevention by dexrazoxane. Cancer Res. 2007;67:8839–46.
45. Lipshultz SE, Rifai N, Dalton VM, et al. The effect of dexrazoxane on myocardial injury in doxorubicin-treated children with acute lymphoblastic leukemia. N Engl J Med. 2004;351:145–53.
46. Lipshultz SE, Scully RE, Lipsitz SR, et al. Assessment of dexrazoxane as a cardioprotectant in doxorubicin-treated children with high-risk acute lymphoblastic leukaemia: long-term follow-up of a prospective, randomised, multicentre trial. Lancet Oncol. 2010;11:950–61.
47. Seymour L, Bramwell V, Moran LA. Use of dexrazoxane as a cardioprotectant in patients receiving doxorubicin or epirubicin chemotherapy for the treatment of cancer. The Provincial Systemic Treatment Disease Site Group. Cancer Prev Control. 1999;3:145–59.
48. Speyer JL, Green MD, Zeleniuch-Jacquotte A, et al. ICRF-187 permits longer treatment with doxorubicin in women with breast cancer. J Clin Oncol. 1992;10:117–27.
49. Swain SM, Vici P. The current and future role of dexrazoxane as a cardioprotectant in anthracycline treatment: expert panel review. J Cancer Res Clin Oncol. 2004;130:1–7.
50. Yu Y, Kalinowski DS, Kovacevic Z, et al. Thiosemicarbazones from the old to new: iron chelators that are more than just ribonucleotide reductase inhibitors. J Med Chem. 2009;52:5271–94.
51. van Dalen EC, Caron HN, Dickinson HO, Kremer LC. Cardioprotective interventions for cancer patients receiving anthracyclines. Cochrane Database Syst Rev. 2011;(6):CD003917.
52. Schuchter LM, Hensley ML, Meropol NJ, Winer EP, American Society of Clinical Oncology C, Radiotherapy Expert P. 2002 update of recommendations for the use of chemotherapy and radiotherapy protectants: clinical practice guidelines of the American Society of Clinical Oncology. J Clin Oncol. 2002;20:2895–903.
53. Kalay N, Basar E, Ozdogru I, et al. Protective effects of carvedilol against anthracycline-induced cardiomyopathy. J Am Coll Cardiol. 2006;48:2258–62.
54. Seicean S, Seicean A, Alan N, Plana JC, Budd GT, Marwick TH. Cardioprotective effect of beta-adrenoceptor blockade in patients with breast cancer undergoing chemotherapy: follow-up study of heart failure. Circ Heart Fail. 2013;6:420–6.
55. Kaya MG, Ozkan M, Gunebakmaz O, et al. Protective effects of nebivolol against anthracycline-induced cardiomyopathy: a randomized control study. Int J Cardiol. 2013;167:2306–10.
56. Bosch X, Rovira M, Sitges M, et al. Enalapril and carvedilol for preventing chemotherapy-induced left ventricular systolic dysfunction in patients with malignant hemopathies: the OVERCOME trial (preventiOn of left Ventricular dysfunction with Enalapril and caRvedilol in patients submitted to intensive ChemOtherapy for the treatment of Malignant hEmopathies). J Am Coll Cardiol. 2013;61:2355–62.

57. Heck SL, Gulati G, Ree AH, et al. Rationale and design of the prevention of cardiac dysfunction during an Adjuvant Breast Cancer Therapy (PRADA) Trial. Cardiology. 2012;123:240–7.
58. Gulati G, Heck SL, Ree AH, et al. Prevention of cardiac dysfunction during adjuvant breast cancer therapy (PRADA): a 2 × 2 factorial, randomized, placebo-controlled, double-blind clinical trial of candesartan and metoprolol. Eur Heart J. 2016;37(21):1671–80.
59. Cardinale D, Colombo A, Sandri MT, et al. Prevention of high-dose chemotherapy-induced cardiotoxicity in high-risk patients by angiotensin-converting enzyme inhibition. Circulation. 2006;114:2474–81.
60. Jensen BV, Skovsgaard T, Nielsen SL. Functional monitoring of anthracycline cardiotoxicity: a prospective, blinded, long-term observational study of outcome in 120 patients. Ann Oncol. 2002;13:699–709.
61. Lipshultz SE, Lipsitz SR, Sallan SE, et al. Long-term enalapril therapy for left ventricular dysfunction in doxorubicin-treated survivors of childhood cancer. J Clin Oncol. 2002;20:4517–22.
62. Silber JH, Cnaan A, Clark BJ, et al. Enalapril to prevent cardiac function decline in long-term survivors of pediatric cancer exposed to anthracyclines. J Clin Oncol. 2004;22:820–8.
63. Barry E, Alvarez JA, Scully RE, Miller TL, Lipshultz SE. Anthracycline-induced cardiotoxicity: course, pathophysiology, prevention and management. Expert Opin Pharmacother. 2007;8:1039–58.
64. Sieswerda E, van Dalen EC, Postma A, Cheuk DK, Caron HN, Kremer LC. Medical interventions for treating anthracycline-induced symptomatic and asymptomatic cardiotoxicity during and after treatment for childhood cancer. Cochrane Database Syst Rev. 2011;(9):CD008011.
65. Cadeddu C, Piras A, Mantovani G, et al. Protective effects of the angiotensin II receptor blocker telmisartan on epirubicin-induced inflammation, oxidative stress, and early ventricular impairment. Am Heart J. 2010;160:487.e1–7.
66. Nakamae H, Tsumura K, Terada Y, et al. Notable effects of angiotensin II receptor blocker, valsartan, on acute cardiotoxic changes after standard chemotherapy with cyclophosphamide, doxorubicin, vincristine, and prednisolone. Cancer. 2005;104:2492–8.
67. Dessi M, Madeddu C, Piras A, et al. Long-term, up to 18 months, protective effects of the angiotensin II receptor blocker telmisartan on Epirubin-induced inflammation and oxidative stress assessed by serial strain rate. Springplus. 2013;2:198.
68. Akpek M, Ozdogru I, Sahin O, et al. Protective effects of spironolactone against anthracycline-induced cardiomyopathy. Eur J Heart Fail. 2015;17:81–9.
69. Seicean S, Seicean A, Plana JC, Budd GT, Marwick TH. Effect of statin therapy on the risk for incident heart failure in patients with breast cancer receiving anthracycline chemotherapy: an observational clinical cohort study. J Am Coll Cardiol. 2012;60:2384–90.
70. Acar Z, Kale A, Turgut M, et al. Efficiency of atorvastatin in the protection of anthracycline-induced cardiomyopathy. J Am Coll Cardiol. 2011;58:988–9.
71. Cardinale D, Colombo A, Lamantia G, et al. Anthracycline-induced cardiomyopathy: clinical relevance and response to pharmacologic therapy. J Am Coll Cardiol. 2010;55:213–20.
72. Hassan SB, Banchs J. Monitoring cardiotoxicity with left ventricular ejection fraction; MD Anderson Practices in Onco-Cardiology. 2016 by Department of Cardiology, The University of Texas MD Anderson Cancer Center. ISBN;978-1-944785-94-9.
73. Yarden Y. The EGFR family and its ligands in human cancer. signalling mechanisms and therapeutic opportunities. Eur J Cancer. 2001;37 Suppl 4:S3–8.
74. Slamon DJ, Leyland-Jones B, Shak S, et al. Use of chemotherapy plus a monoclonal antibody against HER2 for metastatic breast cancer that overexpresses HER2. N Engl J Med. 2001;344:783–92.
75. Chen B, Peng X, Pentassuglia L, Lim CC, Sawyer DB. Molecular and cellular mechanisms of anthracycline cardiotoxicity. Cardiovasc Toxicol. 2007;7:114–21.
76. Bird BR, Swain SM. Cardiac toxicity in breast cancer survivors: review of potential cardiac problems. Clin Cancer Res. 2008;14:14 24.
77. Hudis CA. Trastuzumab—mechanism of action and use in clinical practice. N Engl J Med. 2007;357:39–51.
78. Yavas O, Yazici M, Eren O, Oyan B. The acute effect of trastuzumab infusion on ECG parameters in metastatic breast cancer patients. Swiss Med Wkly. 2007;137:556–8.
79. Keefe DL. Trastuzumab-associated cardiotoxicity. Cancer. 2002;95:1592–600.
80. Perez EA, Rodeheffer R. Clinical cardiac tolerability of trastuzumab. J Clin Oncol. 2004;22:322–9.
81. Ewer MS, Vooletich MT, Durand JB, et al. Reversibility of trastuzumab-related cardiotoxicity: new insights based on clinical course and response to medical treatment. J Clin Oncol. 2005;23:7820–6.
82. de Azambuja E, Bedard PL, Suter T, Piccart-Gebhart M. Cardiac toxicity with anti-HER-2 therapies: what have we learned so far? Target Oncol. 2009;4:77–88.
83. Zhao YY, Sawyer DR, Baliga RR, et al. Neuregulins promote survival and growth of cardiac myocytes. Persistence of ErbB2 and ErbB4 expression in neonatal and adult ventricular myocytes. J Biol Chem. 1998;273:10261–9.
84. Crone SA, Zhao YY, Fan L, et al. ErbB2 is essential in the prevention of dilated cardiomyopathy. Nat Med. 2002;8:459–65.
85. Junttila TT, Akita RW, Parsons K, et al. Ligand-independent HER2/HER3/PI3K complex is disrupted by trastuzumab and is effectively inhibited by the PI3K inhibitor GDC-0941. Cancer Cell. 2009;15:429–40.
86. De Keulenaer GW, Doggen K, Lemmens K. The vulnerability of the heart as a pluricellular paracrine organ: lessons from unexpected triggers of heart failure in targeted ErbB2 anticancer therapy. Circ Res. 2010;106:35–46.
87. Badache A, Hynes NE. A new therapeutic antibody masks ErbB2 to its partners. Cancer Cell. 2004;5:299–301.
88. Cameron DA, Stein S. Drug Insight: intracellular inhibitors of HER2—clinical development of lapatinib in breast cancer. Nat Clin Pract Oncol. 2008;5:512–20.
89. Rusnak DW, Lackey K, Affleck K, et al. The effects of the novel, reversible epidermal growth factor receptor/ErbB-2 tyrosine kinase inhibitor, GW2016, on the growth of human normal and tumor-derived cell lines in vitro and in vivo. Mol Cancer Ther. 2001;1:85–94.
90. Xia W, Mullin RJ, Keith BR, et al. Anti-tumor activity of GW572016: a dual tyrosine kinase inhibitor blocks EGF activation of EGFR/erbB2 and downstream Erk1/2 and AKT pathways. Oncogene. 2002;21:6255–63.
91. Cardinale D, Colombo A, Torrisi R, et al. Trastuzumab-induced cardiotoxicity: clinical and prognostic implications of troponin I evaluation. J Clin Oncol. 2010;28:3910–6.
92. Jones AL, Barlow M, Barrett-Lee PJ, et al. Management of cardiac health in trastuzumab-treated patients with breast cancer: updated United Kingdom National Cancer Research Institute recommendations for monitoring. Br J Cancer. 2009;100:684–92.
93. Rock CL, Flatt SW, Newman V, et al. Factors associated with weight gain in women after diagnosis of breast cancer. Women's Healthy Eating and Living Study Group. J Am Diet Assoc. 1999;99:1212–21.

94. Koelwyn GJ, Khouri M, Mackey JR, Douglas PS, Jones LW. Running on empty: cardiovascular reserve capacity and late effects of therapy in cancer survivorship. J Clin Oncol. 2012;30:4458–61.
95. Irwin ML, Crumley D, McTiernan A, et al. Physical activity levels before and after a diagnosis of breast carcinoma: the Health, Eating, Activity, and Lifestyle (HEAL) study. Cancer. 2003;97:1746–57.
96. Gulati M, Pandey DK, Arnsdorf MF, et al. Exercise capacity and the risk of death in women: the St James Women Take Heart Project. Circulation. 2003;108:1554–9.
97. Giallauria F, Fattirolli F, Tramarin R, et al. Clinical characteristics and course of patients with diabetes entering cardiac rehabilitation. Diabetes Res Clin Pract. 2015;107:267–72.
98. Giallauria F, Maresca L, Vitelli A, et al. Exercise training improves heart rate recovery in women with breast cancer. Springplus. 2015;4:388.
99. Mishra SI, Scherer RW, Snyder C, Geigle PM, Berlanstein DR, Topaloglu O. Exercise interventions on health-related quality of life for people with cancer during active treatment. Cochrane Database Syst Rev. 2012;(8):CD008465.
100. Curigliano G, Cardinale D, Suter T, et al. Cardiovascular toxicity induced by chemotherapy, targeted agents and radiotherapy: ESMO Clinical Practice Guidelines. Ann Oncol. 2012;23 Suppl 7:vii155–66.
101. Lang RM, Bierig M, Devereux RB, et al. Recommendations for chamber quantification: a report from the American Society of Echocardiography's Guidelines and Standards Committee and the Chamber Quantification Writing Group, developed in conjunction with the European Association of Echocardiography, a branch of the European Society of Cardiology. J Am Soc Echocardiogr. 2005;18:1440–63.
102. Moja L, Tagliabue L, Balduzzi S, et al. Trastuzumab containing regimens for early breast cancer. Cochrane Database Syst Rev. 2012;(4):CD006243.
103. Plana JC, Galderisi M, Barac A, et al. Expert consensus for multimodality imaging evaluation of adult patients during and after cancer therapy: a report from the American Society of Echocardiography and the European Association of Cardiovascular Imaging. Eur Heart J Cardiovasc Imaging. 2014;15:1063–93.
104. Virani SA, Dent S, Brezden-Masley C, et al. Canadian Cardiovascular Society Guidelines for Evaluation and Management of Cardiovascular Complications of Cancer Therapy. Can J Cardiol. 2016;32:831–41.
105. Zamorano JL, Lancellotti P, Rodriguez Munoz D, et al. 2016 ESC Position Paper on cancer treatments and cardiovascular toxicity developed under the auspices of the ESC Committee for Practice Guidelines: The Task Force for cancer treatments and cardiovascular toxicity of the European Society of Cardiology (ESC). Eur Heart J. 2016;37:2768–801.
106. Vaz-Luis I, Keating NL, Lin NU, Lii H, Winer EP, Freedman RA. Duration and toxicity of adjuvant trastuzumab in older patients with early-stage breast cancer: a population-based study. J Clin Oncol. 2014;32:927–34.
107. Yeboah J, Rodriguez CJ, Stacey B, et al. Prognosis of individuals with asymptomatic left ventricular systolic dysfunction in the multi-ethnic study of atherosclerosis (MESA). Circulation. 2012;126:2713–9.

Radiation Related Cardiovascular Disease

7

S. Wamique Yusuf

Abstract
Cardiovascular disease, is a well known complication of radiation therapy. This is especially seen in Hogdkin's lymphoma survivors, who have received mediastinal therapy.

In this chapter, we present some of the common conditions associated with radiation induced heart disease.

Keyword
Radiation • Vascular • Heart disease

Improvement in cancer therapy has led to an increasing number of survivors of childhood malignancy. In the United States alone, nearly 14.5 million children and adults with a history of cancer were alive on January 1, 2014 and it is estimated that by 2024, the population of cancer survivors will increase to almost 19 million [1]. Some of these cancer survivors are afflicted with long term side effects of therapy. One well recognized late secondary effect in patients receiving mediastinal and chest wall radiation is cardiovascular disease (CVD) [2].

The data for possible causal association of radiation and heart disease mainly comes from studies of Hodgkin's lymphoma (HL) and breast cancer patients undergoing radiation therapy (RT).

Amongst long term survivors of HL, previously treated with radiation, CVD is one of the most common cause of death [3]. Patients with HL treated with mediastinal radiation, have a 3.0 times higher relative risk of death from myocardial infarction [4]. Patients previously treated with mediastinal radiation are at increased risk for the development of coronary artery disease (CAD), valvular heart disease, congestive heart failure (CHF), pericardial and conduction system disease [1, 5]. The incidence of cardiac events increases with time, can affect younger adults and is related to the radiation dose to the heart [5, 6].

A meta-analysis of eight randomized trials of patients with breast cancer found a 62% increase in cardiac deaths among women who were treated with RT [7]. The curve for development of cardiac diseases and subsequent cardiac procedures rises steeply after 10 years of RT [8].

The basic mechanism behind radiation induced vascular damage is endothelial dysfunction, with activation of inflammatory mechanism, release of cytokines and growth factors with cellular infiltration, fibrin leak into the tissues promoting collagen deposition, which may eventually lead to fibrosis [9].

This chapter illustrates some common CVD encountered in patients with history of previous RT.

RT can affect the pericardium, myocardium, coronary vessel, valves and the conduction system. Pericardium is most frequently involved (Table 7.1).

Acute Pericarditis

Patients with acute pericarditis during RT, frequently present with chest pain, low grade fever and non- specific ECG changes. Sometimes classic ECG finding is seen, as illustrated in the case (Fig. 7.1).

Patients are treated with conventional therapy which includes non-steroidal anti-inflammtory drugs (NSAID), cochicine and steroids (in resistant cases). Treatment of underlying malignancy is usually continued. Echocardiogram

S.W. Yusuf
Department of Cardiology, University of Texas MD Anderson Cancer Center, Houston, TX, USA
e-mail: syusuf@mdanderson.org

S.W. Yusuf, J. Banchs (eds.), *Cancer and Cardiovascular Disease*, https://doi.org/10.1007/978-3-319-62088-6_7

Table 7.1 Clinical manifestations of radiation related cardiovascular disease

Tissue involved	Clinical presentation	Histology
Pericardium	Acute pericarditis	Fibrous pericardial thickening, fibrinous adhesions, chronic inflammatory infiltrate
	Chronic pericardial effusion	
	Constrictive pericarditis	
Myocardium	Myocarditis	Increased collagen (especially Type 1), interstitial fibrosis, myocardial perfusion defects
	Cardiomyopathy	
	Congestive heart failure	
	Diastolic dysfunction	
Vascular tree	Coronary artery disease	Intimal proliferation of fibrous tissue, media destroyed with adventia markedly thickened and fibrotic
	Vascular occlusion	
	Carotid stenosis	
Conduction system	Heart block	Fibrosis of the conduction system
Endocardium	Valvular disease (Stenosis/Regurgitation)	Leaflets/cusps fibrosis, calcification, thickening

CMP Cardiomyopathy, *CHF* Congestive heart failure, *CAD* Coronary artery disease

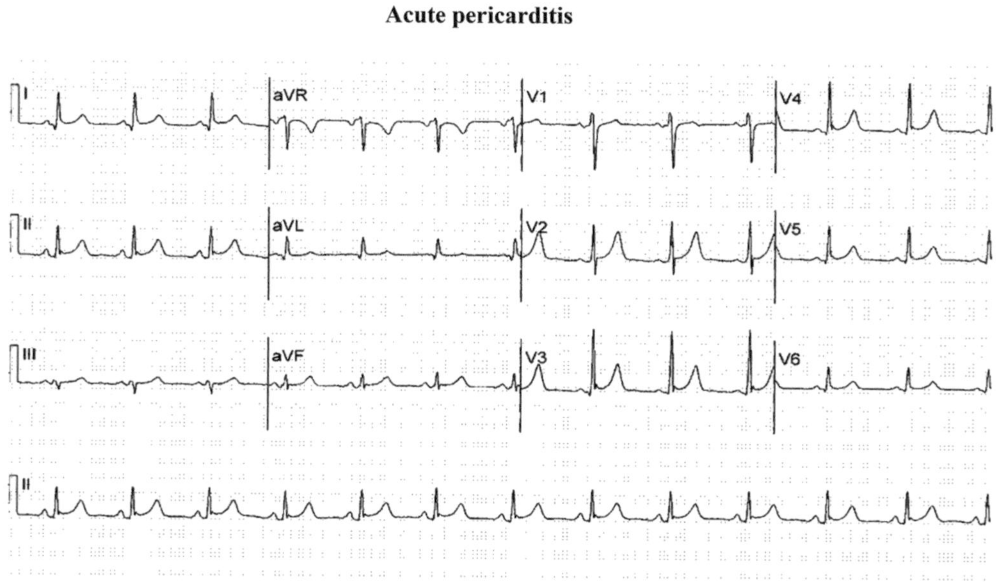

Fig. 7.1 A 12 lead ECG shows concave ST elevation in all leads with ST depression in lead aVR, suggestive of acute pericarditis. The patient presented with pericardial chest pain during RT for carcinoma of the lung

may or may not show minimal to small pericardial effusion. Cases with pericardial effusion should be followed up by a limited echocardiogram in 4–6 weeks. In most cases the effusion resolves with medical therapy. Patients who develop pericardial effusion after radiation, even if minimal should be followed up by periodic echocardiogram, as rarely it may lead to chronic pericardial effusion.

Chronic Pericardial Effusion

Chronic pericardial effusion can develop months or years after completion of radiation therapy. The development of chronic pericardial effusion is usually discovered by the incidental finding of enlarged cardiac silhouette on chest–X-ray or development of pericardial effusion on CT scan, which is done routinely for follow up purposes (Figs. 7.2 and 7.3). Some of these patients may develop symptoms of fatigue, dyspnea on exertion and leg edema.

Following case illustrates the development of chronic pericardial effusion due to RT.

A 49 year old man, stage 3 lung carcinoma, who had received a total of 70 Gy radiation to the chest, completed in Jan 2006. When seen in the clinic on 3rd Dec 2007, he was well and walking 5 miles/day with minimal shortness of breath. A chest-X-ray showed enlarging cardiac silhouette (Fig. 7.2). Review of CT scans showed a slowly increasing pericardial effusion (Fig. 7.3)

This led to an echocardiogram showing a large pericardial effusion, with tamponade physiology, for which he underwent successful pericardiocentesis. The pericardial fluid showed only inflammatory cells with no malignant pathology. Subsequent follow up echocardiograms shows no re-accumulation of the fluid. When seen last in clinic in 2014, he was asymptomatic and doing well.

Constrictive Pericarditis

Pericardial constriction can develop many years after completion of radiation therapy. Patients usually present with fatigue, dyspnea and signs of heart failure.

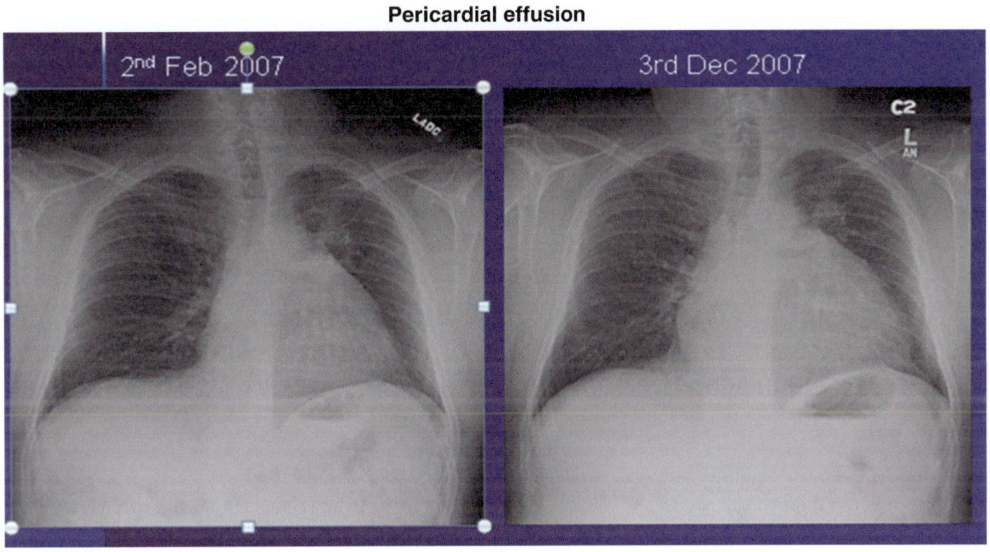

Fig. 7.2 Chest-X-ray (C-x-R) on 2nd Feb 2007, shows minimal cardiomegaly due to a small pericardial effusion. C-x-R on 3rd Dec 2007 shows a significantly enlarged cardiac silhouette due to a large pericardial effusion

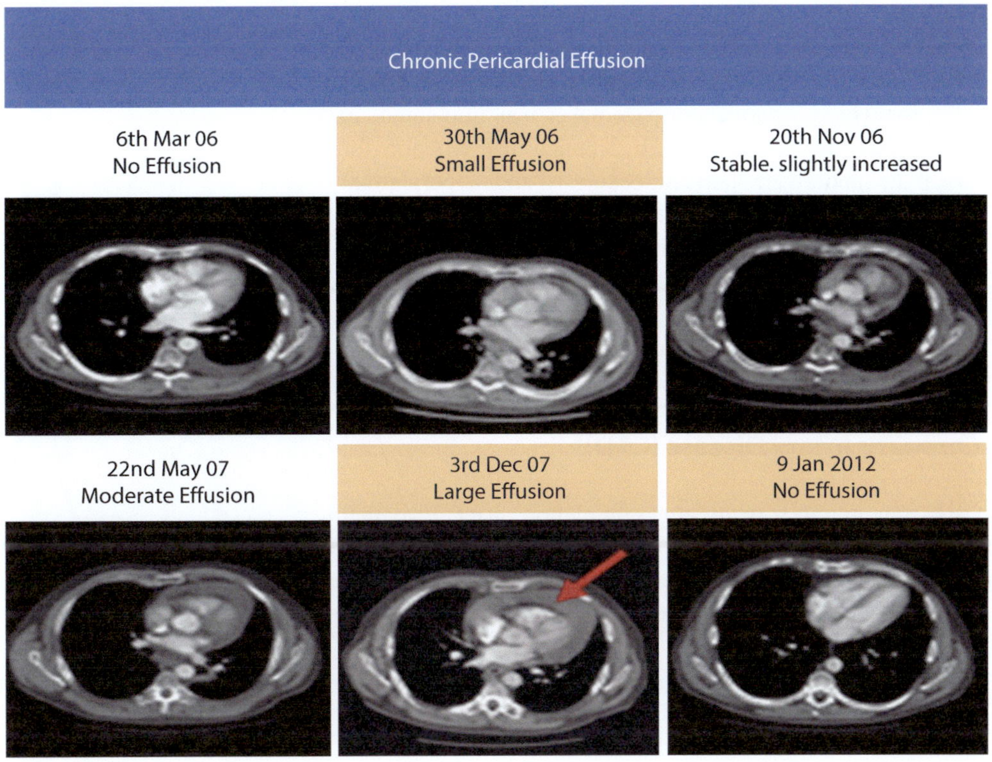

Fig. 7.3 CT scans shows development of chronic pericardial effusion. A CT scan on 6th Mar 2006 showed no pericardial effusion. Subsequent CT scan on 30th May 2006 shows small pericardial effusion, which progressively increases to become large in Dec 2007, necessitating a pericardial drainage. CT scan on 9th Jan 2012, shows no re-accumulation of pericardial fluid. The red arrow points to the large pericardial effusion

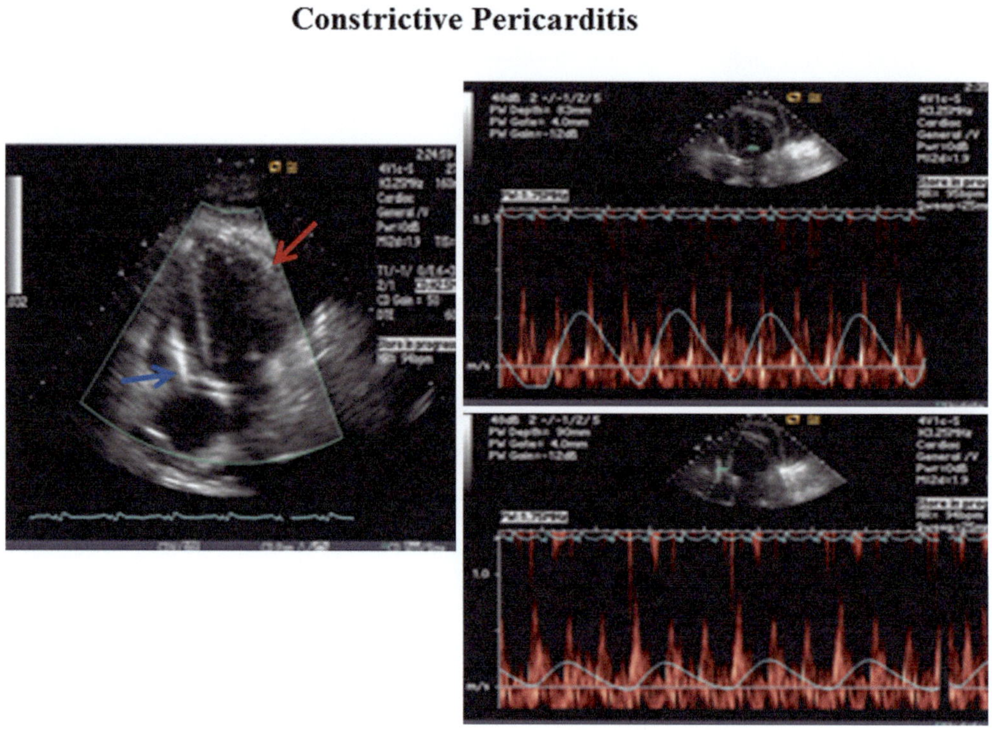

Fig. 7.4 Echocardiogram shows pericardial thickening, respiratory variation in mitral, tricuspid inflow and a permanent pacemaker in the right ventricle. The *red arrow* points to the thickened pericardium and the *blue arrow* points to the pacemaker lead in right ventricle

Figure 7.4 illustrates the case of a young man who completed his radiation therapy 40 Gy to mediastinum and neck for HL in 1984. He presented with complete heart block in 2005 for which a permanent pacemaker was implanted. In March 2007 he presented with a pericardial effusion for which he underwent pericardiocentesis and a pericardial window. His symptoms persisted and further evaluation confirmed a pericardial constriction for which he underwent a pericardial stripping in April 2007. The coronary angiogram also showed a 50% LAD. Figure 7.5 shows hemodynamic findings of constrictive pericarditis.

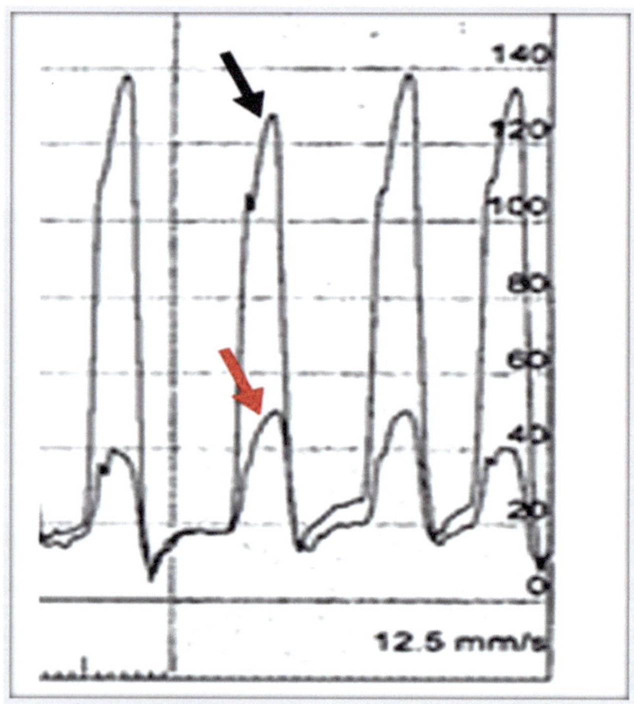

Fig. 7.5 Constrictive pericarditis: Hemodynamics showing venticular discordance (interdependence) with an increase in right venticular (RV) pressure and a simultaneous decrease in left venticular (LV) pressure during inspiration in a patient with constrictive pericarditis due to previous thoracic surgery (The *red arrow* points to the RV and the *black arrow* points to the LV)

Coronary Artery Disease (CAD)

CAD may manifest many after completion of RT. Proximal vessels which are in the field of RT are frequently affected. However radiation is also known to affect the small vessels. Asymptomatic cardiac perfusion defects are seen in about 50% of breast cancer patients treated with RT and can occur as early as early as 6 months after radiotherapy [10].

Following cases illustrates the development of symptomatic and asymptomatic radiation induced CAD (Figs. 7.6 and 7.7).

Patients with radiation induced CAD are treated as per ACC/AHA guidelines, with aggressive medical therapy for stable disease and per-cutaneous intervention for unstable disease. Surgical intervention can sometimes be challenging

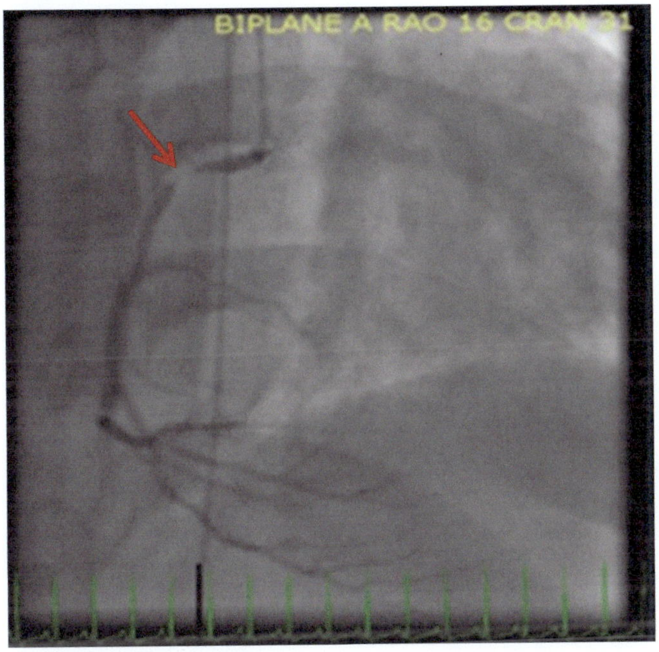

Fig. 7.6 A 34 year female with history of diabetes mellitus and no other risk factors. She completed RT for HL in Nov 2005. In Jan 2014 she presented with a Non ST elevation myocardial infarction (NSTEMI). A coronary angiogram showed a significant proximal right coronary artery (RCA) disease for which she underwent successful percutaneous intervention. The *red arrow* points to the proximal RCA lesion (Image courtesy of Dr. C. Iliescu)

due to significant mediastinal fibrosis and involvement of the internal mammary arteries.

Valvular Heart Disease

There is a high prevalence of asymptomatic valvular disease (particularly aortic), following mediastinal irradiation [11]. Most of the lesions are regurgitant and mild [11]. Rarely severe valvular disease may occur. Fig. 7.8 illustrates the case of radiation induced valvular disease.

Vascular Calcification and Stenosis

Following cases illustrates the development of calcification and stenosis in major vessels (Figs. 7.9, 7.10 and 7.11).

Cardiomyopathy

Cardiomyopathy is also a known complication, and myocardial strain imaging is a novel method to detect myocardial abnormality in patients with RT [12] (Fig. 7.12).

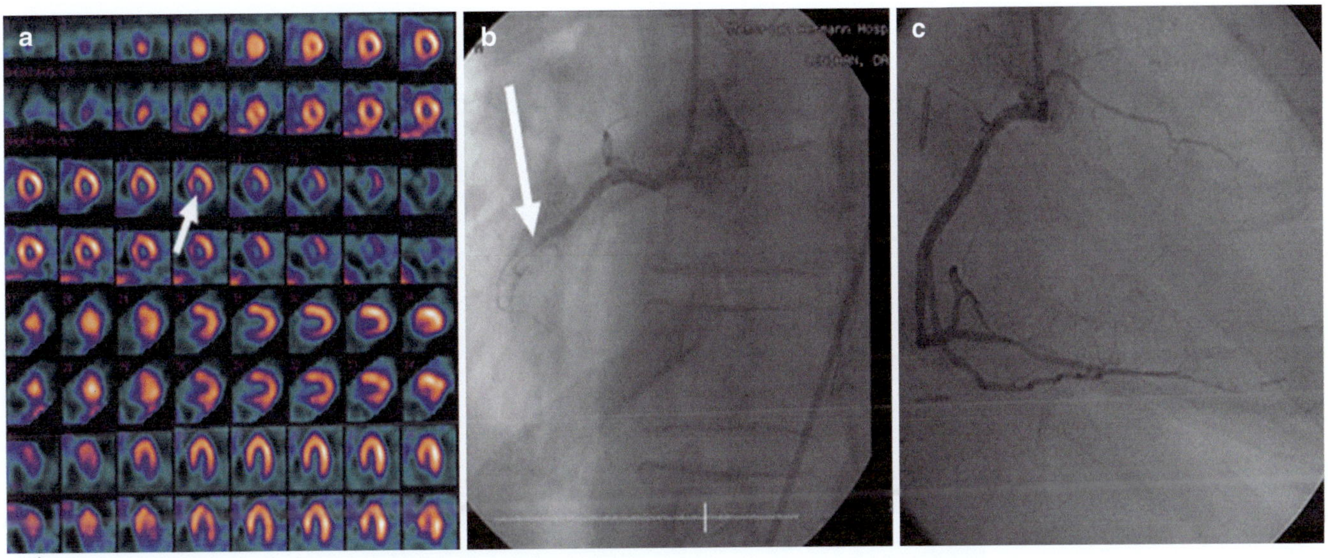

Fig. 7.7 Coronary artery disease: A 50 year old man with previous history of mesothelioma and radiation in the cardiac field, fully asymptomatic. A routing pre-op tress test shows severe ischemia in the inferior wall (in the region of previous radiation). (**a**) A nuclear scan showing inferior wall ischemia. (**b**) A coronary angiogram shows significant RCA disease. (**c**) Following successful coronary intervention and stenting

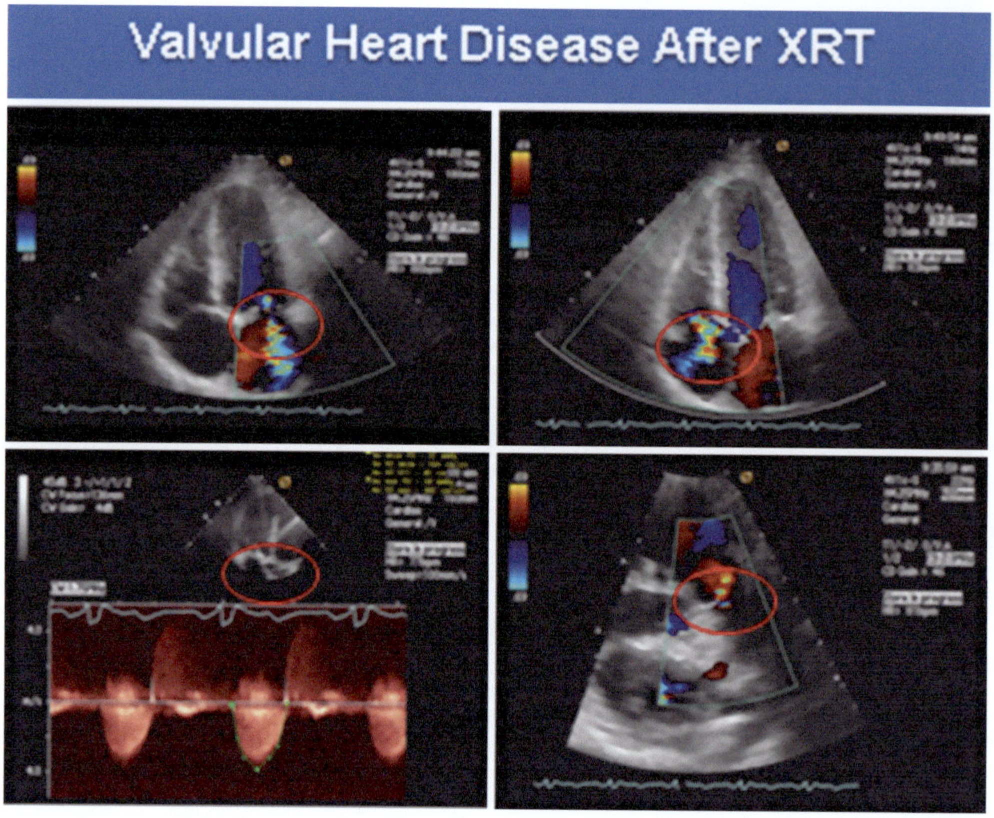

Fig. 7.8 Illustrates the case of a 46 year asymptomatic female, who had completed 30 Gy radiation to the mediastinum and neck for HL in 1976. Following echocardiogram in 2005 (29 years after completion of radiation therapy) was obtained for routine follow up. The echocardiogram shows mild regurgitation of all valves with moderate aortic stenosis

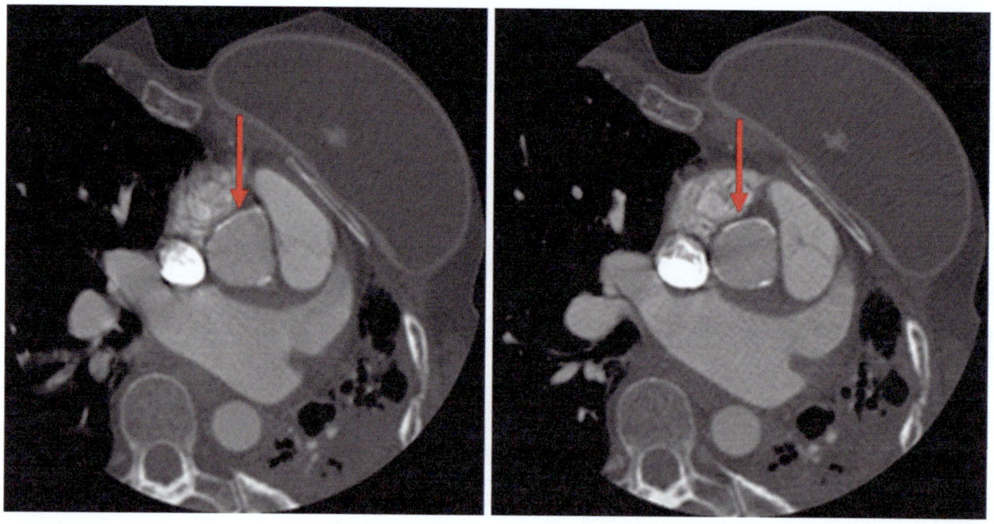

Fig. 7.9 Shows aortic calcification in a childhood lymphoma survivor with non-ischemic cardiomyopathy who had received 48 Gy radiation, 36 years ago. The *red arrow* points to the calcification in the aorta (Images courtesy of Dr. I. Daher)

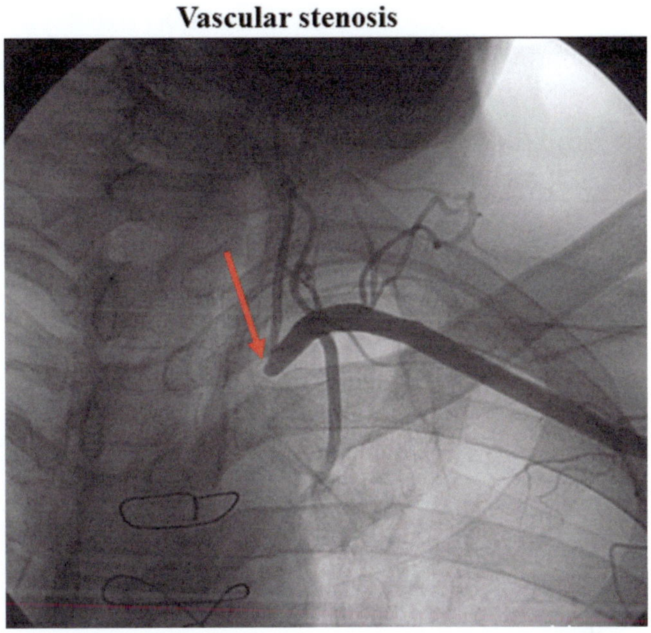

Fig. 7.10 Shows complete occlusion of the left subclavian artery (radial approach) in a 66 year old man with history of radiation in the region of subclavian artery for a hypopharyxngeal tumor. He had a previous history of CABG in 2000. The coronary angiogram was done in Nov 2008 for an abnormal stress test obtained for a pre-operative evaluation. The patient was otherwise asymptomatic, with finding of absent left radial and a barely palpable left brachial pulse. Image shows complete occlusion of the left subclavian artery (*red arrow*) (left brachial artery approach). Left Internal mammary artery (LIMA) is visible. In addition there is about 50% stenosis at the origin of the left vertebral artery. Slide courtesy of Dr. Iliescu

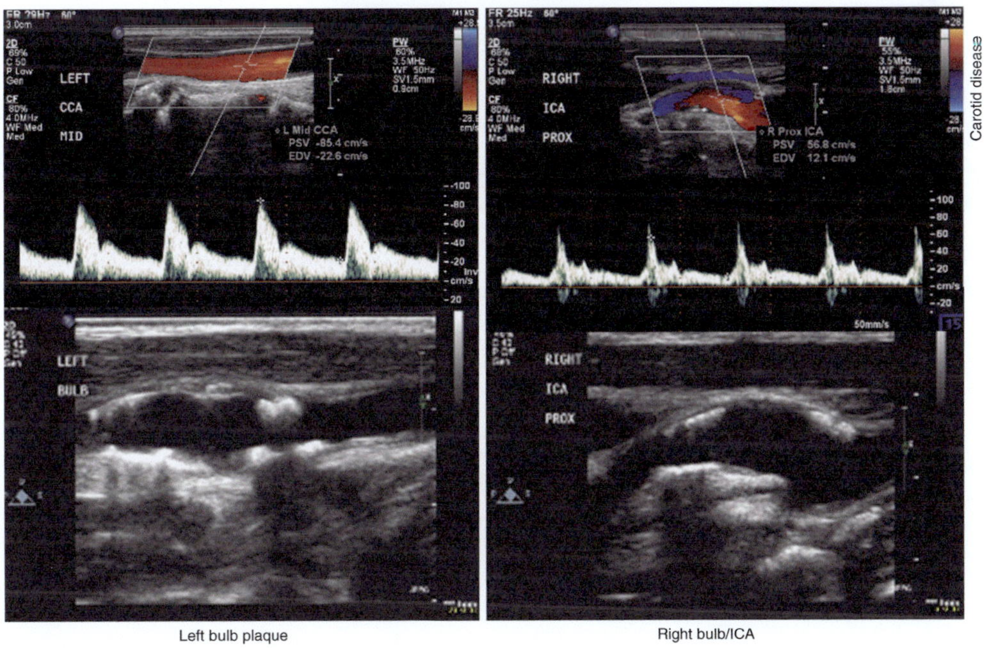

Fig. 7.11 The following image shows carotid atherosclerosis/stenosis in a patient who has received radiation for nasopharyngeal carcinoma more than 25 years ago. This 77 year old man was physically active, with no neurological symptoms and had no history of other vascular disease. A carotid Doppler showed calcified plaques in the right and left bulbs with secondary 50–69% stenosis of the left internal carotid artery segment and <50% stenosis of the right internal carotid artery segment. Normal forward flow was present in the right and left vertebral arteries

Conduction System Disorder

Heart block can occur many years after completion of the RTand is due to fibrosis of the conduction system (Fig. 7.13).

Discussion

As illustrated by cases above, radiation causes pericardial, valvular, vascular, myocardial and conduction system disease.

Effort should be made to prevent the development of these complications. With advancement in radiation and decreasing dose the incidence may decrease over a period of time, but globally still many patients will be afflicted with these cardiovascular side effects of RT.

For patients undergoing mediastinal radiation, at baseline evaluation clinical risk factors like smoking, hyperlipidemia, diabetes mellitus and hypertension should be identified and treated according to existing guidelines. At baseline a lipid profile, thyroid function, 12 lead ECG and an echocardiogram should also be obtained.

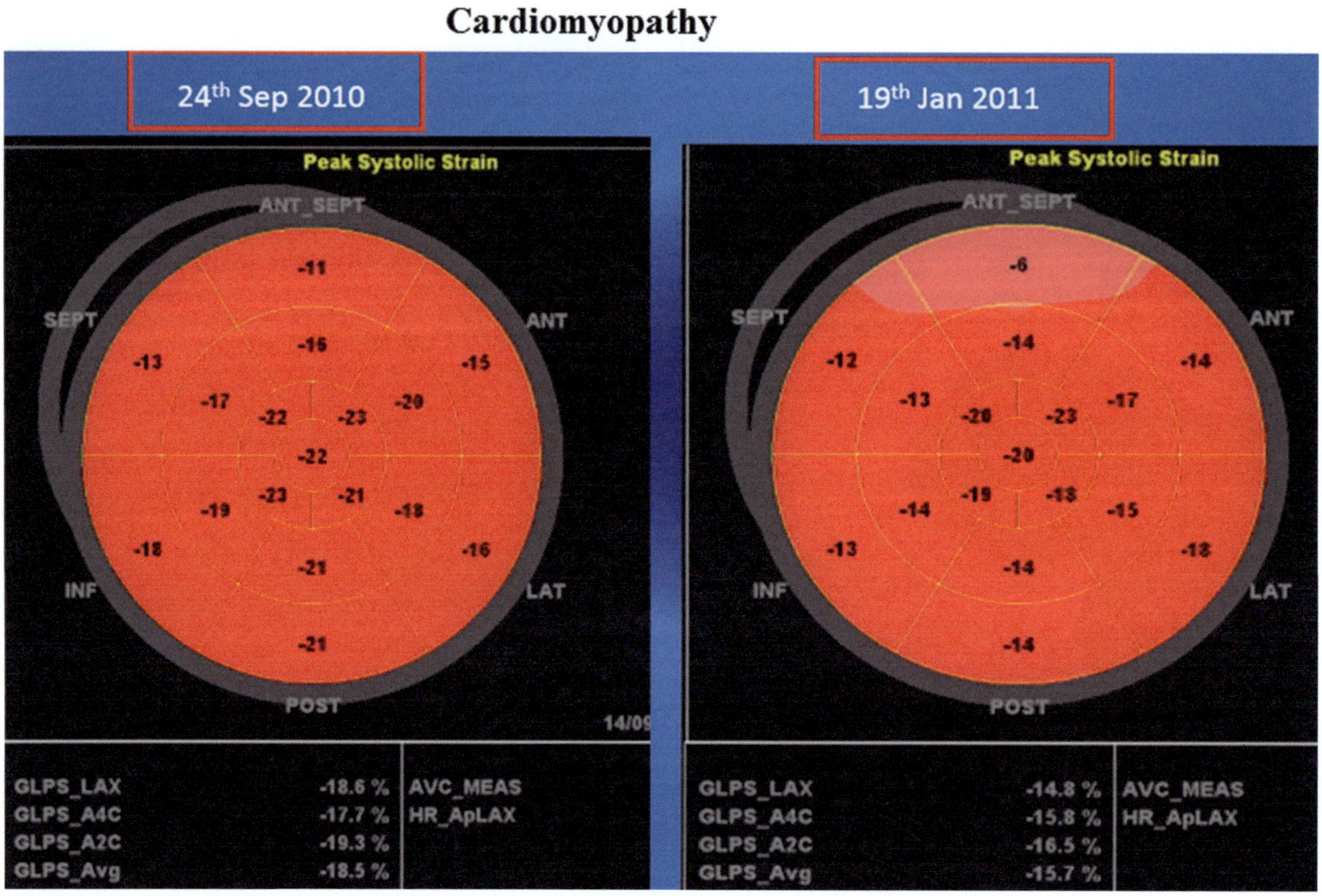

Fig. 7.12 The above image is of a 35 year old man with mediastinal lymphoma, ex-smoker, Chol = 234, LDL = 150, who had received a total of 39.6 Gy radiation between Sep and Oct 2010. The initial global strain (GLPSAvg) (24th Sep 2010) was −18.5, which decreased to −15.7 (19th Jan 2011) with RT, indicating abnormal myocardial strain due to RT(normal myocardial strain is >−18.5)

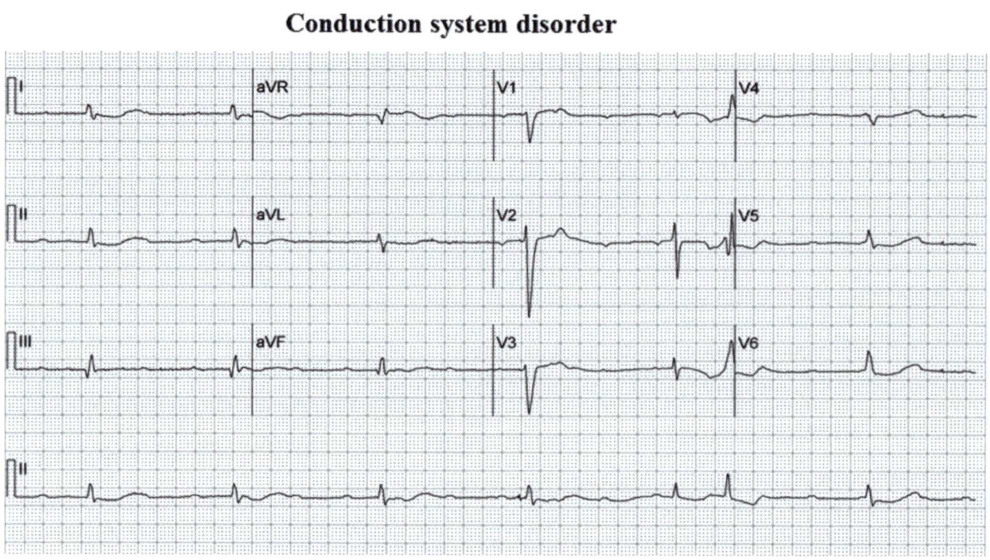

Fig. 7.13 Shows the ECG of a patient who presented with complete heart block 29 years after completion of RT. The patient presented underwent RT for HL (when aged 16 years) in 1978. In 1998 she was found to have moderate aortic regurgitation. In 2001 she under Aortic Valve replacement (AVR) with coronary artery bypass grafting (CABG). In 2009 (aged 47 years), she presented with syncope and was found to be in complete heart block for which she underwent a permanent pacemaker placement

The prevalence and development of radiation associated valve disease (RAVD) is related to the time following RT e.g. in one study the prevalence of moderate to severe aortic regurgitation was 1.1% amongst those who had undergone RT 2–10 years earlier, which increased to 15% amongst the group receiving RT > 20 years ago [11]. Hence a follow up echocardiogram should be done at least at a minimum of 10 year interval after radiation therapy.

Likely due to tumor location, radiation related CAD primarily has been described to involve the proximal vessels, the coronary ostia and left main artery [13, 14]. Patients with radiation induced CAD commonly present with angina, myocardial infarction or syncope related to complete heart block [14]. Rarely, sudden death may be the initial presentation in these patients [14]. Myocardial perfusion defects, in irradiated portion of left ventricle in asymptomatic patients also suggest small vessel damage due to RT [15]. In one study, which included patients who had received more than 35 gray of RT, about 8.4% of patients had some sort of perfusion defect on their stress test. Of these only 5% had received RT within 2–10 years of being enrolled in this study, compared to 20% who had received radiation therapy >20 years ago [16]. In this study, in the group that had received RT within 5–10 years of being enrolled in the study only 1.7% of the total patients enrolled underwent coronary angiogram based on the result of the stress test [16].

A functional non-invasive stress test is recommended 5–10 years after completion of RT, in high risk asymptomatic patients. (patients who have undergone anterior or left sided chest radiation with >1 risk factors for radiation induced heart disease) [17].

Carotid stenosis, is recognosed complication of radiation therapy to the neck. Long segement of the carotid artery may be affected. In one study in which patients received a mean cumulative radiation dose of 6420 cGy (range 5500–7680), with a mean duration of 10.2 years since their last radiation treatment, 16 patients (40%) had significant carotid artery stenosis [18]. Based on little data, a firm conclusion cannot be made for Doppler screening in these patients, but it is not unreasonable to have a screening Doppler of the carotid arteries, at >10 years after completion of radiation, or earlier if any clinical finding of bruit.

Key Points

- Hodgkin's lymphoma and breast cancer survivors treated with radiation therapy are at increased risk of development of cardiovascular disease.
- Radiation related damage to the heart affects the pericardium, myocardium, valves, and coronary vessels, with pericardium being most frequently involved.
- Asymptomatic cardiac perfusion defect are seen in about 50% of breast cancer patients treated with radiation therapy and can occur as early as early as six months after radiotherapy.
- Due to improvement in radiation techniques, the risk of cardiovascular complications in relation to radiation may have declined over time, but the risk of death from myocardial infarction in patients with HL remains increased even amongst those treated after 1985. Recently, population based case-control study of major coronary events in women who received radiation therapy for invasive breast cancer between 1958 and 2001, reported that the subsequent rate of ischemic heart disease was proportional to the mean dose to the heart, with the relative risk increasing by 7.4% per Gray (Gy) [19].
- Endothelial damage is an early sign of radiotherapy induced vascular injury.
- Radiation induced fibrosis seems to be the result of multicellular interactions mediated by inflammatory cytokines, vascular inflammation and endothelial cell dysfunction.
- Prevention of radiation induced heart disease should be the main goal of all clinicians involved in the care of these patients.
- Risk factors like smoking, hypertension, diabetes mellitus, and hyperlipidemia should be aggressively targeted and treated as per current guidelines.
- Echocardiogram should be done at 5–10 years follow up, or earlier if clinically indicated.
- A functional non-invasive stress test is recommended 5–10 years after completion of radiation, in high-risk patients.

References

1. American Cancer Society. Cancer treatment and survivorship facts & figures 2014–2015. 2014. http://www.cancer.org/
2. Yusuf SW, Sami S, Daher IN. Radiation-induced heart disease: a clinical update. Cardiol Res Pract. 2011;2011:317659. doi:10.4061/2011/317659.
3. Ng AK, Bernardo MP, Weller E, et al. Long-term survival and competing causes of death in patients with early-stage Hodgkin's disease treated at age 50 or younger. J Clin Oncol. 2002;20(8):2101–8.
4. Hancock SL, Tucker MA, Hoppe RT. Factors affecting late mortality from heart disease after treatment of Hodgkin's disease. JAMA. 1993;270(16):1949–55.
5. Mulroney DA, Easel MW, Kawashima T, et al. Cardiac outcomes in a cohort of adult survivors of childhood and adolescent cancer: retrospective analysis of the childhood cancer survivor study cohort. BMJ. 2009;339:b4606.
6. Swerdlow AJ, Higgins CD, Smith P, et al. Myocardial infarction mortality risk after treatment for Hodgkin disease: a collaborative British cohort study. J Natl Cancer Inst. 2007;99(3):206–14.
7. Cuzick J, Stewart H, Rutqvist L, et al. Cause-specific mortality in long-term survivors of breast cancer who participated in trials of radiotherapy. J Clin Oncol. 1994;12(3):447–53.
8. Galper SL, Yu JB, Mauch PM, et al. Clinically significant cardiac disease in patients with Hodgkin lymphoma treated with mediastinal irradiation. Blood. 2011;17(2):412–8.

9. Stone HB, Coleman CN, Anscher MS, McBride WH. Effects of radiation on normal tissue: consequences and mechanisms. Lancet Oncol. 2003;4:529–3.
10. Hardenberg PH, Munley MT, Bentel GC, et al. Cardiac perfusion changes in patients treated for breast cancer with radiation therapy and doxorubicin; preliminary results. Int J Radiation Oncol Biol Phys. 2001;49(4):1023–8.
11. Heidenreich PA, Hancock SL, Lee BK, Mariscal CS, Schnittger I. Asymptomatic cardiac disease following mediastinal irradiation. J Am Coll Cardiol. 2003;42(4):743–9.
12. Thavendiranathan P, Poulin F, Lim KD, et al. Use of myocardial strain imaging by echocardiography for the early detection of cardiotoxicity in patients during and after cancer chemotherapy: a systematic review. J Am Coll Cardiol. 2014;63(25 Pt A):2751–68. doi:10.1016/j.jacc.2014.01.073. Epub 2014 Apr 2
13. Brosius FC 3rd, Waller BF, Roberts WC. Radiation heart disease. Analysis of 16 young (aged 15 to 33 years) necropsy patients who received over 3,500 rads to the heart. Am J Med. 1981;70(3):519–30.
14. Orzan F, Brusca A, Conte MR, Presbitero P, Figliomeni MC. Severe coronary artery disease after radiation therapy of the chest and mediastinum: clinical presentation and treatment. Br Heart J. 1993;69(6):496–500.
15. Gyenes G, Fornander T, Carlens P, Glas U, Rutqvist LE. Myocardial damage in breast cancer patients treated with adjuvant radiotherapy: a prospective study. Int J Radiat Oncol Biol Phys. 1996;36(4):899–905.
16. Heidenreich PA, Schnittger I, Strauss HW, et al. Screening for coronary artery disease after mediastinal irradiation for Hodgkin's disease. J Clin Oncol. 2007;25(12):43–9.
17. Lancellotti P, Nkomo VT, Badano LP, BerglerKlein J, Bogaert J, Davin L, et al. Expert consensus for multi-modality imaging evaluationof cardiovascular complications of radiotherapy in adults: a report from the European Association of Cardiovascular Imaging and the American Society of Echocardiography. J Am Soc Echocardiogr. 2013;26(9):1013–32.
18. Steele SR, Martin MJ, Mullenix PS, et al. Focused high-risk population screening for carotid arterial stenosis after radiation therapy for head and neck cancer. Am J Surg. 2004;187:594–8.
19. Darby SC, Ewertz M, McGale P, et al. Risk of ischemic heart disease in women after radiotherapy for breast cancer. N Engl J Med. 2013;368:987–98.

Acute Coronary Syndrome in Patients with Cancer

8

Ezequiel Munoz, Dana Elena Giza, Ricardo Bellera, and Cezar Iliescu

Abstract

Therapeutic management of the cancer patients with symptoms of acute coronary syndrome has to be tailored to patient's comorbidities while balancing potential risks of invasive revascularization. Careful selection of patients with ischemia-inducing stenosis necessitating cardiac catheterization is required to avoid hazardous complications in cancer patients with good prognosis. In general in patients with acute coronary syndrome, an early invasive strategy (coronary angiography and percutaneous coronary intervention or coronary artery bypass graft) is superior to a conservative strategy of optimum medical treatment alone. Intraprocedural tools for lesion assessment (intravascular ultrasonography, optical coherence tomography) allow a better characterization of the luminal processes and assessment of the hemodynamic impact of the lesion. A fractional flow reserve of >0.75 permits postponing stent placement and prompt continuation on anticancer therapy with no increased mortality risk. Special considerations have to be made in respect to primary or acquired thrombocytopenia, the increased propensity to thrombosis associated with cancer as a pro-inflammatory state, and the potential drug interactions. The use of percutaneous coronary angiography with either bare metal stents or drug eluting stents requires combined antiplatelet therapy (aspirin and P2Y12 inhibitors) to prevent early stent thrombosis. Significant collaborative efforts between cardiologists and hematologists/oncologists is of prime importance in order to optimize the care of oncology patients and increase overall survival.

Keywords

Coronary artery disease (CAD) • Cancer • Thrombocytopenia • Percutaneous coronary intervention (PCI) • Fractional flow reserve (FFR) • Intravascular ultrasound (IVUS) • Optical coherence tomography (OCT) • Coronary artery bypass graft (CABG) • Cardiotoxicity • Takotsubo syndrome

Abbreviations

ACS	Acute coronary syndrome
BMS	Bare metal stents
CABG	Coronary artery bypass graft surgery
CAD	Coronary artery disease
DAPT	Dual antiplatelet therapy (aspirin and a thienopyridine)
DES	Drug eluting stents
FFR	Fractional flow reserve

E. Munoz • D.E. Giza • C. Iliescu, M.D. (✉)
Department of Cardiology, University of Texas MD Anderson Cancer Center, 1515 Holcombe Blvd., Unit 1451, Houston, TX 77030, USA
e-mail: ciliescu@mdanderson.org

R. Bellera
Department of Cardiology, The University of Texas Health Science Center, Houston, TX, USA

S.W. Yusuf, J. Banchs (eds.), *Cancer and Cardiovascular Disease*, https://doi.org/10.1007/978-3-319-62088-6_8

IVUS	Intravascular ultrasonography
NSTEMI	Non ST elevation myocardial infarction
PCI	Percutaneous coronary intervention
POBA	Plain balloon angioplasty
UA	Unstable angina

Introduction

Ischemic heart disease in cancer patients can either be long-standing or as consequence of the exposure to "cardiotoxic" therapies (chemotherapy, radiation) along with the hypercoagulable state created by malignancies [1].

Unique issues arise when this patient population develops the need for interventional cardiovascular procedures such as indications, timing of the procedure, additional comorbidities including thrombocytopenia and paraneoplastic disease, vascular access choice, etc. Often, a combined medical and interventional approach is required in order to best balance the risk-benefit profile of these patients [2].

This chapter highlights the treatment approaches to cancer patients with acute myocardial infarction, giving emphasis to percutaneous coronary interventions (PCI) and the importance of intraprocedural tools to improve outcomes in this patient population.

In this chapter we will focus on the following:

1. Management of Myocardial Infarction in Cancer Patients: General Considerations
2. Coronary Interventions
   - Intraprocedural tools for lesion assessment
     - Fractional Flow Reserve (FFR)
     - Intravascular Ultrasound (IVUS)
     - Optical Coherence Tomography (OCT)
   - Left main coronary artery disease
3. Takotsubo stress cardiomyopathy
4. Special considerations in patients with thrombocytopenia

Management of Myocardial Infarction in Cancer Patients: General Considerations

Therapeutic management of the cancer patients with symptoms of acute myocardial infarction (MI) pose significant challenges. Tailored treatment to patient's comorbidities and balancing potential risks are recommended. The available treatment options for MI in cancer patients (aspirin, β blockers, statins, percutaneous coronary intervention (PCI) without stenting, PCI with bare metal stent or drug eluting stent, CABG) rely on studies done in general population, as evidence-based treatments lack for this particular group of patients [2]. In one study in which very few patients underwent coronary intervention, medical therapy with aspirin and beta blockers improved survival [3]. In another study, cardiac death at 1-year was found to be similar in cancer patients and non-cancer patients, probably as result of early reperfusion therapy with coronary intervention [4].

Early invasive approach versus conservative management provide conflicting results and controversies still persist in the literature [4]. The traditional approach in cancer patients with symptoms of acute coronary syndrome (ACS) includes an intense medical management and risk stratification using non-invasive means to identify patients who may need coronary angiography [2]. However, reports have shown that higher risk patients appear to benefit from an early invasive strategy [5]. Results of a recently published randomized controlled multicenter trial including only patients aged ≥80 years presenting with non-ST elevation myocardial infarction (NSTEMI) or unstable angina (UA), showed an early invasive strategy (coronary angiography and subsequent treatment with percutaneous coronary intervention, coronary artery bypass graft) being superior to a conservative strategy of optimum medical treatment alone in the reduction myocardial infarction, need for urgent revascularization, stroke, or death [6]. Early angiography (within 24 h) speeds revascularization, prevents occurrence of further complications of ACS, and facilitates early discharge [7].

Current guidelines in general population recommend early invasive strategy for higher risk patients based on TIMI score and/or GRACE (Global Registry of Acute Coronary Events) risk predictor model [8]. Additional recommendations include [8]:

- Patients with NSTEMI who have refractory angina or hemodynamic or electrical instability.
- Signs or symptoms of heart failure or new or worsening mitral regurgitation.
- Sustained ventricular tachycardia or ventricular fibrillation

The initial step embraces risk stratification by MDACC Risk Score. Presence of ≥3 of these factors favors early angiography (ideally within 24 h) with possible revascularization by percutaneous intervention or bypass surgery. If none of the above, patients should begin intensive medical management according to current cardiovascular guidelines. The MD Anderson Cancer Center approach in cancer patients is shown in Fig. 8.1.

Placement of IABP should be considered in patients with cardiogenic shock or with hemodynamic instability until revascularization can be done or in patients with recurrent ischemia despite maximal medical treatment [2]. Recent data from MD Anderson Cancer Center on patients

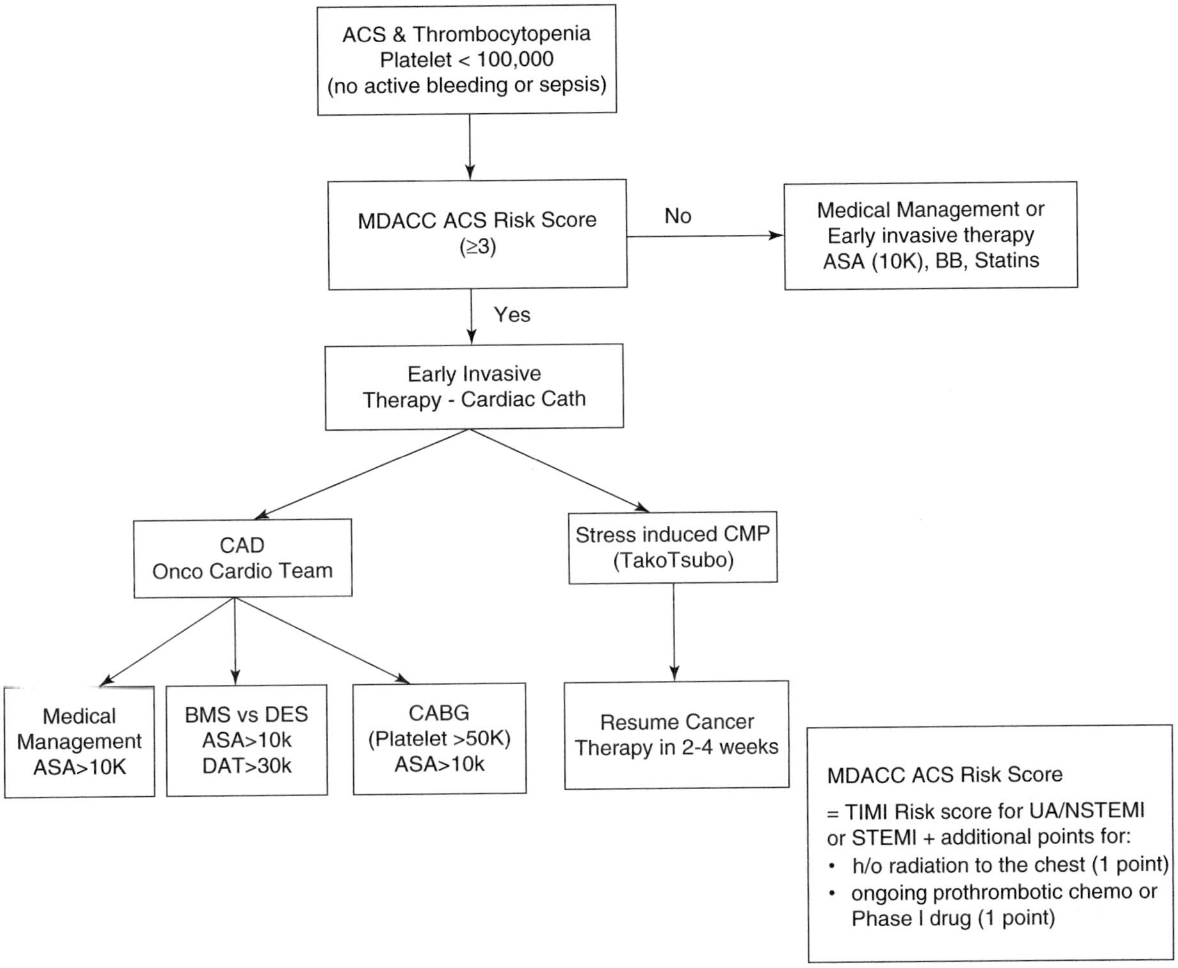

Fig. 8.1 The MD Anderson Cancer Center approach in cancer patients with ACS and thrombocytopenia

diagnosed with acute myocardial infarction showed that cancer patients are more likely to benefit from aggressive medical therapy, with a significant overall survival improvement with the use of aspirin and beta-blockers [3]. The study also reported that patients with hematological malignancies have worse outcomes than patients with solid tumors [3].

If angina symptoms cannot be controlled with optimal medical therapy and further pain palliation is required, PCI or Coronary artery bypass graft (CABG) should be considered as further options (Figs. 8.2 and 8.3). When invasive revascularization is considered, the choice between PCI and CABG is a matter of debate. The general condition of the patient, stage of malignancy and severity of the cardiac disease are factors that influence the decision. CABG is preferred when patients have a good outcome and a potentially curable malignancy, while PCI is reserved for more aggressive disease [2]. If PCI is the option, balloon angioplasty, stenting with implantation of BMS (bare metal stent) or DES (drug eluting stent) are possibilities available. However, cancer patients with coronary artery disease and BMS placed have an increased risk of stent thrombosis compared to general population [9]. In cancer patients with normal platelet counts and no other contraindications, dual antiplatelet therapy with Aspirin and Clopidogrel is recommended for all patients with acute MI [10]. Early discontinuation of Clopidogrel has been associated with subacute and late stent thrombosis and recurrent myocardial infarction. Cancer patients with bare metal stents (BMS) appear to have a higher risk of stent thrombosis compared to the general population with most events in patients on DAPT. This risk could be enhanced by the pro-inflammatory state in cancer and susceptibility for clotting. Some of the chemotherapeutic drugs are thrombogenic (cisplatinum and thalidomide) or might induce thrombocytopenia causing concerns about the need to use the platelet-suppressing agents [11]. Moreover, re-endothelialization after implantation of stent can take longer in cancer patients under chemotherapeutic regimen. Postponement of any non-cardiac surgery is suggested to be done for 6 weeks up 3 months after implantation of BMS and 6–12 months after DES [2].

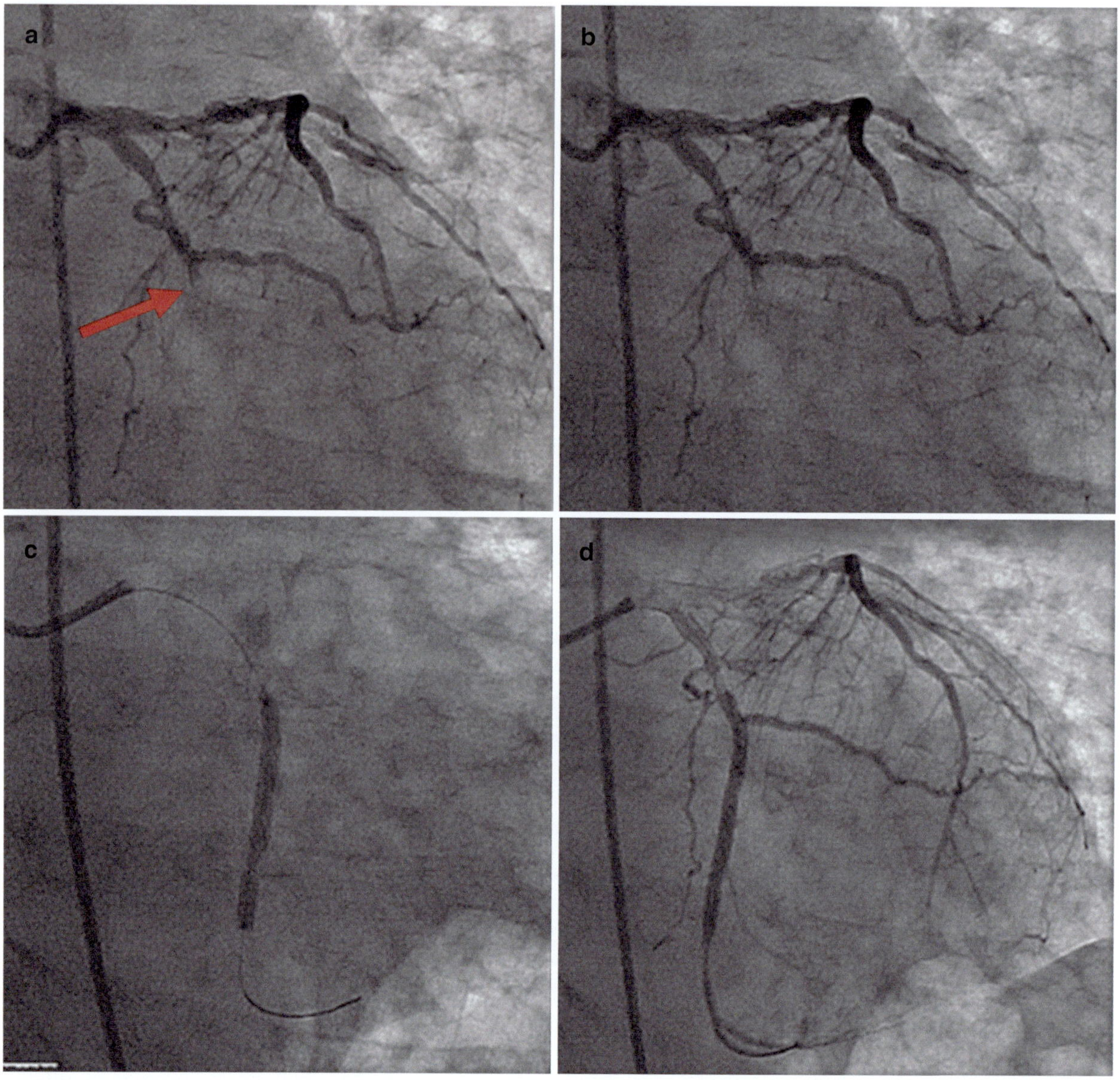

Fig. 8.2 (Panel **a–d**) Sixty-eight year old man with stage IIIB non-small cell lung cancer on chemo-radiation therapy was admitted with chest pain and elevated troponin levels. (**a**) A complete total occlusion (CTO) of the Left Circumflex artery; (**b**) left circumflex artery angioplasty; (**c**) stent deployment in the left coronary artery; (**d**) flow restoration of the left coronary artery

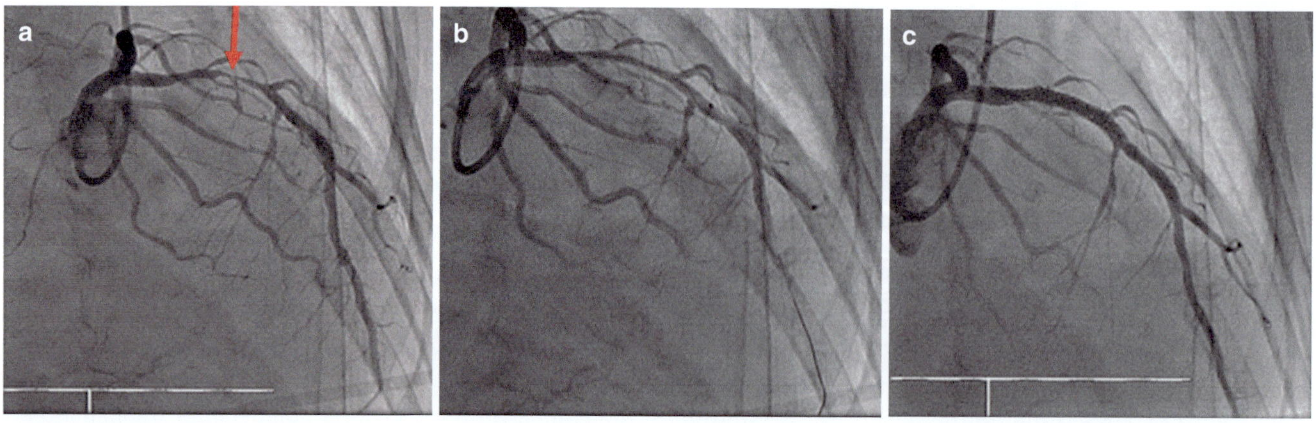

Fig. 8.3 (Panel **a–c**) Sixty-one-year-old male with a past medical history of hypertension, multiple sclerosis, nonsmall-cell lung cancer diagnosed in 2004, status post multiple chemotherapy regimens with variable response, who was started on experimental chemotherapy. (**a**) A subtotal occlusion of the proximal to mid left descending artery (LAD); (**b**) LAD with residual >60% stenosis after balloon angioplasty (POBA), stenting was required; (**c**) flow restoration of the LAD with <10% residual stenosis after post dilation of the stent

Coronary Interventions: Intraprocedural Tools for Lesion Assessment

Fractional Flow Reserve

Interventional treatment of moderate lesions based on angiographic findings alone can be influenced by the patient's symptoms, and stenosis severity can be overestimated [12]. There is suboptimal overlap between the degree of stenosis and coronary blood flow. Hyperemic flow may be limited in stenosis as low as 45% diameter as other factors, such as residual cross-sectional area, lesion length, and collateral circulation influence resistance and flow, and therefore, symptomatology [13].

Fractional flow reserve (FFR) represents a lesion-specific index defined as the maximum achievable blood flow in the presence of a stenosis divided by maximum flow if there was no obstructive epicardial coronary disease [14] (Fig. 8.4). FFR guided PCI is associated with less coronary events when compared with revascularization driven by angiographic aspect. FAME trial results have shown, in general population, a decreased primary composite end point of death, myocardial infarction, and repeat revascularization at 1 year, by quantifying the hemodynamic significance of the lesion by FFR [15]. The combined rate of death and myocardial infarction was also significantly reduced. Justification of FFR guided-PCI use in ischemic coronary disease has been provided by several studies; a recent meta-analysis by Nascimento et al. [16] looked at a total of 19 studies and highlights the safety in deferral of patients with normal FFR and in those receiving intervention with an abnormal FFR.

Controversy in cancer patients regarding the extent of the benefit from PCI exists. Careful selection of patients with ischemia-inducing stenosis requiring revascularization and balancing risks is required in order to avoid hazardous complications in patients with good prognosis. A fractional flow reserve (FFR) of 0.80 or less in non-cancer patients reflects a hemodynamically significant stenosis with an accuracy of 90% [15].

Previous results from unpublished data on cancer patients who underwent coronary angiography and FFR measurement have shown that deferring cancer patients with FFR > 0.75 allows prompt continuation on anticancer therapy and is not related with increased mortality risk. Recommendation is to measure FFR when possible to assess hemodynamic involvement of the lesion.

Intravascular Ultrasound

Intravascular ultrasound (IVUS) due to its higher special resolution is superior to angiography alone in determining lesion severity and allows for better characterization of luminal processes (Fig. 8.5) [17]. It provides information on pre-intervention related to lesion characteristics, including vulnerable plaques, lesion severity, length, and morphology; on post-intervention optimal stent implantation for stent

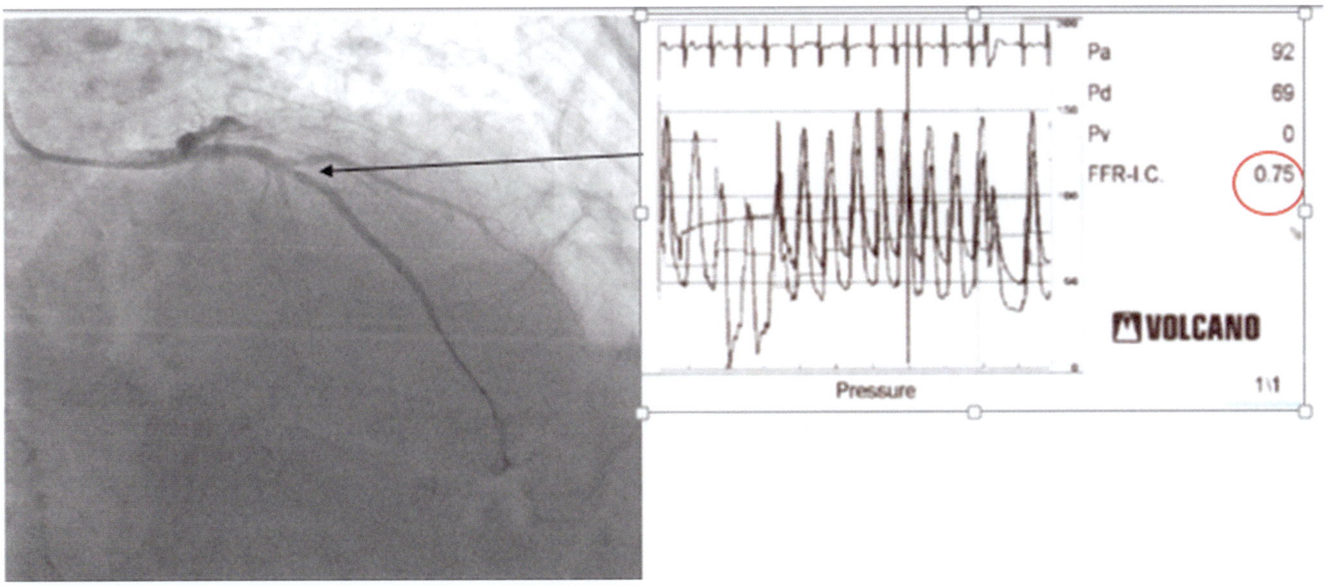

Fig. 8.4 FFR measurement in 72-year-old gentleman with a longstanding history of progressive myelodysplasia syndrome and history of non-ST segment elevation myocardial infarction. Echocardiographic findings showed hypokinesis in the LAD territory. Platelet count was 15 × 10⁹/L. Special considerations were taken to decrease bleeding risk such as radial approach and the use of micro puncture needle. Initial angiographic findings revealed a distal LAD lesion corresponding with 80% stenosis. We proceeded to measure FFR, which showed non-significant hemodynamic compromise. The patient was medically managed and was able to resume cancer therapy

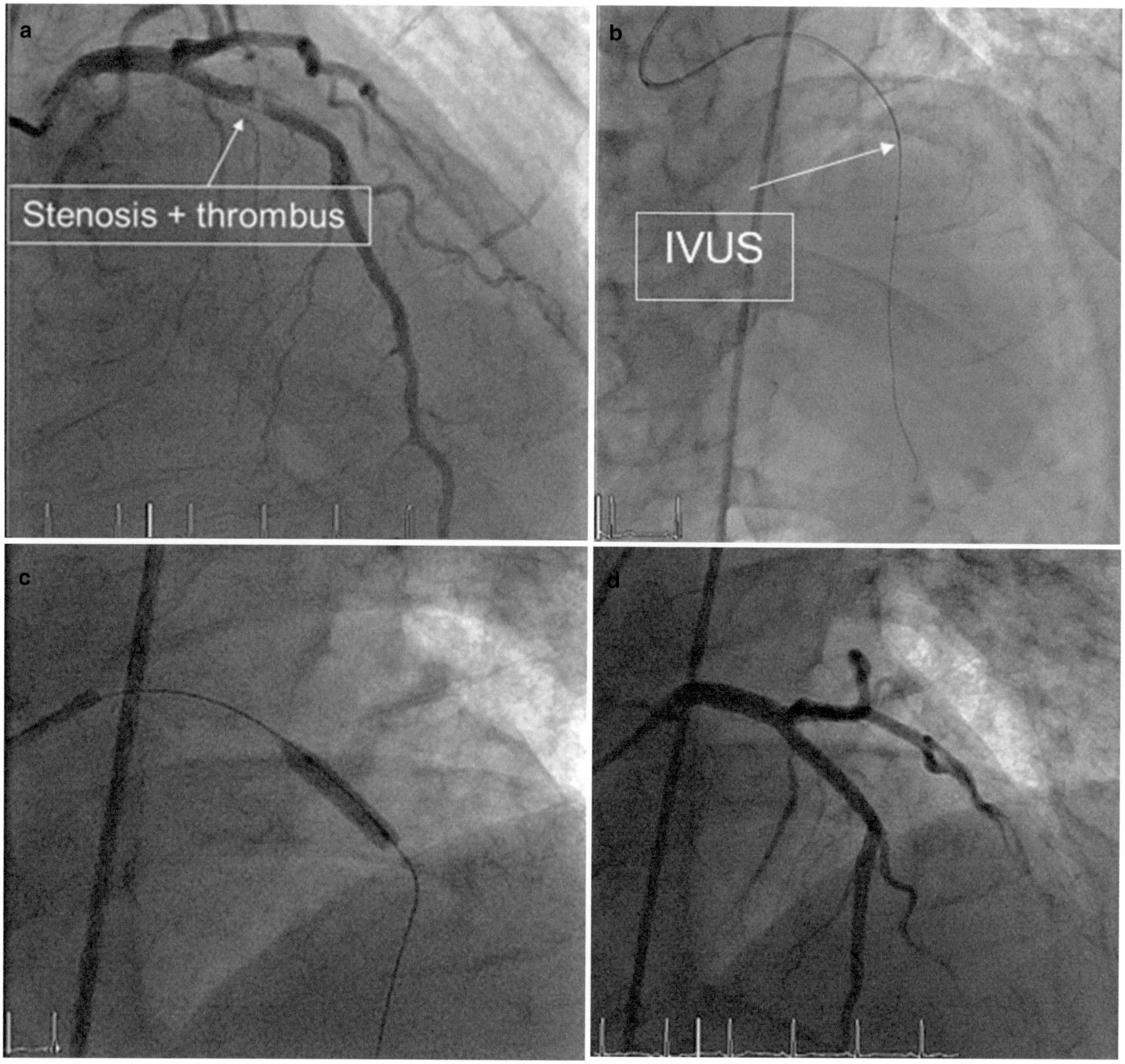

Fig. 8.5 IVUS guided stent placement in a patient with metastatic melanoma. Patient was treated with Carboplatin and Taxol with Avastin for a year and then with GSK-MEK inhibitor. The primary cancer was located in the left neck area, for which he had a surgery and postoperative radiation. Patient had left sided neck discomfort and the troponin level was elevated. Panel **a**—coronary angiography shows stenosis of the proximal segment of LAD; Panel **b**—IVUS assessment before stent placement; Panel **c**—**IVUS** guided stent placement, Panel **d**—restoration of blood flow in LAD

expansion, extension, and apposition; and on possible complications after stent implantation [18]. Recent published data suggest that IVUS-guided DES implantation decreases the rates of major cardiac events, stent thrombosis and target lesion revascularization when compared to angiography-guided PCI [19]. The use of FFR and IVUS have significantly improved detection of coronary stenosis and are frequently used to assess the severity of left main coronary coronary artery stenosis.

Optical Coherence Tomography

Optical coherence tomography (OCT) is a high-resolution imaging modality that uses infrared light emission to provide cross-sectional images of tissue with a resolution of ≤10–20 μm [20]. Due to its high resolution, it enables the differentiation of the various layers of the coronary arterial vessel wall to accurately classify the tissue characteristics and identify morphological features of vulnerable plaque, such as a thin

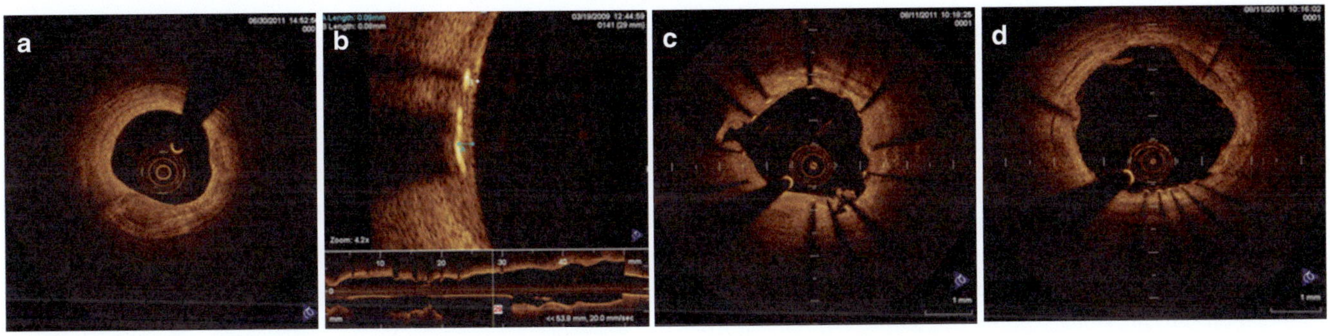

Fig. 8.6 (Panel **a–d**) OCT images for preoperative evaluation in a 60 year old female with breast cancer with multiple PCI and recurrent chest pain. Panel **a**—Optical coherence tomography (OCT) appearance of lipid pool with overlying thin fibrous cap—the lipid core has a diffuse border and high light attenuation resulting in poor tissue penetration. This is the typical appearance of thin cap fibro-atheroma (TCFA). Panel **b**—OCT appearance of calcified plaques—calcified regions with a sharp border, low signal, low attenuation, permitting deeper penetration. Panel **c**—OCT appearance of overlying thrombus on some of the stent struts. Panel **d**—Optical coherence tomography images of common neointima and neoatherosclerosis. Common neointima is recognized by its high-signal. Common neointima is recognized by its high-signal intensity and homogeneous region inside stent struts. All the images were obtain from the same patient, who developed neoatherosclerosis after stent implantation

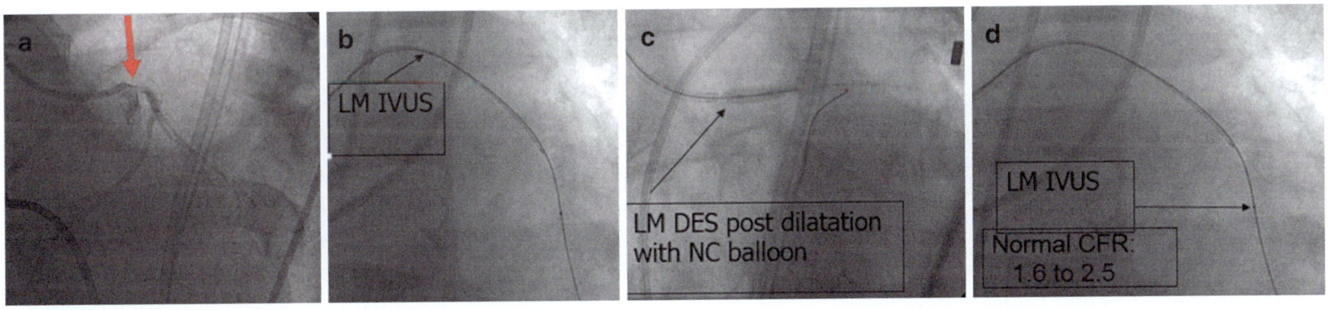

Fig. 8.7 IVUS-guided LM stenosis assessment in a 45-year-old gentleman with metastatic melanoma to the lung and liver and recurrent pulmonary edema. At that time, left heart catheterization revealed an ostial left main stenosis. The *arrow* points to the stenosis (Panel **a**). Patient was considered high-risk for bypass surgery. Decision was made to proceed with left main stenting with a drug-eluting stent (DES). Left main was stented with a Cypher drug-eluting stent 35 × 8 deployed at 14 atmospheres post-dilatation was performed using a quantum 40 × 18 inflated at 14 atmospheres with flare-up of the ostium (Panel **b**, **c**). Intravascular ultrasound post-procedure confirmed good stent apposition (Panel **d**). Patient was transferred to the ICU with intraaortic balloon pump and Swan Ganz catheter

fibrous cap, lipid-rich plaque, and thrombus formation [21]. Ex vivo studies of the coronary arteries have demonstrated the accuracy of optical coherence tomography imaging for definition of plaque characteristics (revealing nearly identical images when compared with the histology) [22] (Fig. 8.6).

OCT has great utility in cancer patients identifying stents with adequate strut apposition and endothelialization [2]. Such findings support a decreased risk of in stent thrombosis and help guide temporary discontinuation of antiplatelet therapy to continue cancer treatment without experiencing adverse cardiovascular effects.

OCT also allows visualization of the key components of the atherosclerotic plaque that appear to confer vulnerability to rupture thickness of the fibrous cap, size of the necrotic core, and the presence of macrophages [23]. Thin fibrous cap cutoff by OCT is <65 μm [24]. Necrotic core (and the broader histopathological category of a lipid pool) is seen as a signal-poor region with poorly defined borders and fast OCT signal drop-of [23, 25]. Macrophage accumulations can sometimes be seen at the border of the fibrous cap and necrotic core, and can appear as punctate signal-rich spots that exceed the background noise of the image [25].

Left Main Coronary Assessment and Therapeutic Strategies

Left main coronary stenosis has become increasingly common in cancer survivors due to mediastinal exposure to radiation therapy [26]. Assessment of the lesion includes coronary angiography in addition to FFR and IVUS to improve the diagnostic accuracy (Fig. 8.7). There is no current data is available for invasive assessment of left main disease in cancer patients. In our experience on patients that underwent coronary angiography we have used a FFR value of >0.80 or absolute cross sectional area by IVUS of >7 mm^2 for symptomatic and >6 mm^2 for asymptomatic patients as cutoff criteria to defer further revascularization strategies. Interventions were deferred in 50% of patients and cancer care was resumed without interruptions.

Stent vs. CABG

Left main stenting has been adopted among clinical practices as a response to previously published studies which reported comparable outcomes when compared to coronary artery bypass graft (CABG) revascularization [27].

Current guidelines of LMCA disease in general population recommend PCI (class IIa recommendation) in patients with ostial or shaft disease, those with low SYNTAX score (<23), or those where PCI can be performed more rapidly and safely than CABG [28].

Takotsubo Stress Cardiomyopathy

Takotsubo stress cardiomyopathy (TSC) is a syndrome characterized by transient myocardial dysfunction with unknown etiology [29]. It represents a clinical syndrome that mimics acute myocardial infarction, with indistinguishable electrocardiographic findings, as well as non-specific biomarker elevation. Recently studied data at MD Anderson Cancer Center found that almost 10% of patients with cancer who exhibited clinical characteristics of NSTEMI had TSC [30]. Physical and psychological stress have been identified as most common triggers in general population, mostly due to sympathetic activation [31] . Takotsubo syndrome is also considered to be a side effect of chemotherapeutic use for antineoplastic agents such as 5-FU, Sunitinb, Daunorubicin, Cytarabine [32]. However, in cancer patients, surgical procedures account for most of the cases (Fig. 8.8).

Researchers at the Mayo Clinic proposed the following diagnostic criteria for TSC [33]:

1. Transient hypokinesis, akinesis, or dyskinesis in the left ventricular mid segments with or without apical involvement;
2. Regional wall motion abnormalities that extend beyond a single epicardial vascular distribution; and frequently, but not always, a stressful trigger;
3. Absence of obstructive coronary disease or angiographic evidence of acute plaque rupture;
4. New ECG abnormalities (ST-segment elevation and/or T-wave inversion) or modest elevation in cardiac troponin; and,
5. Absence of pheochromocytoma and myocarditis.

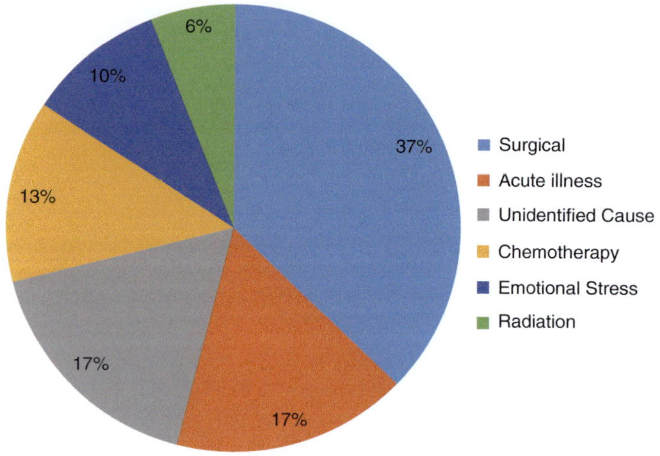

Fig. 8.8 Takotsubo Triggering Factors in Cancer Patients

The gold standard for definitive differentiation between AMI and TSC is cardiac catheterization (Fig. 8.9). Identifying TSC in cancer patients is essential since they may represent a subgroup of patients that could promptly resume cancer therapy with complete ejection fraction recovery. Also identifying TSC may allow withholding antiplatelet therapy in patients who are at risk of bleeding and in the absence of confirmed diagnosis of TSC would otherwise may receive antiplatelet therapy. In absence of significant underlying comorbidities the prognosis is good. Cancer therapy should be resumed in 2–4 weeks and for long term treatment β-blockers can be used to reduce the sympathetic heart stimulation. Past experience have shown that 95% of the patients who required further oncologic treatment were able to continue it without recurrent TSC with a mean time of 21 days [34].

Studies on long-term prognosis of TSC have found no difference in terms of survival when compared to AMI [29], suggesting that this clinical syndrome is less benign than previously thought. Physicians should be aware and low threshold for cardiac catheterization should be considered in highly suspicious patients.

Special Considerations in Patients with Thrombocytopenia

Prevalence of thrombocytopenia (TP) varies from 10 to 25% among cancer patients, approximately 10% having platelet counts less than 100 × 10^9/L [35].Thrombocytopenia may be a feature of the underlying malignancy or may result from the treatment of cancer itself, and increases the risk of bleeding and other cardiac events. Chemotherapy-induced thrombocytopenia triggers spontaneous bleeding (not life threatening or intracranial) in patients with platelet counts

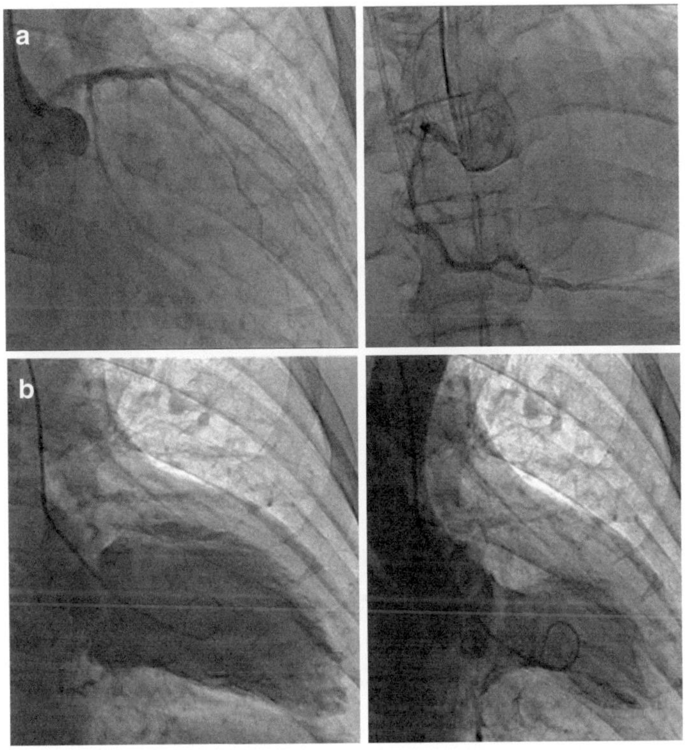

Fig. 8.9 Angiographic study in a 70-year-old Caucasian woman with a history of marginal cell lymphoma who had undergone threecycles of Fludarabine with Mitoxantrone and presented with progressive dyspnea on exertion. She was found to have new onset systolic heart failure with regional wall motion abnormalities and elevated cardiac enzymes. (**a**) Coronary angiography showing clean coronaries without any signs of obstruction and (**b**) LV gram showing apical balloon. A diagnosis of Takotsubo cardiomyopathy was made and the patient made an unremarkable recovery and was discharged home without any sequelae

less than 10×10^9/L [36]. .Bleeding risk in patients with TP is increased, however, low platelet counts does not protect against thrombotic events (Fig. 8.10).

A platelet count of $40–50 \times 10 \times 10^9$/L should be sufficient to perform most of the interventional procedures. Safety measures during the procedure include ultrasound guidance, micro puncture needles, and fluoroscopic guidance, may contribute to the best possible outcomes [2]. 30–50 U/kg unfractionated heparin is the initial recommended dose for thrombocytopenic patients undergoing PCI who have platelets $<50 \times 10^9$/L with ACT monitoring during the procedure and additional heparin administration if ACT < 250 s.

The use of antiplatelet therapy remains controversial; however, experience at MD Anderson Cancer Center in patients with thrombocytopenia and ischemic heart disease showed a significant improvement in survival among the patient cohort when therapy with ASA was added to the treatment regimen, and no bleeding complications were found [37]. This finding implies that regardless of the platelet count, antiplatelet therapy should be considered Administration of Aspirin can be used in patients with platelet counts more than 10,000/mL. Given the high risk of early stent thrombosis, dual antiplatelet therapy with Aspirin or Clopidogrel is recommended when platelet counts are $>30–50 \times 10^9$/L. Usually, in cancer patients with thrombocytopenia, Clopidogrel can be administered with a 75 mg oral dose daily, after an initial loading dose of 150–300 mg [38].

DAPT may be restricted to 2 weeks following PTCA alone, 4 weeks after bare-metal stent (BMS), and 6 months after second or third generation drug-eluting stents (DES) if platelet counts are more than 50×10^9/L. Consultation with hematology/oncology specialists is recommended for severely thrombocytopenic cancer patients with MI undergoing cardiac catheterization. In MD Anderson Cancer Experience, no patient with thrombocytopenia has received GPIIb/IIIa inhibitors [10]. There is a lack of data on the use of Abciximab, Eptifibatide, Tirofiban in association with medical and invasive treatment in cancer patients with MI, while in general population a low risk of bleeding (<25%) and of thrombocytopenia (<0.5%) has been reported.

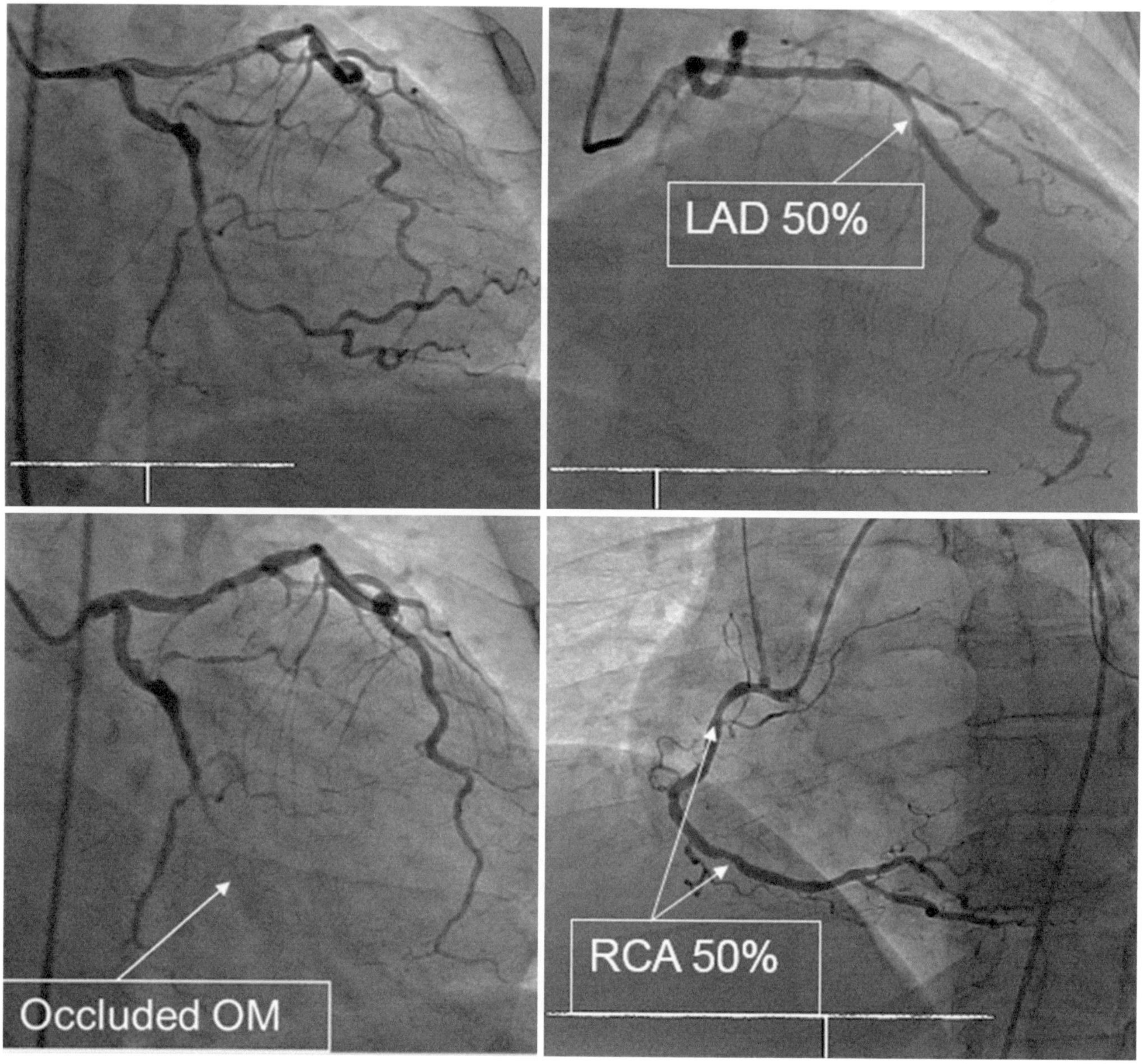

Fig. 8.10 Coronary angiography images with multiple vessels stenosis in a 39 year old female with acute myeloid leukemia, in remission. She presented 2 weeks prior to SCT, with acute myocardial infarction and was found to thrombocytopenic, with a platelet count of 32×10^9/L

Conclusions

In cancer patients with stable coronary disease, symptoms can be managed conservatively, with medical treatment only as with general population. In contrast, in patients with severe three vessel disease involving left anterior descending artery and symptoms of UA/MI there is a critical need for revascularization. Data on the outcomes after performing invasive procedures in cancer patients with concomitant active coronary artery disease are lacking, as major clinical trials have excluded this particular group of patients. Special considerations have to be made in respect to cancer' comorbidities such as thrombocytopenia, the increased propensity to thrombosis, and the potential drug interactions between drugs commonly used in the management of coronary disease and antineoplastic agents in cancer treatment. In order for patients to receive an appropriate treatment and avoid hazardous consequences of invasive treatment proper selection of patients who will benefit from revascularization has to be made. Detection of angiographically significant coronary disease can be made by using FFR or intravascular ultrasound (IVUS) in order to identify patients in whom interventions can be deferred. If FFR or IVUS are unavailable, optical coherence tomography (OCT) or noninvasively using cardiac PET may be considered. The use of PCI with either bare metal stents or drug eluting stents requires combined antiplatelet therapy (aspirin and P2Y12 inhibitors) to prevent early stent thrombosis. Significant collaborative efforts between cardiologists and hematologists/oncologists is of prime importance in order to optimize the care of oncology patients and increase overall survival.

References

1. Whitlock MC, Yeboah J, Burke GL, Chen H, Klepin HD, Hundley WG. Cancer and its association with the development of coronary artery calcification: an assessment from the multi-ethnic study of atherosclerosis. J Am Heart Assoc. 2015;4(11).
2. Iliescu CA, Grines CL, Herrmann J, et al. SCAI expert consensus statement: evaluation, management, and special considerations of cardio oncology patients in the cardiac catheterization laboratory (endorsed by the Cardiological Society of India, and Sociedad Latino Americana de Cardiologia Intervencionista). Catheter Cardiovasc Interv. 2016;87(5):E202–23.
3. Yusuf SW, Daraban N, Abbasi N, Lei X, Durand JB, Daher IN. Treatment and outcomes of acute coronary syndrome in the cancer population. Clin Cardiol. 2012;35(7):443–50.
4. Kurisu S, Iwasaki T, Ishibashi K, Mitsuba N, Dohi Y, Kihara Y. Comparison of treatment and outcome of acute myocardial infarction between cancer patients and non-cancer patients. Int J Cardiol. 2013;167(5):2335–7.
5. Pratap P, Gupta S, Berlowitz M. Routine invasive versus conservative management strategies in acute coronary syndrome: time for a "hybrid" approach. J Cardiovasc Transl Res. 2012;5(1):30–40.
6. Tegn N, Abdelnoor M, Aaberge L, et al. Invasive versus conservative strategy in patients aged 80 years or older with non-ST-elevation myocardial infarction or unstable angina pectoris (After Eighty study): an open-label randomised controlled trial. Lancet. 2016;387(10023):1057–65.
7. Patel MR, Dehmer GJ, Hirshfeld JW, Smith PK, Spertus JA. ACCF/SCAI/STS/AATS/AHA/ASNC/HFSA/SCCT 2012 appropriate use criteria for coronary revascularization focused update: a report of the American College of Cardiology Foundation Appropriate Use Criteria Task Force, Society for Cardiovascular Angiography and Interventions, Society of Thoracic Surgeons, American Association for Thoracic Surgery, American Heart Association, American Society of Nuclear Cardiology, and the Society of Cardiovascular Computed Tomography. J Am Coll Cardiol. 2012;59(9):857–81.
8. Amsterdam EA, Wenger NK, Brindis RG, et al. 2014 AHA/ACC guideline for the management of patients with non-ST-elevation acute coronary syndromes: a report of the American College of Cardiology/American Heart Association Task Force on Practice Guidelines. J Am Coll Cardiol. 2014;64(24):e139–228.
9. Gross CM, Posch MG, Geier C, et al. Subacute coronary stent thrombosis in cancer patients. J Am Coll Cardiol. 2008;51(12):1232–3.
10. Iliescu C, Durand JB, Kroll M. Cardiovascular interventions in thrombocytopenic cancer patients. Tex Heart Inst J. 2011;38(3):259–60.
11. Krone RJ. Managing coronary artery disease in the cancer patient. Prog Cardiovasc Dis. 2010;53(2):149–56.
12. Takashima H, Waseda K, Gosho M, et al. Severity of morphological lesion complexity affects fractional flow reserve in intermediate coronary stenosis. J Cardiol. 2015;66(3):239–45.
13. Abbott JD. More than addition the use of fractional flow reserve in serial stenoses. J Am Coll Cardiol Interv. 2012;5(10):1019–20.
14. Pijls NHJ, Van Gelder B, Van der Voort P, et al. Fractional flow reserve: a useful index to evaluate the influence of an epicardial coronary stenosis on myocardial blood flow. Circulation. 1995;92(11):3183–93.
15. Tonino PAL, De Bruyne B, Pijls NHJ, et al. Fractional flow reserve versus angiography for guiding percutaneous coronary intervention. New Engl J Med. 2009;360(3):213–24.
16. Nascimento BR, Belfort AF, Macedo FA, et al. Meta-analysis of deferral versus performance of coronary intervention based on coronary pressure-derived fractional flow reserve. Am J Cardiol. 2015;115(3):385–91.
17. Cheneau E, Leborgne L, Mintz GS, et al. Predictors of subacute stent thrombosis: results of a systematic intravascular ultrasound study. Circulation. 2003;108(1):43–7.
18. Hong SJ, Kim BK, Shin DH, et al. Effect of intravascular ultrasound-guided vs angiography-guided everolimus-eluting stent implantation: the IVUS-XPL randomized clinical trial. JAMA. 2015;314(20):2155–63.
19. Jang JS, Song YJ, Kang W, et al. Intravascular ultrasound-guided implantation of drug-eluting stents to improve outcome: a meta-analysis. JACC Cardiovasc Interv. 2014;7(3):233–43.
20. Khandhar SJ, Yamamoto H, Teuteberg JJ, et al. Optical coherence tomography for characterization of cardiac allograft vasculopathy after heart transplantation (OCTCAV study). J Heart Lung Transplant. 2013;32(6):596–602.
21. Jang IK, Tearney GJ, MacNeill B, et al. In vivo characterization of coronary atherosclerotic plaque by use of optical coherence tomography. Circulation. 2005;111(12):1551–5.
22. Otsuka F, Joner M, Prati F, Virmani R, Narula J. Clinical classification of plaque morphology in coronary disease. Nat Rev Cardiol. 2014;11(7):379–89.
23. Sinclair H, Bourantas C, Bagnall A, Mintz GS, Kunadian V. OCT for the identification of vulnerable plaque in acute coronary syndrome. JACC Cardiovasc Imaging. 2015;8(2):198–209.
24. Miyamoto Y, Okura H, Kume T, et al. Plaque characteristics of thin-cap fibroatheroma evaluated by OCT and IVUS. JACC Cardiovasc Imaging. 2011;4(6):638–46.
25. Tearney GJ, Regar E, Akasaka T, et al. Consensus standards for acquisition, measurement, and reporting of intravascular optical coherence tomography studies: a report from the International Working Group for Intravascular Optical Coherence Tomography Standardization and Validation. J Am Coll Cardiol. 2012;59(12):1058–72.
26. Yusuf SW, Sami S, Daher IN. Radiation-induced heart disease: a clinical update. Cardiol Res Pract. 2011;2011:317659. doi:10.4061/2011/317659.
27. Buszman PE, Buszman PP, Banasiewicz-Szkróbka I, et al. Left main stenting in comparison with surgical revascularization: 10-year outcomes of the (Left Main Coronary Artery Stenting) LE MANS Trial. JACC: Cardiovasc Interv. 2016;9(4):318–27.
28. Dash D, Chen SL. Stenting of left main coronary artery stenosis: data to clinical practice. J Cardiovasc Dis Diagn. 2015;3:222.
29. Tornvall P, Collste O, Ehrenborg E, Jarnbert-Petterson H. A case-control study of risk markers and mortality in Takotsubo stress cardiomyopathy. J Am Coll Cardiol. 2016;67(16):1931–6.
30. Munoz E, Iliescu G, Vejpongsa P, et al. Takotsubo stress cardiomyopathy: "good news" in cancer patients? J Am Coll Cardiol. 2016;68(10):1143–4.

31. Akashi YJ, Nef HM, Lyon AR. Epidemiology and pathophysiology of Takotsubo syndrome. Nat Rev Cardiol. 2015;12(7):387–97.
32. Fakhri Y, Dalsgaard M, Nielsen D, Lav Madsen P. 5-Fluorouracil-induced acute reversible heart failure not explained by coronary spasms, myocarditis or takotsubo: lessons from MRI. BMJ Case Rep. 2016;2016.
33. Akashi YJ, Goldstein DS, Barbaro G, Ueyama T. Takotsubo cardiomyopathy: a new form of acute, reversible heart failure. Circulation. 2008;118(25):2754–62.
34. Vejpongsa P, Banchs J, Reyes M, Iliescu G, Akinyemi M, Yusuf SW, Iliescu C. Takotsubo cardiomyopathy in cancer patients. Triggers, recovery, and resumption of therapy. J Am Coll Cardiol. 2015;65(10S):A927.
35. Elting LS, Rubenstein EB, Martin CG, et al. Incidence, cost, and outcomes of bleeding and chemotherapy dose modification among solid tumor patients with chemotherapy-induced thrombocytopenia. J Clin Oncol. 2001;19(4):1137–46.
36. Wang J, Cai X, Cheng X, Song P, Jiang S, Gong J. Acute myocardial infarction caused by tumor-associated thrombotic thrombocytopenic purpura: case report. Med Princ Pract. 2014;23(3):289–91.
37. Sarkiss MG, Yusuf SW, Warneke CL, et al. Impact of aspirin therapy in cancer patients with thrombocytopenia and acute coronary syndromes. Cancer. 2007;109(3):621–7.
38. Yusuf SW, Iliescu C, Bathina JD, Daher IN, Durand JB. Antiplatelet therapy and percutaneous coronary intervention in patients with acute coronary syndrome and thrombocytopenia. Tex Heart Inst J. 2010;37(3):336–40.

9 Arterial Complications in Patients with Cancer

Tam T.T. Huynh, Hue T. Cao, Susana G. Palma, and Karen C. Broadbent

Abstract

Complications of peripheral arterial disease in cancer patients are associated with increased morbidity and mortality. Medical management with modification of vascular risk factors remains the first line of treatment for cancer patients with arterial occlusive disease. Endovascular or surgical revascularization is indicated for patients who have critical limb ischemia or disabling claudication symptoms. In this article, we review the management of peripheral arterial disease in cancer patients, and present a series of common and rare case examples of arterial complications that can occur during or after oncologic therapy.

Keywords

Angiography • Angioplasty • Arterial disease • Cancer • Endarterectomy • Limb ischemia • PAD • Radiation • Stenting • Vascular

Introduction

Cardiovascular complications are a common cause of morbidity and mortality in patients undergoing oncologic treatment. The presence of a malignancy is known to be associated with a state of hypercoagulability and increased risk of venothromboembolism (VTE) in patients diagnosed with cancer [1–3]. Certain chemotherapeutic drugs have known potential deleterious cardiovascular side effects [4, 5]. The field of cardio-oncology has emerged as an important subspecialty in our fight against cancer [5, 6]. However, the management of arterial complications in cancer patients, not directly related to the heart, remains ill defined and controversial.

The prevalence of peripheral arterial disease (PAD) in older patients diagnosed with cancer is estimated to be roughly 15–40% [6]. The incidence of acute arterial thrombosis in cancer patients is infrequent but has been linked to advanced cancer stage and poor prognosis [7, 8]. Some experts have suggested that palliative expectant treatment may be the most appropriate management for cancer patients who develop arterial complications due to their associated dismal survival rate [8–10]. In contrast, other groups have shown good outcome in treating arterial complications in cancer patients [11, 12]. In this article, we review the management of PAD in patients diagnosed with cancer and present a series of common and rare case examples of arterial complications that can occur during or after oncologic therapy.

T.T.T. Huynh, M.D. (✉)
Department of Thoracic and Cardiovascular Surgery, The University of Texas – MD Anderson Cancer Center, 1515 Holcombe Blvd., Unit 1489, Houston, TX 77030-4009, USA

Department of Interventional Radiology, The University of Texas – MD Anderson Cancer Center, 1515 Holcombe Blvd., Unit 1489, Houston, TX 77030-4009, USA
e-mail: tamhuynh@mdanderson.org

H.T. Cao, M.P.A.S.
Department of Thoracic and Cardiovascular Surgery, The University of Texas – MD Anderson Cancer Center, 1515 Holcombe Blvd., Unit 1489, Houston, TX 77030-4009, USA

S.G. Palma, R.N. • K.C. Broadbent, B.S.N., R.N, R.V.T.
Thoracic and Orthopedic Center, The University of Texas – MD Anderson Cancer Center, 1515 Holcombe Blvd., Unit 1489, Houston, TX 77030-4009, USA

S.W. Yusuf, J. Banchs (eds.), *Cancer and Cardiovascular Disease*, https://doi.org/10.1007/978-3-319-62088-6_9

PAD Epidemiology and Clinical Significance

Approximately 8.5 million people over the age of 40 in the United States have atherosclerotic PAD, including 12–20% individuals over the age of 60 [13, 14]. Most patients with chronic PAD are asymptomatic, with a minority presenting with symptoms of classic intermittent claudication, and less than 5% have critical limb ischemia [15, 16]. The lifetime risk of limb-loss for the majority of patients with PAD is less than 5%, reflecting the relative "stable" or "slow-progression" nature of the disease. The clinical importance of PAD is more related to it being a marker of atherosclerotic disease at other sites rather than it causing limb loss. Individuals suffering from PAD are at a much higher risk of morbidity and mortality from complications related to cardiac and cerebrovascular complications than individuals without PAD [17]. In general, studies have shown that antiplatelet and statin therapy can reduce the rate of myocardial and ischemic stroke events in PAD patients [18, 19]. However, there are still no good clinical predictors to indicate PAD progression in the affected limbs.

For the subgroup of patients with chronic critical limb ischemia, the more severe form of the disease, the 1-year risk of limb-loss can exceed 25%. Typically, chronic critical ischemia occurs as a result of multi-level arterial occlusive disease (affecting more than one artery segment), or is due to extensive tibial artery disease. Intervention on the occluded aorto-iliac or femoro-popliteal segments, either by endovascular or surgical techniques, or a combination of both approaches (hybrid), can achieve high limb-salvage rates. Revascularization for patients with tibial arterial occlusive disease remains a challenging task.

Up to 10% of patients with critical limb ischemia can have concomitant malignancy [20]. It is well recognized that patients with critical leg ischemia who also harbor a malignancy have shorter survival than patients with critical leg ischemia who do not have a malignancy. It is unclear whether death in patients with concomitant malignancy and critical leg ischemia is due to the underlying malignancy or related to their cardiovascular co-morbidities. Moreover, the limb-salvage outcome for these patients are not well reported in the literature, and there remains a need for determining the optimal management cancer patients with critical leg ischemia.

Diagnostic Evaluation

The diagnosis of arterial insufficiency in cancer patients can often be delayed, due to the presence of confounding factors such as cancer-related pain or symptoms of peripheral neuropathy caused by chemotherapy drugs. However, a presumptive diagnosis of arterial insufficiency can usually be made after a thorough history and physical examination. The symptoms of intermittent leg claudication in the hip, thigh or calf muscles, precipitated by walking and relieved by rest, are typically reproducible. The symptom of ischemic rest pain in the foot with recumbency, which wakes the patient from sleep and is relieved by dangling of the affected foot, is a reliable indicator of severe arterial insufficiency. On exam, the loss of palpable pulses in the affected extremity is a diagnostic sign of PAD. Typically palpable pulses will be lost below the level of complete arterial occlusion. Other chronic signs of moderate to severe leg ischemia include loss of hair and atrophic muscles in the affected limb. Other chronic signs of severe ischemia include dependent rubor, and tissue loss such as non-healing wound or tissue necrosis. Patients who suffer acute limb-threatening ischemia (ALI) typically complain of new sudden onset of leg pain, coldness, pallor, numbness and weakness.

Measurement of the ankle-brachial index (ABI) can usually confirm and estimate the severity of ischemia, or rule out ischemia if normal (0.9–1.1). Duplex ultrasonography is the fist vascular imaging modality of choice for patients with suspected PAD, as it provides real-time dynamic visualization of the aorto-iliac, femoro-popliteal and tibial arteries. High-resolution CT angiogram can be used for further evaluation when vascular duplex ultrasound is non-diagnostic. In patients with iodine contrast allergy or severe renal insufficiency, we use MR angiogram as an alternative diagnostic imaging modality. Conventional selective contrast arteriography is currently performed primarily as part of a therapeutic endovascular intervention and is rarely required in the diagnostic work-up.

The Trans-Atlantic Society Consensus, also known as the Inter-Societal Consensus, TASC II classification of PAD has been widely adopted, both in clinical practice and research communities, nationally and internationally [21]. The TASC II classification allows for stratification according to the location and severity of disease. TASC II classification divides PAD anatomical involvement into aorto-iliac, femoro-popliteal, and infra-popliteal segments. In TASC II classification, PAD disease extent ranges from A, B, C to D, in increasing severity, and includes single short partial segmental occlusion to multiple long complete occlusions. In addition, the TASC guidelines for the management of PAD have emerged as a valuable resource for vascular specialists from across different disciplines. Currently, medical therapy is still the first line of treatment for patients with PAD. Endovascular interventions are typically considered for symptomatic PAD patients with TASC II A or B lesions. Surgical interventions remain the accepted method of revascularization for TASC II C or D lesions, even though endovascular techniques are increasingly being used for more extensive disease. When endovascular intervention is deemed unsuitable or fails, surgical revascularization remains a good secondary option for limb-salvage.

Medical Management

The recommended medical therapy for PAD in cancer patients follows the same guiding principles as for PAD patients without concomitant cancer diagnosis. Lifestyle modifications are effective and well-validated interventions for symptomatic PAD, with tobacco cessation and supervised exercise demonstrated to improve functional performance, and quality of life scores, while reducing symptoms [22, 23]. In addition, best medical therapy is recommended for all patients with PAD including antiplatelet, statin, and control of blood pressure and diabetes. Optimal medical therapy has been shown to reduce the incidence and fatality of cardiovascular events such as stroke or myocardial infarction in patients with PAD, and should be continued throughout oncologic treatment unless otherwise deemed contra-indicated [24, 25]. For cancer patients undergoing chemotherapy that can cause severe thrombocytopenia, antiplatelet agents can be withheld temporarily to minimize bleeding risk, but should be resumed when the platelet count returns to a level greater than 50,000/μL. Similarly, PAD patients needing oncologic surgical resection can temporarily stop antiplatelet medication but should resume it as soon as the risk of postoperative bleeding subsides. Cilostazol and pentoxifylline are the only two agents specifically approved for the treatment of intermittent claudication in the USA. Both drugs inhibit platelet aggregation, and have rheologic, and vasodilatory effects. Cilostazol and pentoxifylline can be stopped during oncologic treatment without significant increased cardiovascular risk.

In general, we encourage patients with mild to moderate symptoms of intermittent claudication to continue to exercise. In addition, we provide patients with reassurance that the risk of limb loss is minimal and that the claudication pain is harmless. Revascularization can be considered in cancer patients with severe disabling claudication symptoms to relieve symptoms but is best delayed until after completion of oncologic treatment. In contrast, cancer patients who show evidence of critical ischemia, such as ischemic rest pain or tissue loss in the affected extremity, have a high risk of limb loss and should be evaluated urgently for revascularization.

Surgical Versus Endovascular Revascularization

Vascular reconstructive surgery remains the gold-standard treatment for patients with symptomatic PAD and critical leg ischemia. The two most common synthetic graft materials used in vascular bypass reconstruction are polyester (Dacron) and polytetrafluoroehtylene (PTFE); the former is traditionally used as the conduit choice for aorto-femoral bypass and the latter for femoro-popliteal bypass. However, autogenous saphenous vein is still the preferred graft for infra-inguinal reconstruction, as it has higher patency rates when compared to synthetic grafts in this location [26]. In general, long-term patency of aorto-femoral bypass procedure is approximately 80–85% over 5 years [27]. The long-term patency of infra-inguinal bypass reconstructions is roughly 50–80% [26, 28]. Although endovascular interventions have not been shown to produce superior results over open surgical revascularizations, a practice shift toward an "endovascular approach first" has undeniably taken place over the last two decades [29, 30]. It is generally recognized that repeated interventions are more common after endovascular treatment than after surgical revascularization. However, the minimally invasive nature of the endovascular approach, which is associated with less morbidity when compared to surgical bypass, has made the former a more attractive and popular option to patients and providers.

Advances in endovascular techniques and devices have continued to improve the success of endovascular interventions. Endovascular interventions for aorto-iliac occlusive disease are known to produce high success rates and durable results. Comparatively, the reported outcomes of endovascular interventions for infra-inguinal occlusive disease remain variable. Several different types of endovascular tools including balloons, stents, and other devices are now commercially available. The novel drug-coated balloon and drug-eluting stent platforms have shown promising short and intermediate term results in PAD treatment [31–33]. The anti-proliferative effect of paclitaxel and everolimus, (the two drugs currently used in this technology) has been shown to be associated with reduced rates of binary restenosis and target revascularization [31, 34, 35]. Vascular stents are either self-expandable or balloon-expandable. We prefer to use balloon-expandable stents to treat ostial common iliac artery lesions, for their higher radial force, better visibility, and more predictable placement, when compared to self-expandable stents. In contrast, we preferentially use the more flexible self-expandable stents to treat lesions in the external iliac artery, which can be more tortuous and are subject to external forces. Covered stents (also known as stent-graft) are increasingly used in the treatment of PAD. The principal advantages of the covered stents over bare metal stents include the exclusion of thrombus and coverage of vessel rupture. The superior long-term outcome of covered stents over bare metal stents in the treatment of aorto-iliac and femoro-popliteal occlusive disease remains to be proven [36–39]. The presence of graft material (PTFE) on the covered stents is thought to provide a mechanical barrier to prevent intimal proliferation and stent fracture, two factors that have been associated with in-stent restenosis in the femoro-popliteal lesions. The larger diameter of the covered stents (for vessel diameters greater than 6 mm) still require larger size delivery sheath compared to the smaller sheaths for bare metal stents of comparable size.

For patients undergoing concomitant oncologic treatment, the advantage of a quicker recovery after endovascular intervention over surgical bypass is obvious. Patients can typically resume chemotherapy or radiation therapy within 1–2 weeks after endovascular intervention. In contrast, we recommend waiting approximately 3–6 weeks following surgical bypass before resuming or starting chemotherapy to allow adequate time for wound healing. Radiation treatment can usually take place safely away from the operative wounds within 2–3 weeks after surgery. Anti-platelet therapy has become standard adjuvant treatment following endovascular and surgical revascularization, although the anti-platelet agent of choice (aspirin versus clopidogrel) and duration of therapy remains variable. In general, we recommend lifelong aspirin after surgical bypass. On the other hand, we recommend clopidogrel after endovascular stenting for 3–6 months and lifelong aspirin subsequently.

Acute Limb-Threatening Ischemia

The three most common causes of acute limb threatening ischemia are: (1) acute thromboembolism from cardiogenic or other sources, (2) acute arterial graft or stent thrombosis (in patients who had prior vascular intervention), and (3) acute native arterial thrombosis with or without prior chronic atherosclerotic occlusive disease. The initial management of patients who develop ALI remains controversial. The treatment of patients who have concomitant malignancy and acute limb-threatening ischemia is even more debatable. Guarded survival outcomes and higher morbidity rates have been reported for patients who have surgical revascularization for ALI with concomitant malignancy compared to patients without a malignancy diagnosis [8–10]. However, Tsang et al. reported more favorable results in patients with concomitant malignancy who underwent surgical revascularization for ALI [11]. Similarly, we have shown more promising results in patients who develop ALI with concomitant malignancy, using selective treatment strategies including endovascular approach, surgical revascularization, or medical therapy alone or in combination [12].

Our current approach is to tailor treatment to cancer patients who develop ALI based on the severity of ischemia, the patient's performance status, and associated comorbidities. Surgical revascularization generally achieves reperfusion within 3–6 h. It is our preferred method of revascularization for patients who have severe immediately threatened limb ischemia, requiring prompt limb reperfusion. Surgical procedures to restore arterial flow range from simple thrombo-embolectomy for acute thromboembolism, to more extensive endarterectomy and bypass reconstruction for acute on chronic arterial thrombosis. Endovascular approach, including pharmaco-mechanical thrombectomy and catheter directed thrombolysis, usually takes up to 8–24 h to achieve revascularization. We recommend endovascular intervention for patients with ALI in whom the longer time to revascularization is deemed acceptable. Immediately following successful endovascular recanalization, adjuvant balloon and/or stent angioplasty is commonly required to maintain vessel patency. The advantages of endovascular approach over surgical treatment are well recognized, including less morbidity and quicker recovery. In our experience, inconsequential ecchymosis and minor bleeding at access sites are common occurrences with catheter directed thrombolytic therapy, but fortunately the incidence of major bleeding and intra-cranial hemorrhage has been low. In addition to the typical absolute contra-indications to catheter directed thrombolysis including active bleeding, recent major surgery or stroke, we consider thrombocytopenia (platelet count $<100,000/\mu L$), intra-cranial metastatic disease from renal cell cancer, thyroid cancer, or melanoma primary tumors as relative contra-indications to catheter directed thrombolysis.

Following treatment for ALI, long-term therapeutic anticoagulation is recommended to prevent recurrent thromboembolic complications in patients who have chronic atrial fibrillation or valvular heart disease. Long-term anticoagulation is similarly indicated for patients with established hypercoagulability. We have traditionally used subcutaneous low molecular weight heparin injection as the chronic anticoagulation therapy of choice for cancer patients. However, oral direct thrombin inhibitors have recently become available and are emerging as a comparable and more attractive option for patients. The long-term use of anticoagulation after vascular intervention for ALI in patients with a malignancy but without cardiogenic embolic source is not well described. We have empirically recommended a 3–6 month period of anticoagulation for these patients.

Radiation Induced Vasculopathy

Late onset radiation induced vasculopathy can develop several years after high-dose external beam radiation therapy for various kinds of cancer. It is postulated that radiation can cause acute injury to the vasa vasorum and endothelium, that leads to subsequent accelerated atherosclerosis and formation of occlusive plaque in irradiated vessels [40]. Radiation vasculopathy appears to affect the major arteries more frequently than the vein counterparts.

Radiation induced carotid disease is discussed elsewhere in this book. The external iliac artery appears to be the most commonly affected pelvic vessel in women who had radiation treatment for cervical and vulvar cancer [41, 42]. Radiation induced vasculopathy can also involve other any major artery that is within the index radiation field, such as the axillary or femoral artery in the treatment of breast cancer, limb sarcoma, myeloma, lymphoma, and etc. We recommend expectant medical therapy with exercise, aspirin and statin therapy for patients who have non-critical ischemia related to radiation induced vasculopathy.

Vascular intervention is reserved for limb-salvage in patients who have symptoms and signs of critical limb-threatening ischemia. These patients can present with acute, subacute, or chronic insidious ischemic symptoms. Endovascular interventions including catheter directed thrombolysis and arterial stenting have produced satisfactory results, but are associated with high rate of re-interventions. Surgical bypass has resulted in seemingly better long-term graft patency and lower re-intervention rates, and can be offered to patients in whom endovascular interventions have failed or are not feasible. In general, surgical bypass options involving extra-anatomical bypass procedures such as cross-over bypass from the contralateral common femoral artery to ipsilateral common femoral artery, or axillary-femoral artery bypass are preferred to avoid the risks associated with operating in a previously irradiated abdomen or pelvis. However, aorto-bifemoral bypass remains an option for patients with limb-threatening ischemia due to severe bilateral aorto-iliac occlusive disease not amenable to endovascular intervention. Much work lies ahead of us to determine the pathogenesis of radiation-induced vasculopathy in order to improve our management and ultimately prevent its development.

Chemotherapy and Vascular Thrombosis

Several chemotherapy drugs have been reported to increase risk of VTE, arterial thrombosis or both in cancer patients, although the mechanism of causing thrombosis for various agents is yet fully elucidated [4, 43]. Currently, Cisplatin, an alkylating agent, and Bevacizumab, a monoclonal antibody targeting the vascular endothelial growth factor (VEGF) are two widely used drugs in the treatment of solid malignant neoplasms that have been associated with increased risk of myocardial infarction, stroke and peripheral arterial thrombosis [44, 45]. The newer tyrosine kinase inhibitors (TKI), Imatinib, Nilotinib and Ponatinib, recently established as highly effective front-line therapies for chronic myeloid leukemia (CML), have also been linked to increased risk of peripheral arterial thrombosis [46]. However, in a recent case-controlled study using the Surveillance, Epidemiology, End-Results (SEER) cancer registry and Medicare claims data, investigators showed that elderly patients with CML have greater rates of myocardial infarction, stroke, pulmonary embolism and peripheral artery disease than age-matched non-cancer patients from the same region [47]. These event rates were not higher in the TKI-treated patients suggesting that risk for the vascular events in the patients with CML was more related to underlying cardiovascular risk factors of patients with CML and not with TKI treatment.

Treatment of Arterial Complications at the University of Texas-M.D. Anderson Cancer Center

The following are the synopsis of ten patients with critical limb ischemia recently treated at The University of Texas--M.D. Anderson Cancer Center. We review their clinical presentation, management, and outcome. Vascular imaging and photographs of the cases are shown. In addition, we provide brief pertinent expert comments on each case. We selected these ten cases as examples of common and rare arterial complications seen in patients who either have concomitant active malignancy or are cancer survivors.

Case #1. Metastatic Esophageal Cancer and Chronic Critical Leg Ischemia

A fifty-six year-old Caucasian male was referred to our institution for treatment of stage IV distal esophageal adenocarcinoma with distant metastasis to the left arm triceps muscle. The patient was a former smoker and had chronic renal insufficiency. The patient had right external iliac artery stenting and multiple failed left leg bypass graft procedures (Fig. 9.1a–d). Initially, the patient only reported left leg claudication and intermittent symptoms of ischemic rest pain in the left foot. Vascular assessment showed ABI in the severe ischemic range and multilevel arterial occlusive disease. However, the viability of the left ischemic leg was not immediately threatened. We first recommended medical therapy with aspirin, cilastazol, and statin. Chemotherapy with 5-FU and Herceptin was started. Subsequently, the patient showed remarkable oncologic response to systemic chemotherapy, becoming symptom-free from his cancer after approximately 18 months of treatment. The patient remained on maintenance chemotherapy and resumed full-time work.

At 20 months after cancer diagnosis, the patient became more incapacitated by progressive claudication symptoms and experienced worsening ischemic rest pain in the left foot. Vascular work-up showed chronic occlusion of left external iliac, common femoral, and superficial femoral arteries with reconstitution of the distal below-knee popliteal artery via collateral from patent profunda artery (Fig. 9.1e). On the right, there was severe stenosis of the right external iliac artery. The decision was made to proceed with revascularization of the left leg for limb-salvage. We opted for a hybrid procedure with stenting of the right common (using 8 × 27 mm balloon-expandable stent) and external (7 × 10 mm covered self-expandable stent-graft) iliac arteries (Fig. 9.1f), and concomitant redo cross-over right common femoral artery to left profunda artery bypass using an 8 mm heparin-bonded PTFE graft. The patient recovered well after hybrid surgical revascularization with resolution of both ischemic rest symptoms and claudication. Postoperative duplex image of fem-fem PTFE graft and left profunda shows satisfactory appearance and flow (Fig. 9.1g, h). Maintenance chemotherapy was resumed after a 6-week interruption. The patient is currently at 5 months after revascularization without symptoms of leg claudication or rest pain. Unfortunately, a recurrent malignant stricture in the distal esophagus has been diagnosed and further oncologic treatment is being considered at the time of writing this manuscript.

Comments: Even though this patient had severe chronic leg ischemia when he was first diagnosed with metastatic esophageal cancer, we prioritized his cancer treatment to prolong his survival over the limb ischemia. Revascularization was delayed until after the patient showed clinical response to chemotherapy. An alternative revascularization option for this patient would have been an aorto-bifemoral bypass reconstruction, but this would have interrupted the patient's maintenance chemotherapy for a longer post-operative

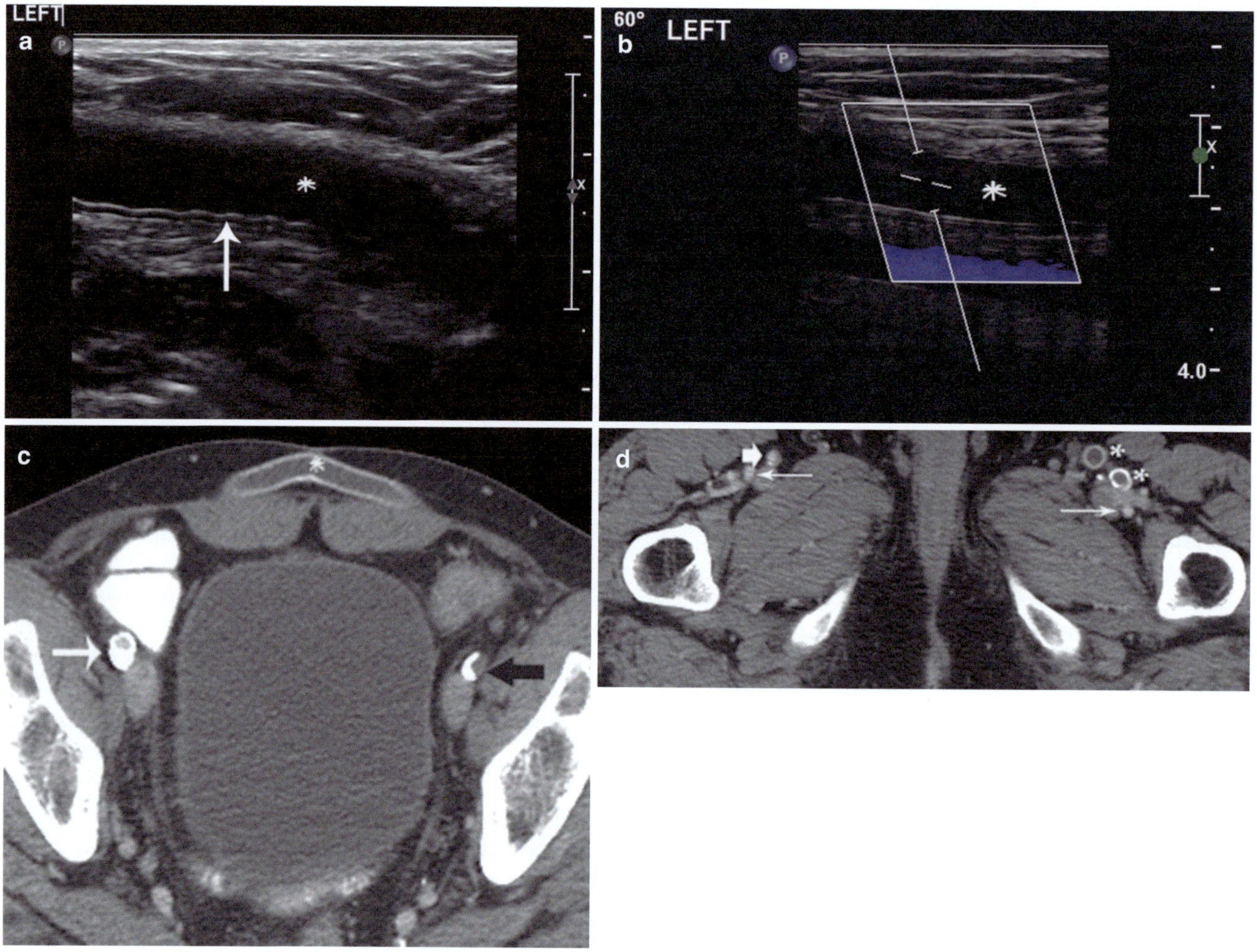

Fig. 9.1 Metastatic esophageal cancer and chronic critical leg ischemia. (**a**) Gray-scale ultrasound image shows an occluded supra-pubic cross-over femoro-femoral synthetic bypass graft; *asterisk*, lumen of graft (filled with hypoechoic thrombus), and *arrow* points to wall of graft. (**b**) Colorflow ultrasound image shows an occluded left femoral-popliteal synthetic graft; *asterisk*, lumen of graft (filled with hypoechoic thrombus). *Blue colorflow* is seen in the native femoral vein adjacent to the graft. (**c**) Axial CT image shows the occluded native left distal external iliac artery (*black arrow*) and a calcified and narrowed distal right external iliac artery (*white arrow*). (**d**) Axial CT image shows the occluded synthetic grafts (*asterisk*) with bright rims in the left groin; *long arrows* point to the respective patent native profunda arteries. The *short arrow* denotes the patent right superficial femoral artery.

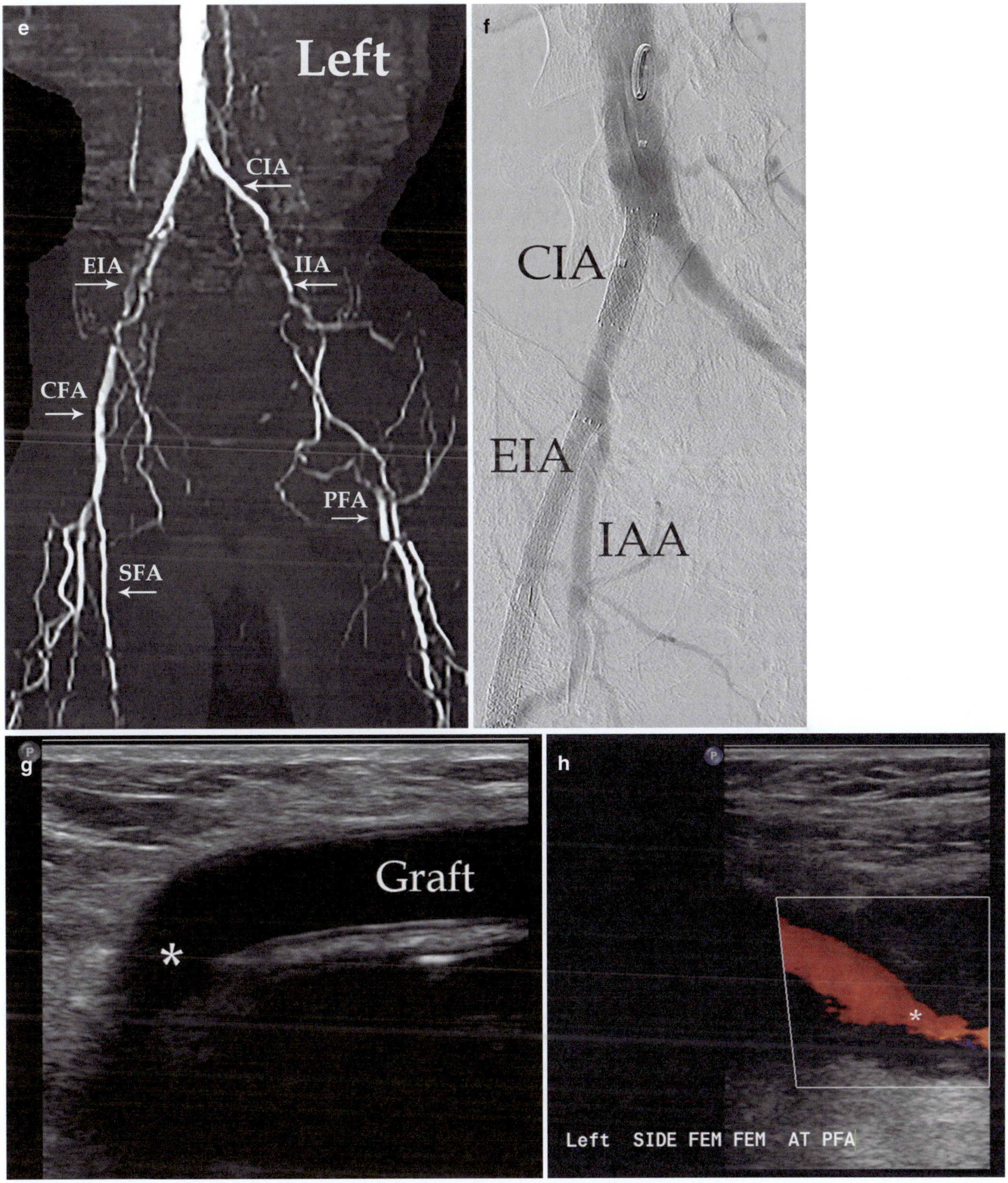

Fig. 9.1 (continued) (**e**) Reformatted MRA image reveals patency of the distal abdominal aorta and bilateral common iliac arteries (CIA). The right external iliac artery (EIA) is severely diseased and the left external iliac and common femoral arteries are occluded. The right common femoral (CFA), profunda and superficial femoral (SFA) are patent. On the left, numerous branches of the internal iliac (IIA) and profunda (PFA) arteries are seen. (**f**) Right iliac stenting was performed as part of a hybrid revascularization procedure to provide inflow to a new cross-over right to left femoro-femoral bypass graft. Stents are shown in the right common iliac (CIA) and external iliac (EIA) arteries; IAA, internal iliac artery. (**g**) Gray-scale ultrasound image shows the new cross-over femoro-femoral synthetic graft showing the right femoral-graft anastomosis (*asterisk*). (**h**) Colorflow ultrasound image shows the new femoro-femoral synthetic graft at the left graft to profunda femoral artery (PFA) anastomosis (*asterisk*)

recovery. It is also noteworthy to mention that the patient's ischemic leg symptoms resolve following the inflow procedure and distal bypass of the left femoral and popliteal artery occlusion was not required.

Case # 2. Acute Femoral Artery Thromboembolism in a Patient with Metastatic Renal Cell Cancer

A fifty-eight year-old Caucasian woman presented to the emergency room with 24-h history of acute right leg ischemic symptoms including pain, numbness and weakness. The patient had started Axitinib (a tyrosine kinase inhibitor—TKI) treatment for progressive metastatic renal cell cancer to the lungs. The patient had radical right nephrectomy 7 years prior and partial left nephrectomy for bilateral renal cell cancer 4 years later. Duplex ultrasound showed acute occlusion of the right common femoral and superficial femoral arteries with distal reconstitution (Fig. 9.2a, b). We performed surgical thromboembolectomy removing occluding clots from the femoral artery bifurcation (Fig. 9.2c, d). Her native iliac, femoral, popliteal and tibial arteries were otherwise normal without significant plaque disease. After successful revascularization, the patient was initiated on long-term anticoagulation, transitioning from unfractionated intravenous heparin to warfarin. Cardiac work-up showed normal sinus rhythm and normal left ventricular ejection fraction without evidence of a thrombus or valvular heart disease. The patient resumed Axitinib few weeks after thromboembolectomy and was kept on warfarin. However, she developed intermittent hemoptysis the following year and systemic anticoagulation was discontinued. Two years after the

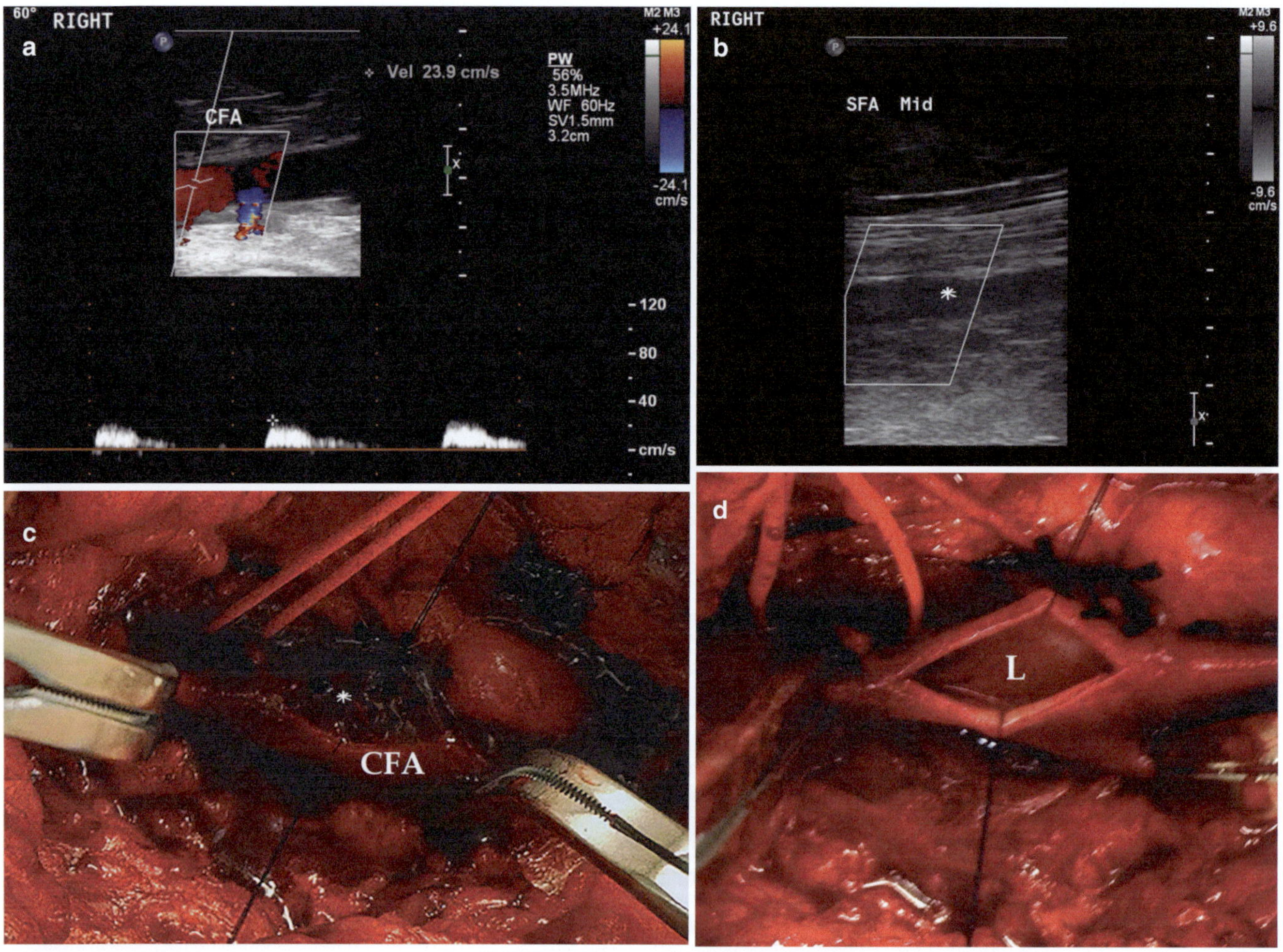

Fig. 9.2 Acute femoral artery thromboembolism in a patient with metastatic renal cell cancer. (**a**) Ultrasound image shows blunted low flow velocity in the common femoral artery. (**b**) Gray-scale ultrasound image shows the occluded superficial femoral artery (SFA) with lumen filled by hypoechoic thrombus (*asterisk*). (**c**) Intra-operative photograph shows fresh clots (*asterisk*) inside the lumen of opened common femoral artery (CFA). Artery is temporarily clamped proximally and distally during thromboembolectomy. (**d**) Intra-operative photograph of the CFA after removal of the clots demonstrates the normal appearance of the luminal surface (L) and vascular wall

acute thromboembolic event, the patient's metastatic disease has progressed to the brain. The patient also developed new onset of atrial fibrillation and cardiomyopathy. She has been started on Cabozantinib (a newer TKI approved for advanced renal cell cancer) and is currently resuming anticoagulation.

Comments: At the time the acute arterial thromboembolic event, it was not clear whether the acute arterial thrombosis was related to hypercoagulability, TKI drug, or an embolism from a cardiogenic source. At that time, the patient had normal echocardiogram and was in sinus rhythm. The patient has had no recurrent arterial thromboembolic event while remaining on TKI, even when anticoagulation was stopped. In this case, the exact cause or source of the thromboembolic event remained undetermined even though the patient subsequently developed atrial fibrillation.

Case # 3. High-Grade Invasive Bladder Cancer and Subacute Left Leg Ischemia After Neoadjuvant Chemotherapy

A sixty-five year-old woman former heavy smoker was referred to our institution for treatment of high-grade invasive urothelial cancer. Prior trans-urethral partial resection of the tumor resulted in bladder perforation and neodajuvant chemotherapy was recommended prior to definitive cystectomy (combination of Methotrexate, Vinblastine, Adriamycin, and Cisplatin). The patient completed five cycles of chemotherapy but developed insidious onset of left leg disabling hip and calf claudication, ischemic rest pain, and left foot numbness toward the end of chemotherapy. The patient denied antecedent claudication symptoms. Prior CT imaging showed non-occlusive arteriosclerotic plaque disease in the aorta and bilateral iliac arteries. Repeat CT imaging demonstrated interval occlusion of the left common and external iliac arteries (Fig. 9.3a). An incidental right lower lobe pulmonary embolus was also found on CT. Cardiac evaluation was negative.

We performed catheter-directed thrombolysis and successfully recanalized the left common and external iliac arteries (Fig. 9.3b). A focal residual stenosis in the left external iliac artery was stented (Fig. 9.3c). The patient was kept on therapeutic low molecular weight heparin and aspirin after revascularization. She underwent radical bladder cystectomy with neo-bladder urinary diversion and bilateral pelvic node dissection 2 weeks after the endovascular intervention. The patient made remarkable progress after oncologic surgery. She completed 4 months of anticoagulation and remained on aspirin. She returned to full-time work within couple of months. One year following her oncologic surgery, the patient developed locally advanced tumor recurrence. She also reported recurrent left leg claudication symptoms. Re-occlusion of the left iliac arteries and stent was confirmed on imaging. As she did not have symptoms or signs of immediate limb-threatening ischemia, the patient declined repeat vascular intervention. Unfortunately, it was deemed that further oncologic treatment would not benefit the patient and she passed away approximately 2 years after the initial cancer diagnosis.

Comments: We postulate that this patient was likely hypercoagulable. The combination of high-grade malignancy and aggressive chemotherapy both contributed to the acute arterial thrombosis. Interestingly, the patient did have a normal duplex ultrasound of the stented left iliac artery at 6–9 months after stent placement, suggesting that the vascular re-occlusion may have been due to cancer-related hypercoagulability state. It is conceivable that re-occlusion of the left iliac arteries and stent could have been prevented if anticoagulation had been maintained.

Case # 4. Renal Cell Cancer and Severe Aorto-Iliac Occlusive Disease

A sixty-seven year-old male presented with chronic progressive disabling hip and calf claudication bilaterally, new onset of severe ischemic rest pain in both feet, and non-healing right toe ulcer. Vascular work up demonstrated chronic occlusion of the infra-renal aorta and bilateral common iliac arteries on CT angiogram (Fig. 9.4a), and an incidental finding of a large exophytic right renal mass. Because of the incapacitating ischemic pain in his legs, the patient was unable to begin oncologic therapy. Therefore, we elected to proceed first with surgical revascularization to relieve the ischemic pain in his legs. Following successful axillary-bifemoral bypass grafting, the patient's pain resolved and his performance status improved rapidly (Fig. 9.4b, c). Although the patient had metastatic disease, the cancer was deemed oncologically "stable", and a debulking radical right nephrectomy was recommended. The patient underwent oncologic resection approximately 3 months after the extra-anatomical surgical bypass without complications. The patient was then kept on surveillance until progression of metastatic disease was noted in imaging approximately 2 years after the initial cancer diagnosis, at which time he was started on Pazopanib. His axillo-bifemoral bypass remains patent at 26 months (Fig. 9.4d, e).

Comments: This patient's chronic aorto-iliac occlusion was not amenable to endovascular intervention. One alternative option would have been concomitant surgical aorto-bifemoral bypass and radical right nephrectomy. However, major concomitant surgery was initially deemed not beneficial, in light of the metastatic disease, uncertain cancer behavior, and poor performance status at presentation. Although primary chemotherapy without oncologic resection was the initial recommended oncologic therapy, because of the observed "stability" of the cancer and patient's improved performance status after surgical revascularization, the oncologic strategy changed to surgical tumor resection.

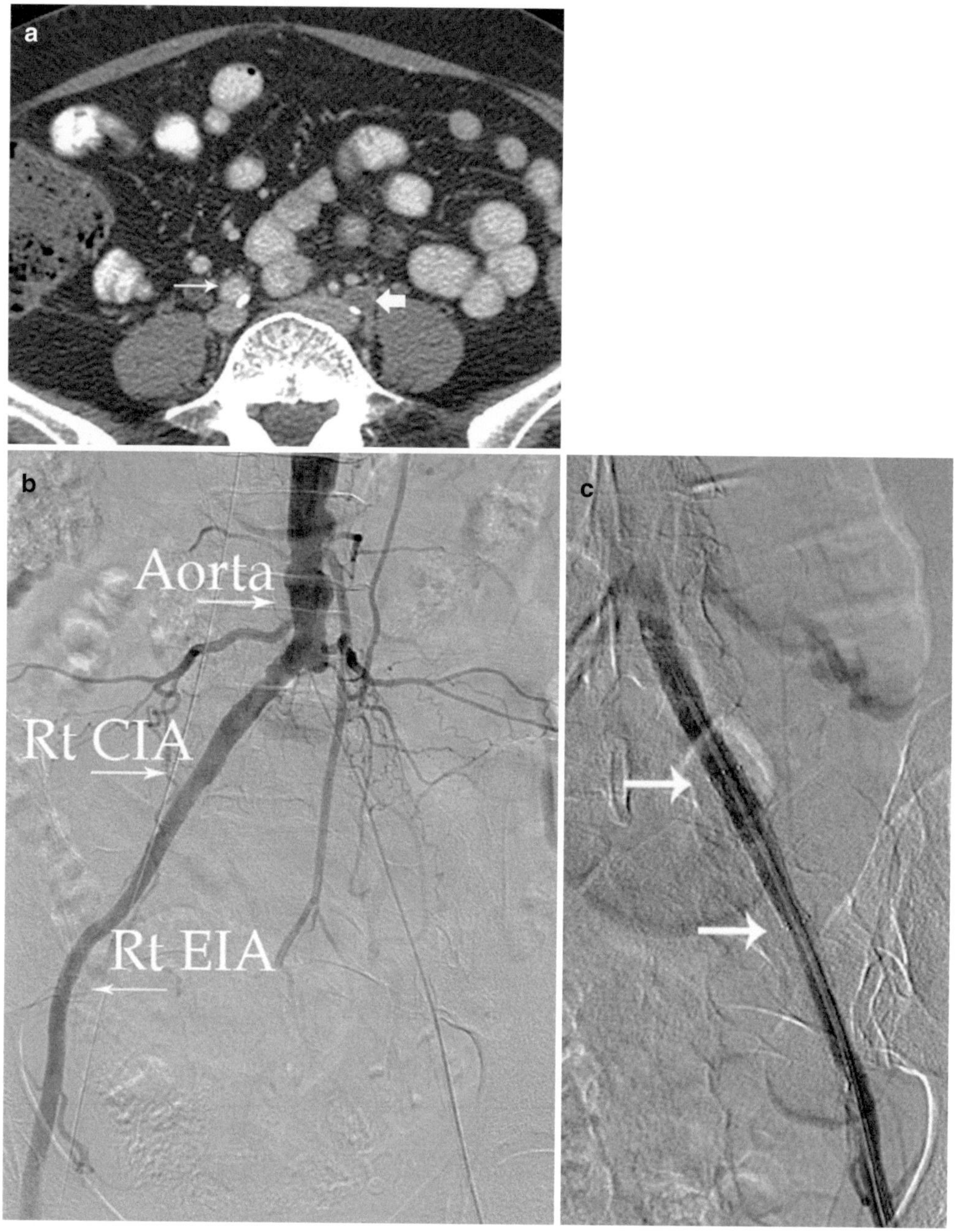

Fig. 9.3 High-grade invasive bladder cancer and subacute left leg ischemia after neoadjuvant chemotherapy. (**a**) Axial CT image shows no contrast filling of the occluded left common iliac artery (*short arrow*) and patent right common iliac artery (*long arrow*); calcified plaque is seen in the posterior wall of both iliac arteries. (**b**) Digital substraction angiographic (DSA) image shows total occlusion of the left common and external iliac arteries (no contrast filling). The distal aorta is irregular with non-occlusive plaque disease. The right (Rt) common (CIA) and external iliac (EIA) arteries are patent without significant luminal stenosis. (**c**) DSA image of the stented left common/external iliac artery (*arrows* point to the proximal and distal edges of stent); no contrast filling of occluded left internal iliac artery

Case # 5. Blue Toe Syndrome and Lung Cancer

A sixty-eight year-old man developed right leg DVT and was started on rivaroxaban. Further work-up found non-small cell lung cancer (NSCLC). The patient underwent right upper lobectomy. Pathological and clinical staging was IIIA with repeat PET/CT showing residual disease in the mediastinum after surgical resection. The patient was scheduled to receive concurrent chemoradiation therapy 6 weeks post-operatively. He developed painful blue toe syndrome involving mostly the first and fifth left toes just prior to starting chemoradiation (Fig. 9.5a, b). Vascular work up revealed normal pedal pulses. CT angiogram showed minimal plaque disease in the aorto-iliac and infrainguinal arteries. Aspirin therapy was added to anticoagulation. The ischemic pain and discoloration in the affected toes resolved with expectant management. Patient tolerated three cycles of Carboplatin and Paclitaxel without further vascular complications (at the time of this writing).

Comments: Blue toe syndrome is typically due to an atheroemboli, or a microemboli occluding a small distal digital vessel. The embolic source is usually an atherosclerotic

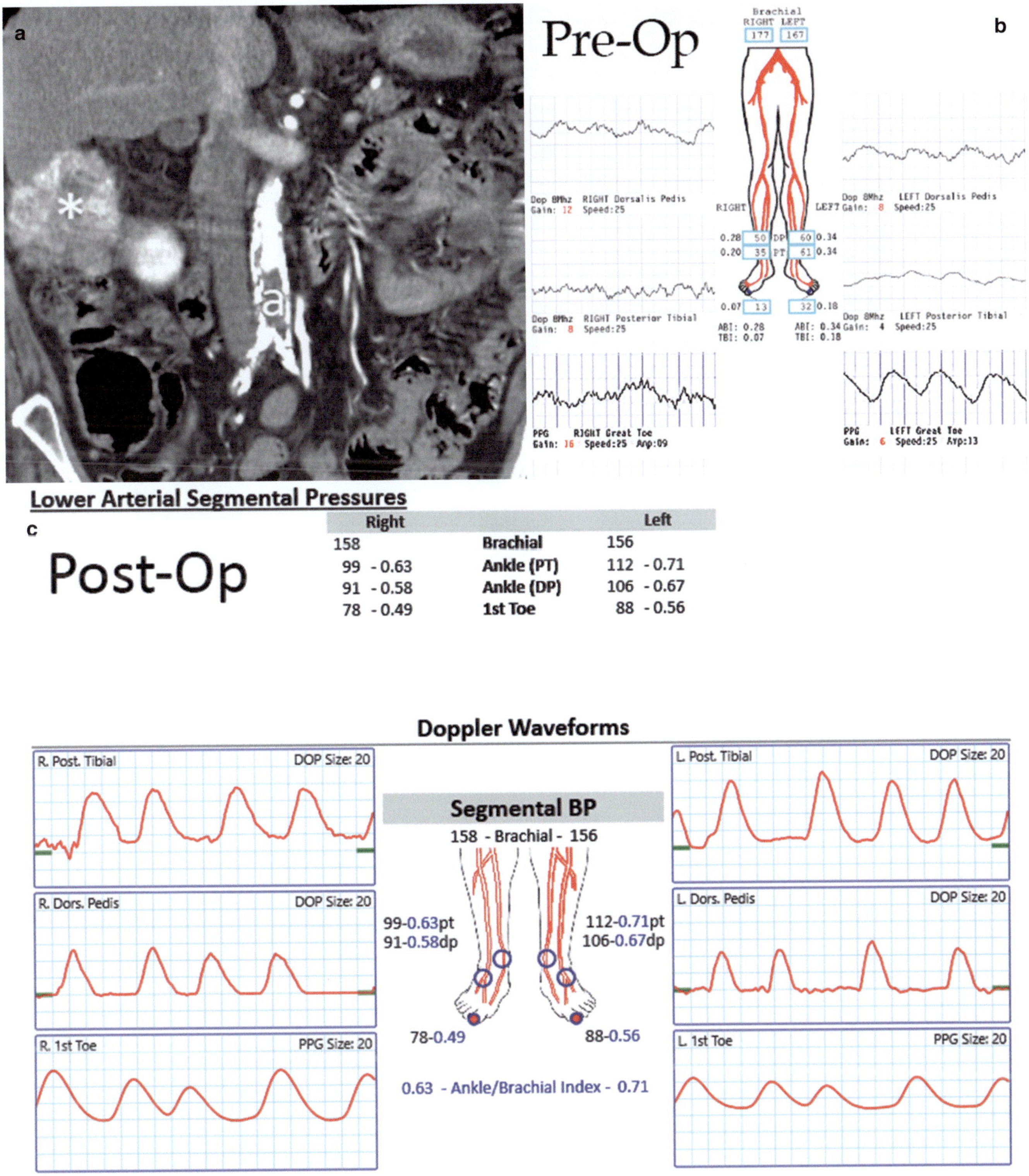

Fig. 9.4 Renal cell cancer and severe aorto-iliac occlusive disease. (**a**) Coronal CT image of abdomen shows heavily calcified occluded aorto-biiliac arteries (**a**) and large exophytic mass (*asterisk*) in superior pole of the right kidney. (**b**) Physiologic arterial testing shows severely reduced preoperative ankle-brachial indexes (ABI): 0.28 on right and 0.34 on left. (**c**) Post-operative ABIs are increased: 0.63 on right and 0.71 on left.

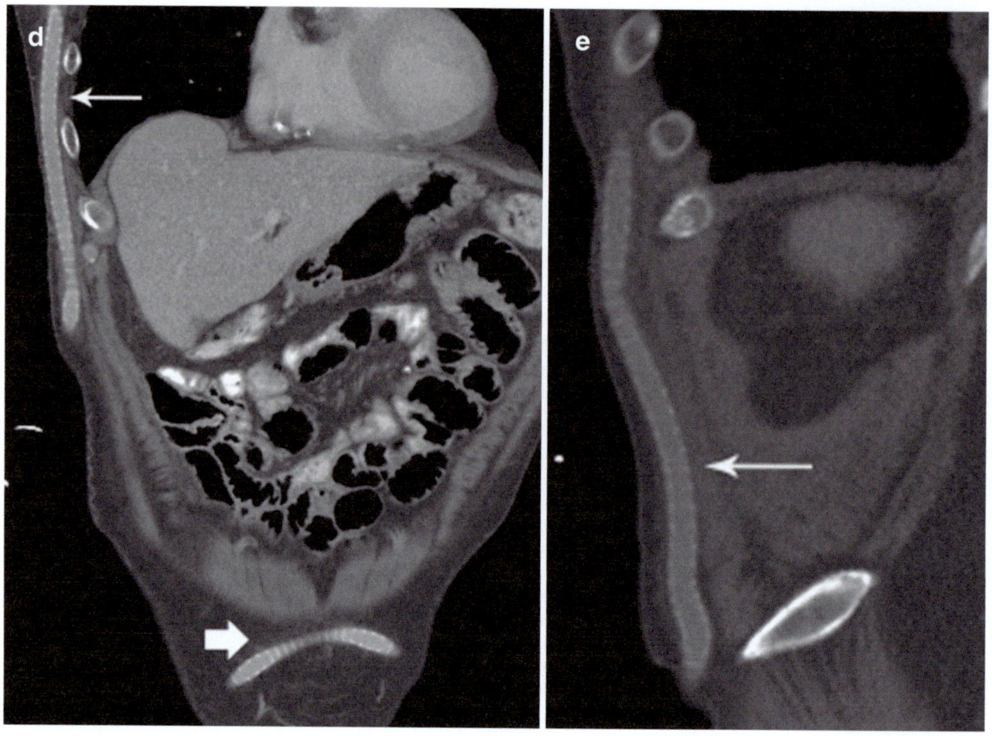

Fig. 9.4 (continued) (**d**) Coronal CT image shows patent axillary (*thin arrow*) and femoral (*short arrow*) segments of the extra-anatomical bypass reconstruction. (**e**) Patent axillary segment of axillo-bifemoral bypass graft (*arrow*) is shown on sagittal CT image

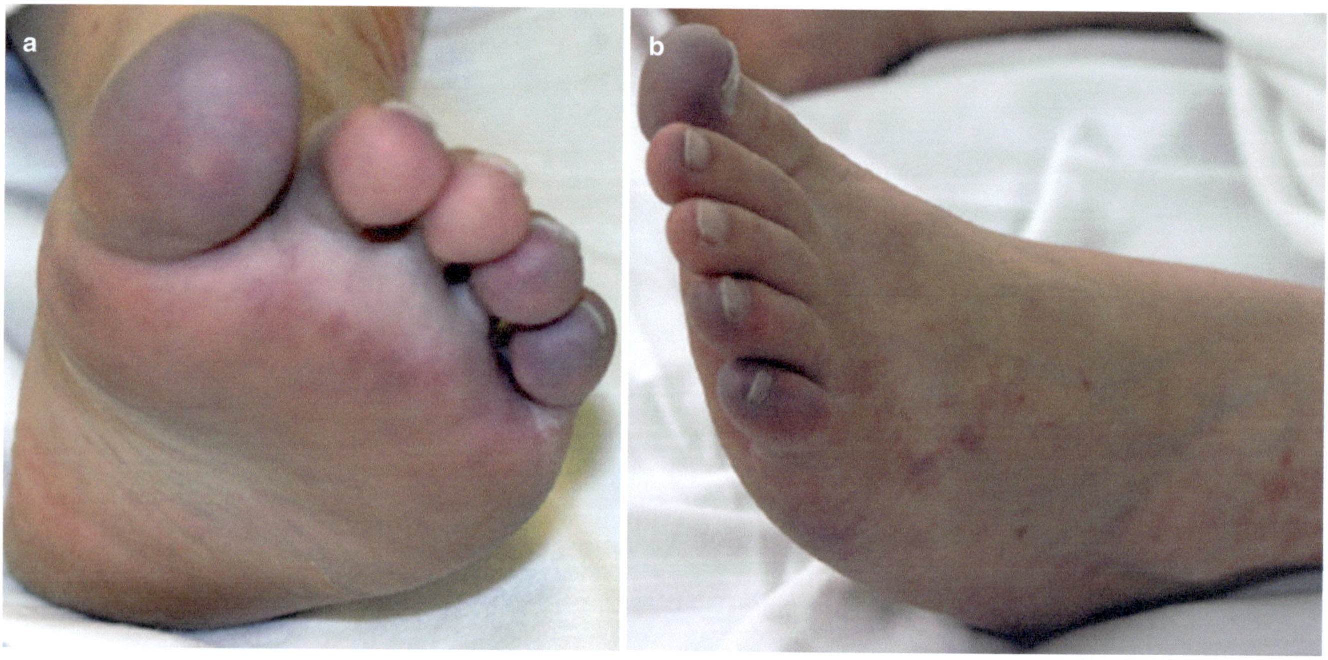

Fig. 9.5 Blue toe syndrome and lung cancer. Photographs of the patient's left foot show blue discoloration of the ischemic first and fifth toes on plantar (**a**) and dorsal (**b**) views

plaque in a proximal large vessel such as the aorta or iliac arteries. The classic description refers to ischemia of one or more toes in the absence of large vessel occlusive disease. We have observed blue toe syndrome in patients with various types of solid tumors. We generally recommend antiplatelet and statin therapy for blue toe syndrome.

Case # 6. Multiple Myeloma and Acute on Chronic Critical Leg Ischemia

This is the case of a Caucasian male diagnosed with multiple myeloma in 1995. The patient had external beam radiation to right hip and sacrum. He received three cycles of mephalan and prednisolone therapy in 1995 and remained on maintenance cyclophosphamide treatment ever since. The patient reported a 15 pack-years history of tobacco smoking but quit in 1990. In addition, he has well-controlled longstanding non-insulin dependent diabetes and essential hypertension. The patient developed an acute right parietal ischemic stroke in 2011, at the age of 66, and had right carotid endarterectomy for severe proximal internal carotid artery stenosis. The patient was kept on aspirin, statin, anti-hypertensive, metformin, and cyclophosphamide maintenance therapy. In 2013, the patient develops insidious onset of right leg ischemic rest pain, numbness, foot drop and a non-healing wound at the base of the fifth toe (Fig. 9.6a), although he had had chronic bilateral leg claudication. Vascular work-up showed severe occlusive disease of the right common femoral artery bifurcation including proximal superficial femoral (SFA) and profunda arteries, and severe distal right SFA stenosis (Fig. 9.6b–f). We performed hybrid revascularization with extensive right common femoral artery bifurcation endarterectomy and reconstruction with patch angioplasty of the proximal profunda and SFA (Fig. 9.6g–j); concomitant stenting of the right mid to distal SFA was done using covered self-expandable stent-graft (Fig. 9.6k–m). The patient recovered well with good revascularization and eventual healing of ischemic toe wound (Fig. 9.6n, o).

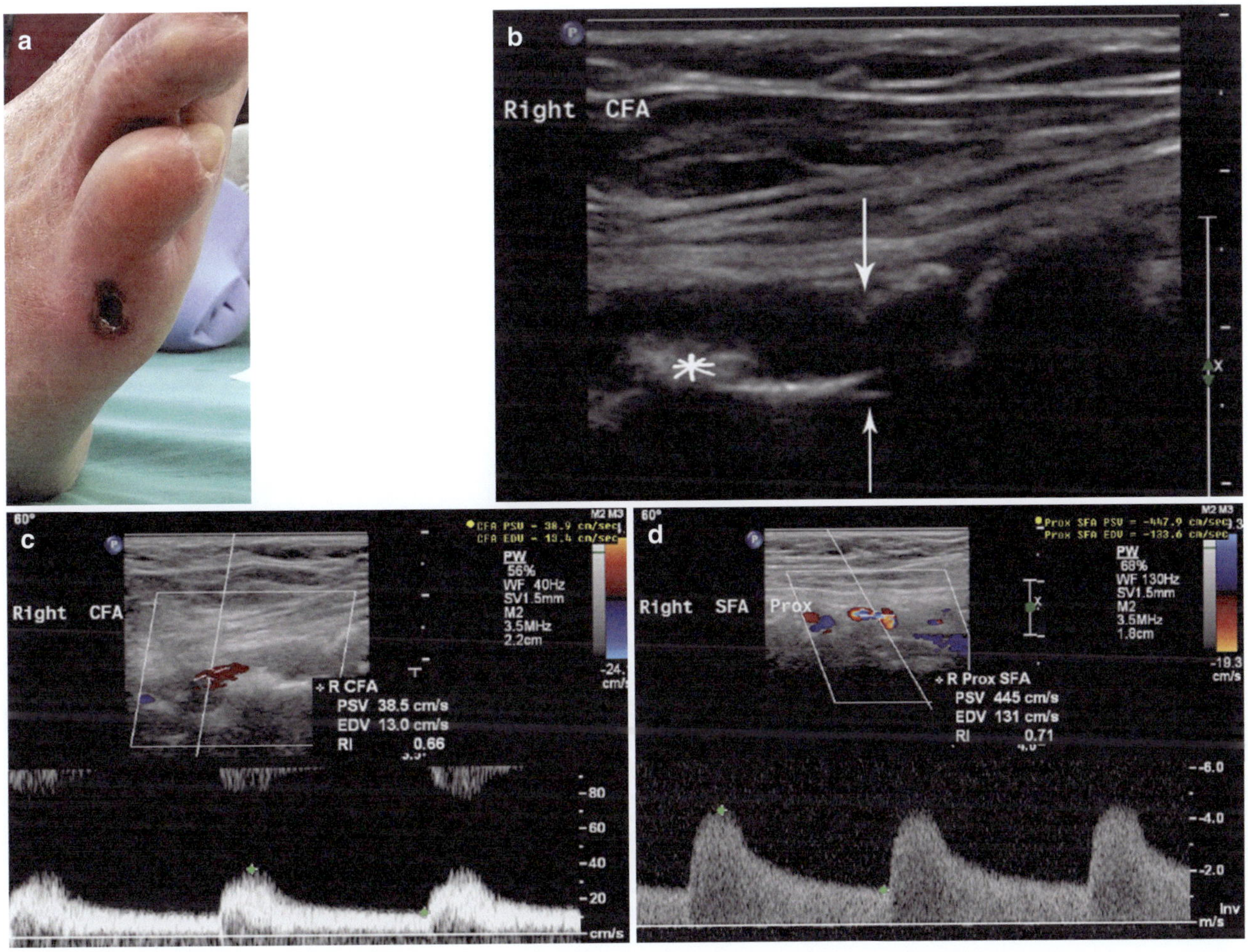

Fig. 9.6 Multiple myeloma and chronic critical leg ischemia. (**a**) Photograph of right foot shows signs of chronic ischemia: non-healing wound at base of the fifth toe, thin skin, muscle atrophy, and toe discoloration. (**b**) Gray-scale image of right common femoral artery (CFA). The *arrows* point to the vessel walls and *asterisk* marks the location of a dense plaque. (**c**) Markedly reduced Doppler flow velocity is shown in the CFA beyond the occluding plaque. (**d**) Increased flow velocities in the proximal superficial femoral artery (SFA) indicate severe vessel stenosis.

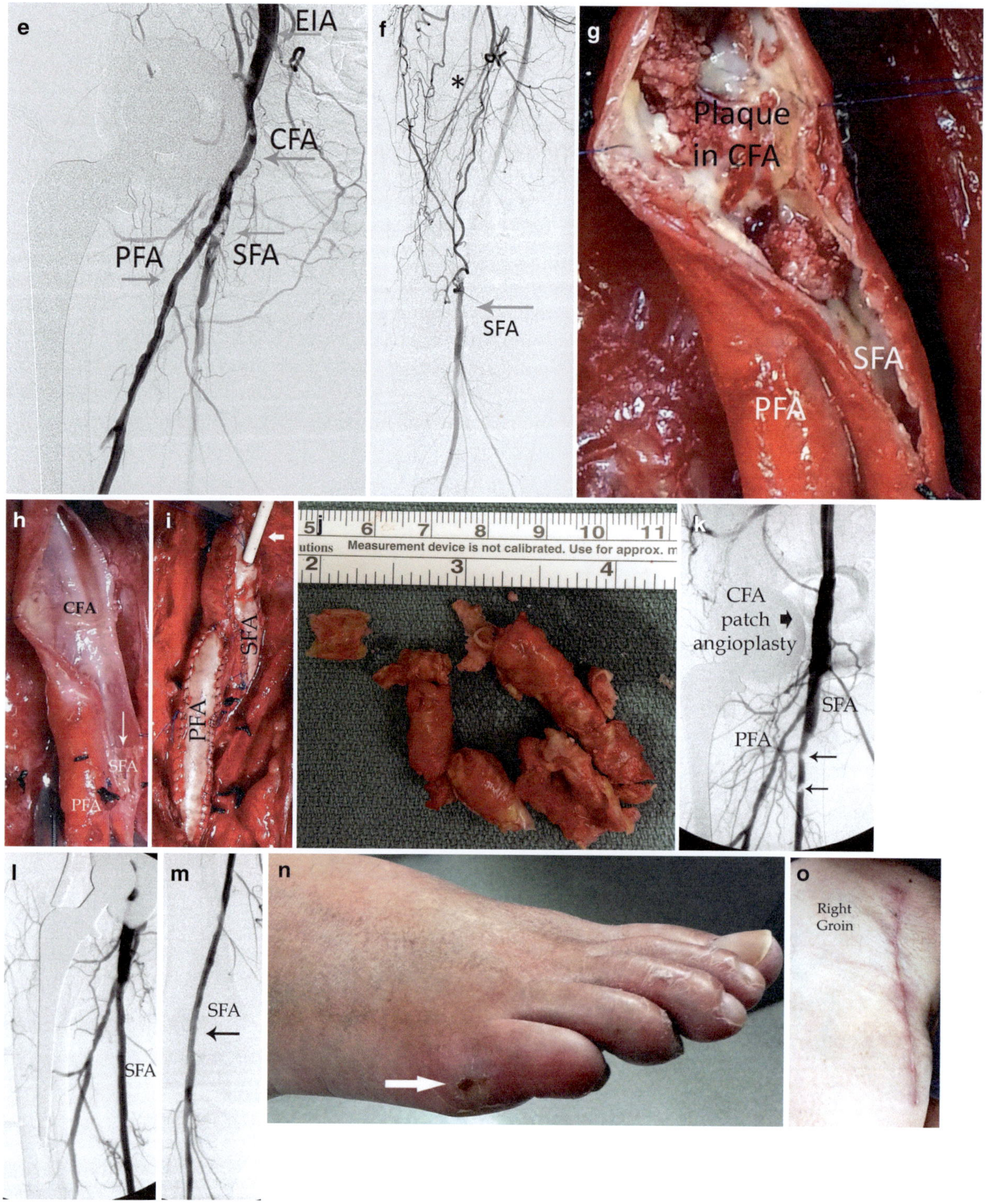

Fig. 9.6 (continued) (**e**) DSA image shows widely patent external iliac artery (EIA), narrowed CFA, nearly occluded proximal SFA, and patent profunda femoral artery (PFA). (**f**) DSA image shows large profunda branches (surrounding *asterisk*) reconstituting flow in the distal SFA. (**g**) Intra-operative photograph depicts an arteriotomy in the CFA extended through the proximal SFA and shows extensive calcified eccentric occluding plaque disease. (**h**) Intra-operative photograph shows luminal surface of CFA after removal of the plaque and endarterectomy; *arrow* points to the distal transition point with residual intimal thickening in the SFA; in this image the PFA is still intact. (**i**) Intra-operative photograph shows reconstructed patch reconstruction of the SFA and PFA after endarterectomy. *Arrow* points to a vascular sheath placed in an antegrade fashion for hybrid endovascular stenting of the remaining SFA stenoses. (**j**) Multiple fragments of the endarterectomized plaque specimen are shown. (**k**) DSA image demonstrates residual severe stenoses in the SFA distal to the patch angioplasty (*arrows*) after patch angioplasty reconstruction of the femoral artery bifurcation. (**l**) Completion DSA image shows satisfactory appearance of proximal to mid SFA stenting. (**m**) Completion DSA image shows satisfactory appearance of distal SFA stenting (*arrow* points to stent). (**n**) Photograph demonstrates healing of toe wound (*arrow*) after revascularization. (**o**) Hybrid revascularization including concomitant femoral endarterectomy and reconstruction and SFA stenting was completed through a single right groin incision

The patient subsequently developed similar symptoms of ischemic rest pain in the left leg and underwent similar hybrid revascularization successfully in 2015. The following year, the patient sustained acute myocardial infarction following right hip redo replacement and had drug-eluting stents placed in the right coronary artery. Dual antiplatelet therapy was added. Just over 12 months after right coronary artery stenting, the patient now reports that he has been recommended to undergo coronary artery bypass for multivessel coronary artery disease.

Comments: This case underscores the systemic nature of atherosclerotic disease. In this patient, the first cardiovascular manifestation was an embolic stroke from severe carotid artery disease. He then had bilateral extremity revascularization for severe multilevel arterial occlusive disease and subsequently coronary revascularization. All these events took place within 5–6 years while the patient remained on maintenance chemotherapy (cyclophosphamide) for multiple myeloma. Anecdotally, this case demonstrates that long-term survival is possible for patients with cardiovascular risk factors and active cancer. Regarding the treatment of severe common femoral bifurcation occlusive disease, surgical endarterectomy and reconstruction remains the treatment of choice. In this case, hybrid revascularization allowed concomitant surgical reconstruction of the common femoral artery bifurcation and stenting of the tandem proximal and distal SFA occlusive lesions. Adjunct femoral artery stenting is less invasive with clear advantages over the traditional femoro-popliteal bypass with less post-operative pain and swelling.

Case # 7. Ulcerated Squamous Cell Skin Cancer in Patient with PAD

A sixty-eight year-old woman presented with cutaneous squamous cell cancer in a chronic painful large ulcerated wound in her right calf (Fig. 9.7a). Work-up showed prior infrarenal aortic graft reconstruction for abdominal aortic aneurysm and chronic occlusion of the right superficial femoral artery with reconstitution of the above-knee popliteal artery and 2–3 vessel run-off (Fig. 9.7b, c). We staged her treatment. First, we performed surgical revascularization with a femoral to popliteal artery bypass using ipsilateral great saphenous vein graft (Fig. 9.7d). Wide surgical resection of the cutaneous cancer was subsequently done with skin engrafting (Fig. 9.7e).

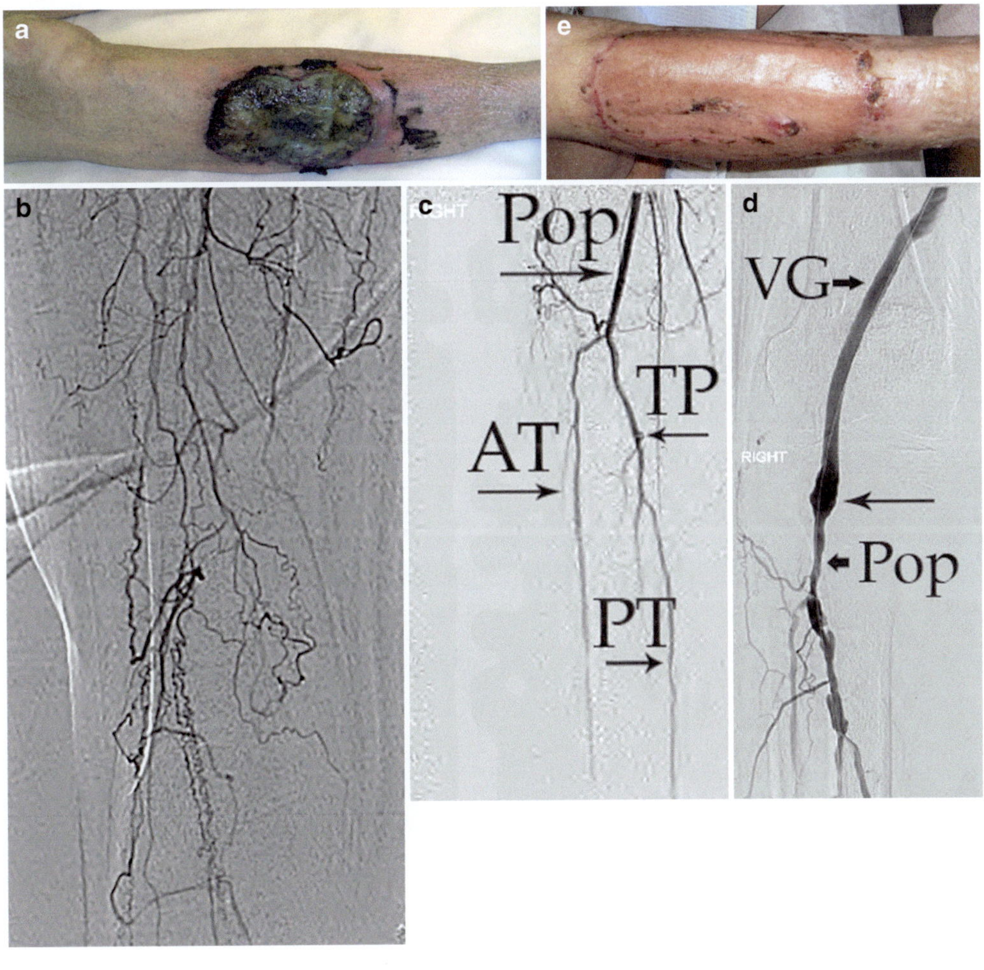

Fig. 9.7 Ulcerated squamous cell skin cancer in patient with PAD. (**a**) Photograph shows the large ulcerated skin growth. (**b**) DSA image of mid thigh demonstrates large collateral network from profunda branches secondary to chronic occlusion of the superficial femoral artery. (**c**) DSA image shows reconstituted popliteal (Pop), patent anterior tibial (AT), tibio-peroneal (TP) trunk, and posterior tibial (PT) arteries. (**d**) Completion DSA image after femoro-popliteal artery bypass shows satisfactory appearance of the vein graft (VG; *short arrow*). *Long arrow* points to the distal anastomosis. (**e**) Photograph shows healed skin graft wound following wide tumor resection

Comments: Endovascular recanalization of the long chronic right superficial femoral artery was not possible. However, staged surgical revascularization and wide oncologic resection allowed for limb-salvage, as opposed to the alternative option of major limb amputation.

Case # 8. Radiation Induced Femoral Artery Occlusion Following Surgical Resection and Radiation Treatment for Extremity Desmoid Tumor

A thirty-seven year-old woman presented with insidious onset of severe left leg pain for several months. Her past history included surgical resection of desmoid tumor in the left posterior thigh and adjuvant high dose external beam radiation at age of 16. Approximately 15 years later, the patient was found to have local recurrence in the left posterior thigh and had a second round of high dose external beam and repeated surgical resection. In addition, multiple subsequent orthopedic interventions were required to treat non-union pathologic fractures of left femur (Fig. 9.8a, b). Meanwhile, the patient continued to receive systemic single agent chemotherapy including Tamoxifen first, then Imatinib (TKI), and lastly Sorafenib (TKI) for recurrent regional disease. At the time of the vascular complication, Sorafenib was on hold due to other side effects. Vascular work-up showed critical ischemia of the left due to radiation induced long occlusion of the left superficial femoral artery with reconstitution of the popliteal artery (Fig. 9.8c–f). We performed left common femoral to below-knee popliteal artery bypass using ipsilateral saphenous vein graft for limb-salvage. The left leg bypass graft is still patent 2 years after reconstruction (Fig. 9.8g, h). The patient remains active and has resumed Sorafenib for progressive regional disease.

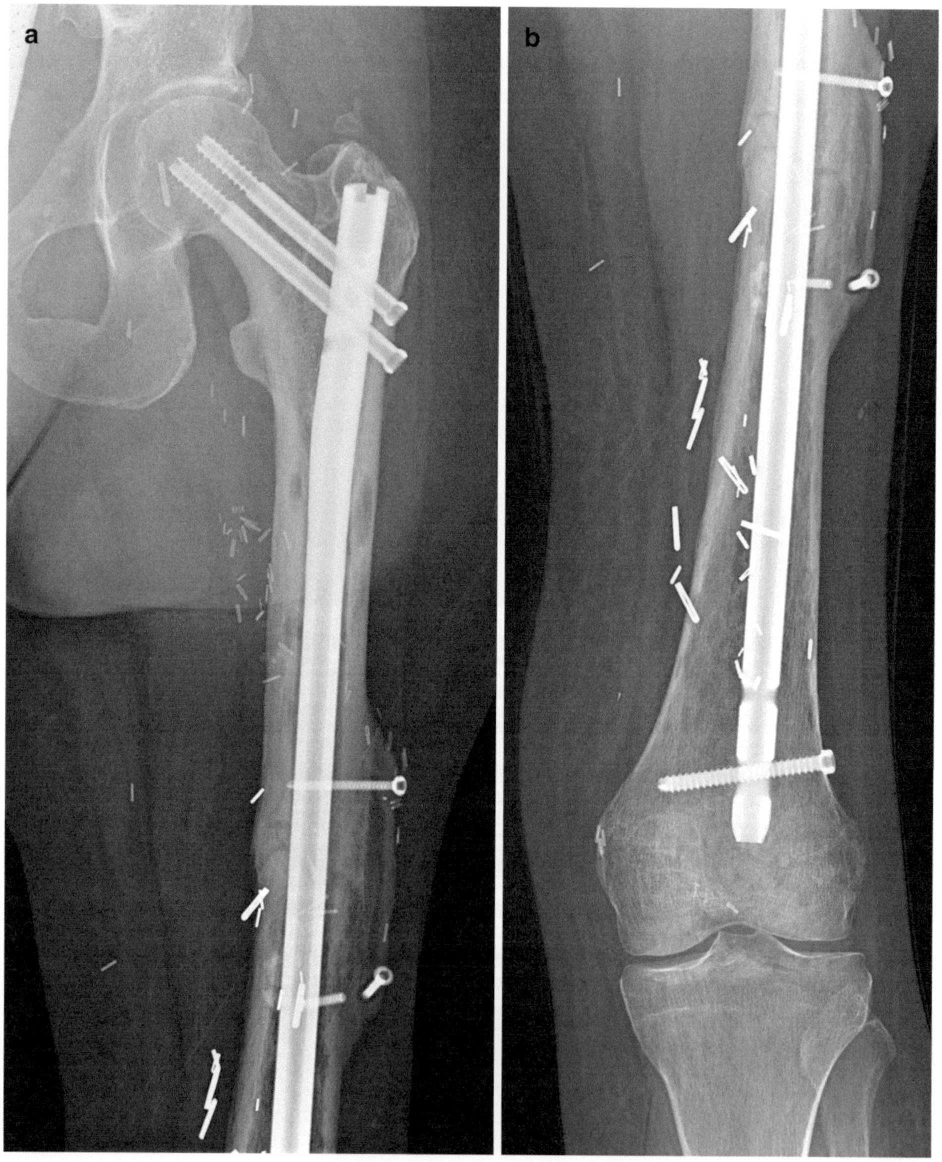

Fig. 9.8 Radiation-induced femoral artery occlusion following surgical resection and radiation treatment for lower extremity desmoid tumor. (**a**) Radiograph shows top part of intramedullary rod fixation of the left femur for non-union. (**b**) Radiograph shows lower part of intramedullary rod fixation of the left femur for non-union.

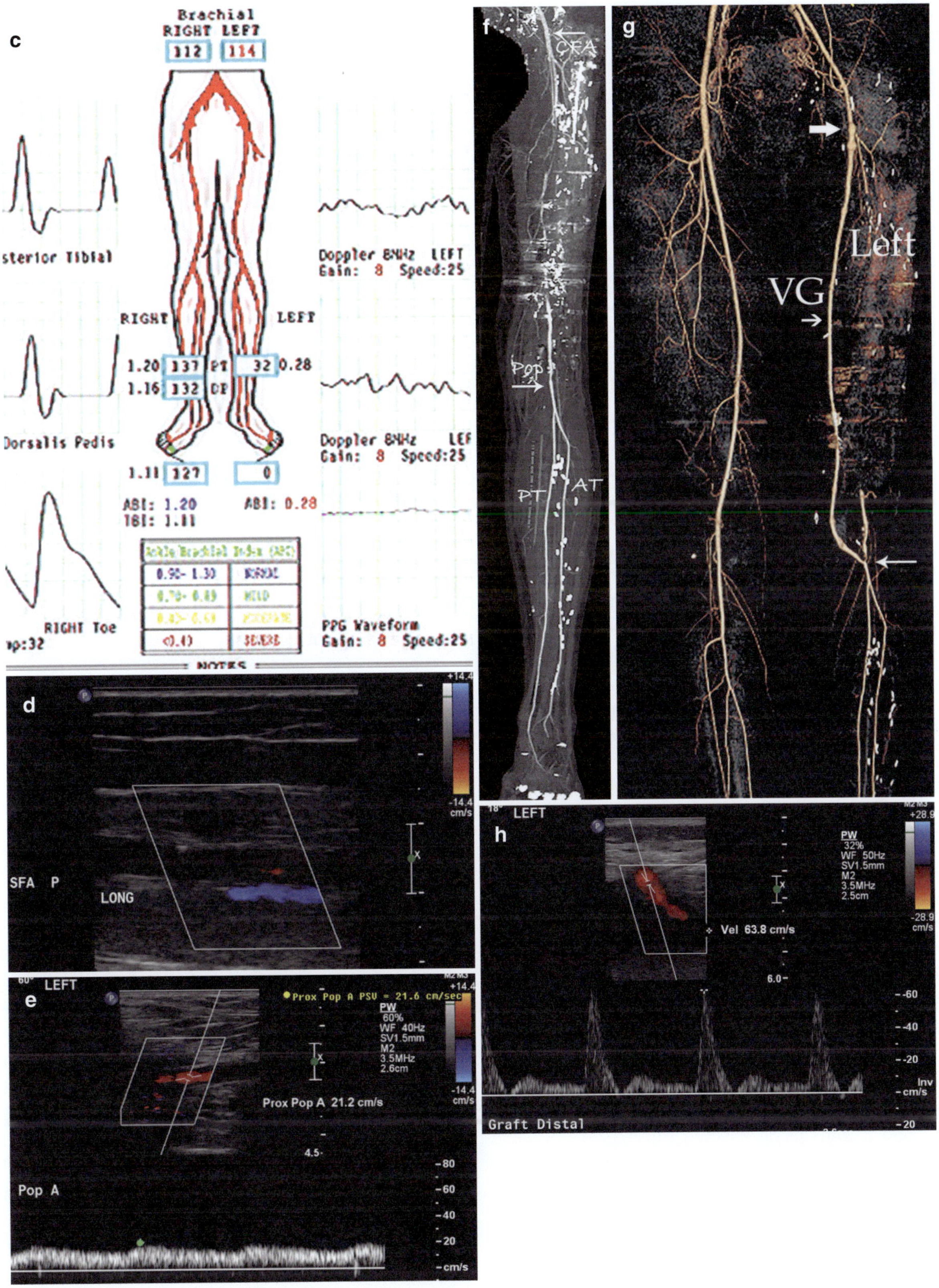

Fig. 9.8 (continued) (**c**) Left ABI is markedly reduced (0.28) indicating severe ischemia. (**d**) Colorflow image of the left superficial femoral artery (SFA) shows no flow in artery; flow is seen (*blue color*) in the adjacent left femoral vein. (**e**) Flow velocity by Doppler is markedly reduced in the reconstituted popliteal artery. (**f**) Reformatted CT angiogram shows chronic occlusion of the left SFA, reconstituted distal SFA and popliteal arteries, and patent AT and PT; numerous metal clips from prior surgeries are seen causing beam artifacts. (**g**) Post-operative reformatted CT angiogram shows satisfactory appearance of the left femoral popliteal artery bypass vein graft (VG). *Short arrow* points to the proximal anastomosis and *long arrow* to the distal anastomosis. (**h**) Colorflow ultrasound image shows satisfactory Doppler flow velocities at the distal femoral-popliteal anastomosis

Comments: Endovascular intervention was not considered in this case because of the long chronic occlusion of the superficial femoral artery and small distal target vessel. Surgical revascularization in the irradiated and scarred operative field was indeed very challenging in this case. Healthy soft tissue coverage of vascular graft is imperative in irradiated field to help promote wound healing and prevent complications. For this patient, we transposed the left sartorius muscle to provide coverage of the vein graft in the irradiated groin wound. We have kept the patient on aspirin and will continue to monitor her leg bypass graft with periodic duplex ultrasound.

Case # 9. Radiation-Induced Iliac Occlusive Disease Following Treatment for Cervical Cancer

A thirty-nine year-old woman had hysterectomy and pelvic node dissection and high dose radiation for uterine cervix squamous cell cancer in 2006. The patient developed recurrent right pelvic wall disease and had further surgical resection including right ureter reconstruction in 2008. Additional targeted Proton radiation therapy was given to the site of the recurrent disease. In 2013, the patient developed insidious ischemic rest pain and numbness in the right leg for about 1 month prior to seeking medical attention. Vascular work-up showed occlusion of the right common and external iliac arteries with reconstitution of the common femoral artery (Fig. 9.9a, b). The patient had no other cardiovascular risk factors. She is a lifelong non-smoker. Pharmaco-mechanical thrombectomy and catheter directed thrombolysis resulted in successful revascularization of the right leg (Fig. 9.9c–e). A focal stenotic plaque in the right external iliac artery was stented using self-expandable 6 mm stent. The patient was maintained on clopidogrel. One year later, the patient developed re-occlusion of the right common and external iliac arteries and stent, and had recurrent ischemic symptoms. Repeat endovascular intervention was again successful with pharmaco-mechanical thrombectomy, catheter directed thrombolysis, and additional stenting of the right external iliac (6 mm), and overlapping stenting of the common iliac artery (7 and 8 mm) using covered self-expandable stent-grafts (Fig. 9.9f–i). Following revascularization, the patient was kept on antiplatelet and anticoagulation. Unfortunately, the patient became symptomatic again about a year later with re-occlusion of overlapping right iliac stents. The decision was made to proceed with surgical revascularization. A cross-over left common femoral to right common femoral artery was constructed using an 8 mm PTFE graft. The patient did well after bypass surgery and was kept on aspirin therapy. Approximately 1 year after surgical revascularization, the patient developed acute ischemic symptoms again with thrombosis of the cross-over femoral bypass graft. Catheter directed thrombolysis restored patency to the bypass graft and normal flow to the right leg (Fig. 9.9j, k). The patient is currently doing well without symptoms at 13 months since the last intervention on aspirin and rivaroxaban.

Comments: Long-term radiation induced vasculopathy is an uncommon disease in cancer survivors. Endovascular treatment is usually preferred over surgical intervention for radiation-induced vasculopathy. However, in-stent restenosis remains an obstacle in the treatment of radiation-induced vasculopathy. Surgical bypass in irradiated field is technically challenging and is associated with higher morbidity than endovascular intervention. In our experience, surgical bypass for radiation-induced vasculopathy appears to require less repeated interventions when compared to endovascular treatment. In this patient, we identified acute dehydration as possible cause of the acute femoral graft thrombosis.

Case # 10. Axillary Artery Occlusion 8 Years After Radiation Treatment for Breast Cancer

A sixty-three year-old woman complained of finger discoloration, pain and numbness in the right hand for several months. Eight years prior to this presentation, the patient had modified radical right mastectomy and post-operative adjuvant high dose external beam radiation to the chest wall and axilla. Although, she had chronic right arm lymphedema, the patient denied prior symptoms of arm claudication. On exam, the patient had distal necrosis of the tip of the fifth finger (Fig. 9.10a). Duplex showed severe stenosis of the right axillary artery and reduced distal flow to the right hand (Fig. 9.10b, c). Selective angiography showed multiple stenoses of right axillary artery with two sites of near occlusion. We deployed two overlapping self-expandable 6 and 5 mm stents with great angiographic result (Fig. 9.10d, e). Revascularization was successful and relieved the patient's ischemic symptoms. The distal fifth finger wound healed without complication (Fig. 9.10f). Since the initial stent angioplasty, the patient has had four

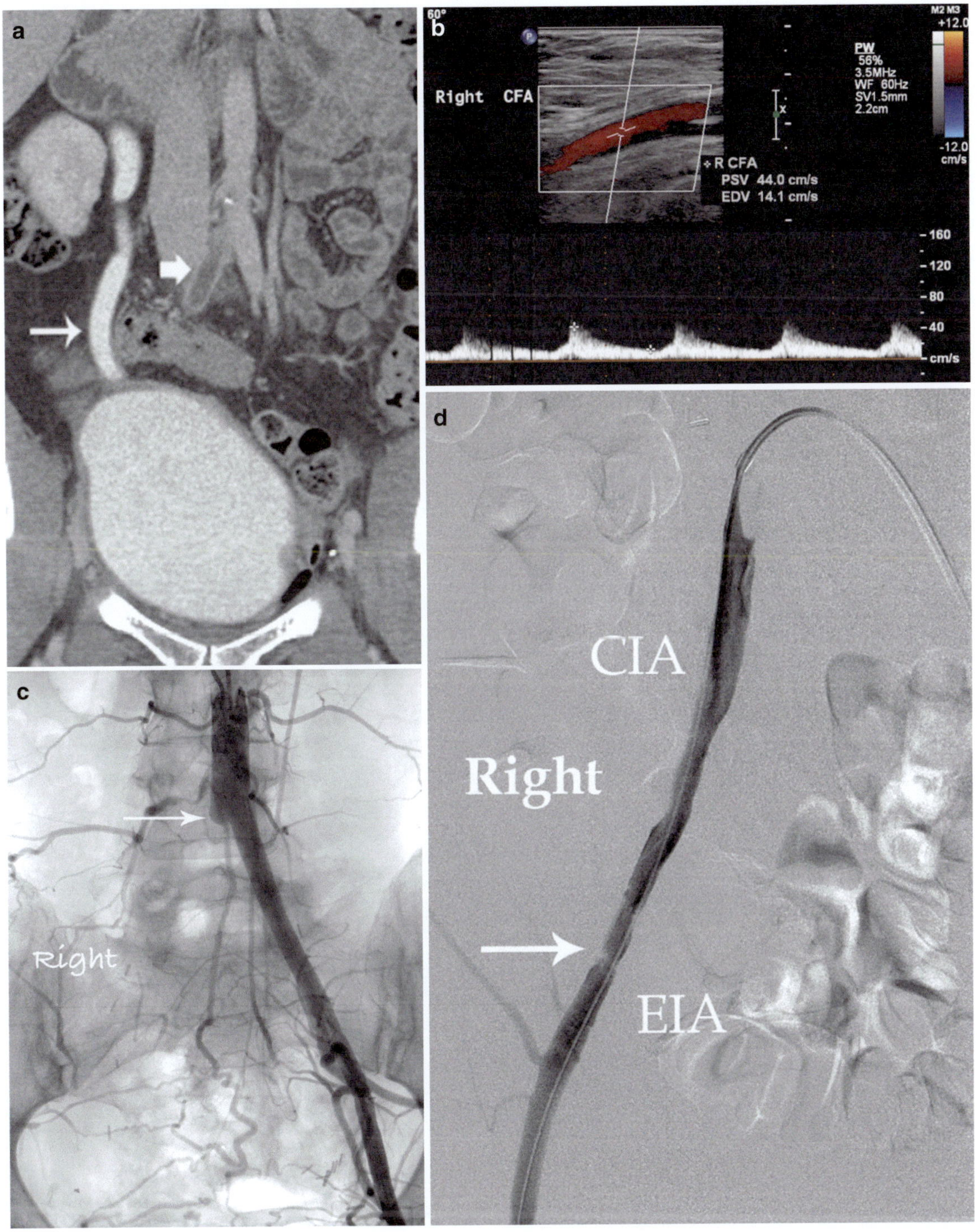

Fig. 9.9 Radiation-induced iliac occlusive disease following treatment for cervical cancer. (**a**) Coronal CT image shows thrombosed right common iliac artery (*short arrow*) and reconstructed right ureter (*long arrow*) to bladder junction. (**b**) Doppler flow velocity is reduced in the reconstituted right common femoral artery (CFA). (**c**) DSA image demonstrates flush occlusion of the right common iliac artery (*arrow*). Left common and external iliac arteries are normal and widely patent. (**d**) Following successful recanalization of the right common (CIA) and external iliac (EIA) arteries, a residual stenosis is seen (*arrow*) in the EIA.

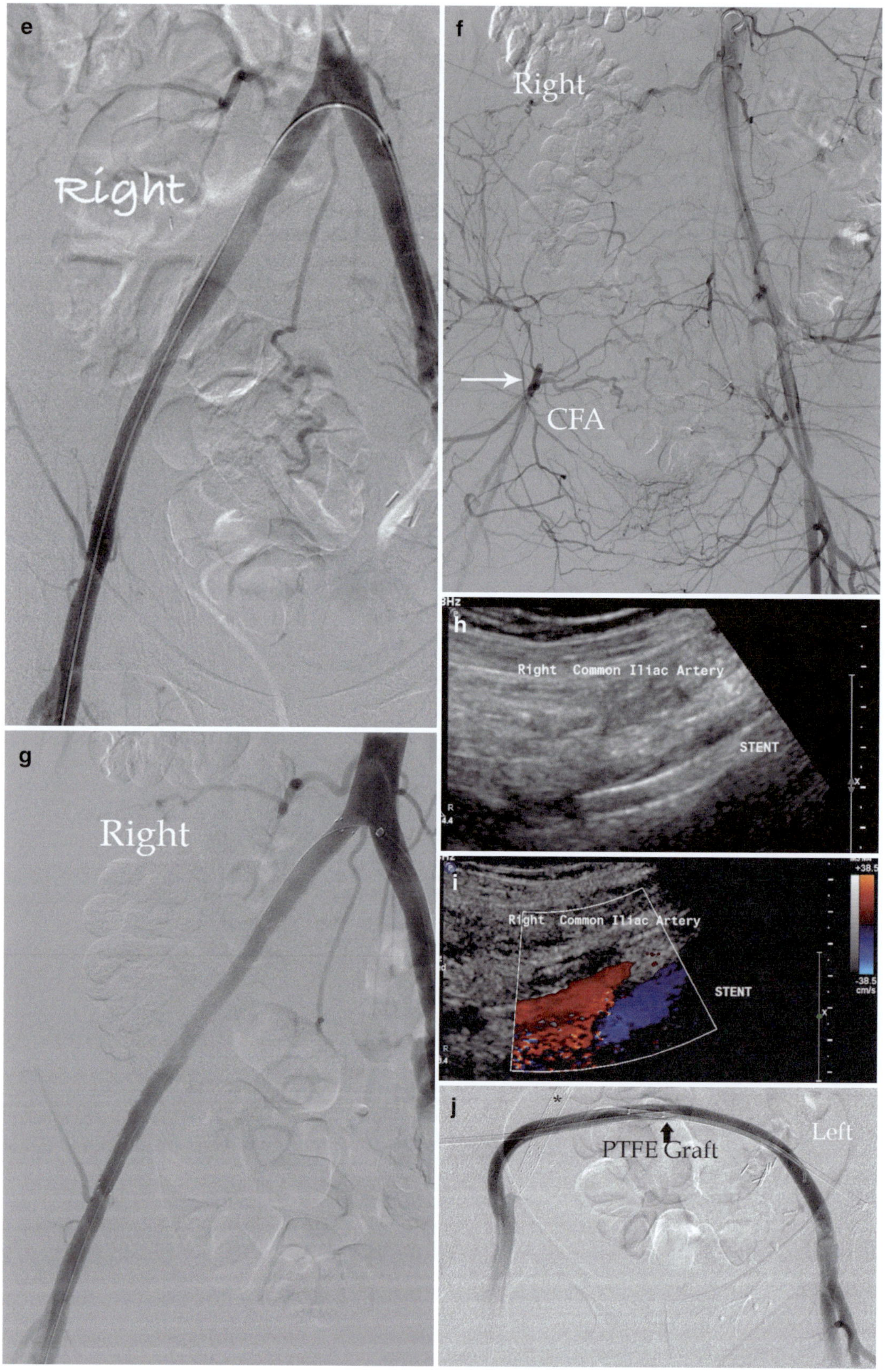

Fig. 9.9 (continued) (**e**) DSA image shows satisfactory result after stenting of the right EIA stenosis. (**f**) DSA image shows re-occlusion of the right CIA and EIA with reconstitution of the CFA (*arrow*). (**g**) Repeat endovascular intervention including pharmaco-mechanical thrombectomy, catheter directed thrombolysis and further stenting of the right CIA and EIA successfully restored flow as shown in this DSA image. (**h**) Gray-scale ultrasound image of right CIA stent demonstrates good apposition of stent to vessel wall. (**i**) Ultrasound color-flow image shows patency of right CIA stent. (**j**) DSA image shows patent cross-over synthetic femoro-femoral bypass graft after repeat endovascular intervention; vascular sheaths are still inside graft (*arrow*). *Asterisk* denotes the old occluded iliac artery stent.

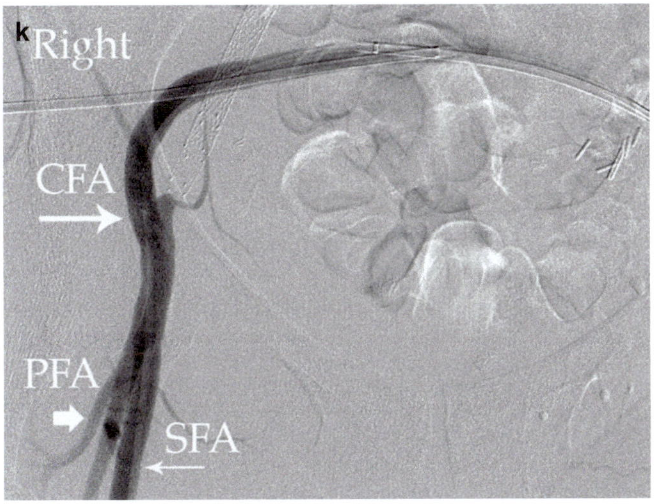

Fig. 9.9 (continued) (**k**) DSA image demonstrates widely patent right CFA anastomosis, profunda femoral (PFA) and superficial femoral (SFA) arteries

additional endovascular interventions and stenting within 16 months (Fig. 9.10g, h). In addition, at 17 months, the patient developed acute right axillary artery thrombosis, which was treated successfully by surgical thromboembolectomy. The patient is currently maintained on clopidogrel and anticoagulation.

Comments: As mentioned in the previous example, high rate of in-stent restenosis remains the Achilles heel of endovascular treatment for radiation-induced vasculopathy. In this patient, the restenotic lesions have occurred primarily at the very distal edge of the stent. Surgical revascularization in this patient would entail a long bypass from the subclavian artery to the brachial artery, traversing chronically edematous tissues in the previously irradiated field, which would be associated with increased risk of wound complication. Should the patient develop re-occlusion of the multiple-times stented axillary artery, surgical bypass will be indicated for limb-salvage.

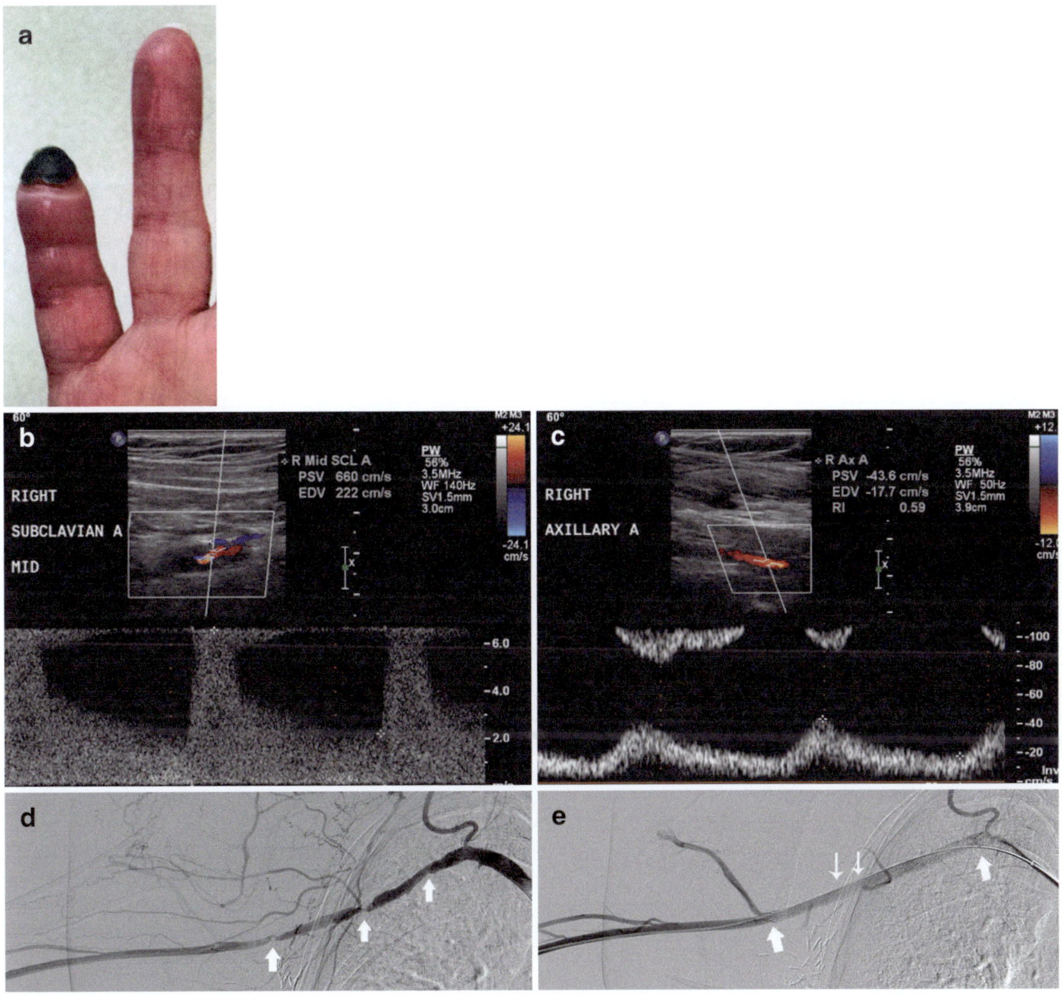

Fig. 9.10 Axillary artery occlusion 8 years after radiation treatment for breast cancer. (**a**) Photograph depicts dry necrosis of the distal tip of right fifth finger, consistent with chronic digital ischemia. (**b**) Ultrasound image of the right axillary artery shows markedly increased Doppler flow velocities indicating focal severe stenosis of the vessel. (**c**) Reduced monophasic Doppler flow velocities are shown in the right axillary artery distal to the stenotic lesion. (**d**) DSA image reveals multiple in tandem stenotic lesions (*arrows*) of the right axillary artery associated with prominent collateral vessels. (**e**) Post-stenting DSA image shows satisfactory appearance of stented axillary artery; *thick arrows* denote the proximal and distal edge of the overlapping self-expandable uncovered stents (6 and 5 mm diameters, respectively), and *thin arrows* point to the overlapping part of the stents.

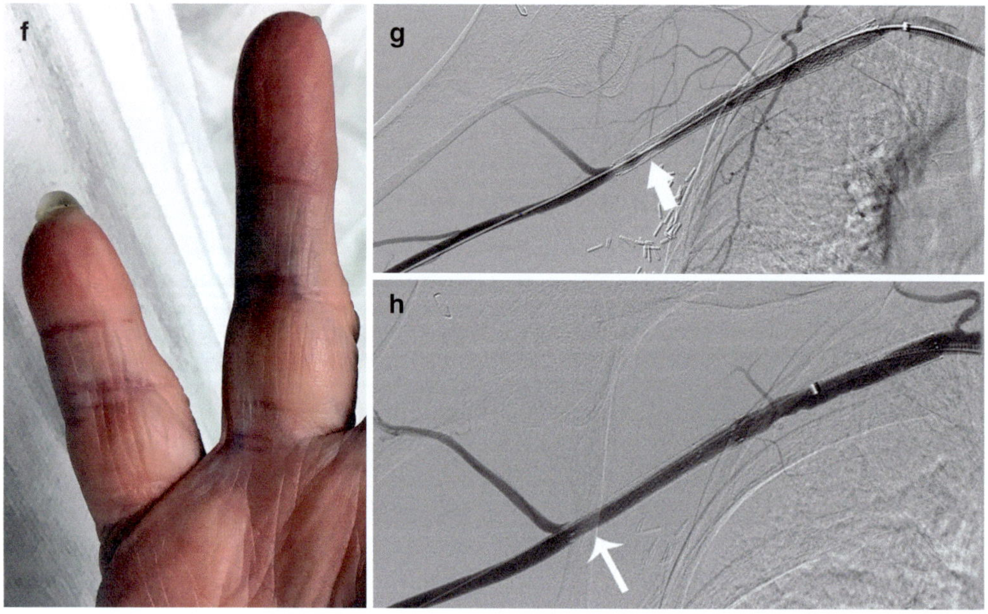

Fig. 9.10 (continued) (**f**) Photograph shows complete healing of the fifth digit after 3 months after successful revascularization. (**g**) DSA image demonstrates in-stent restenosis (*arrow*) in the distal stented axillary artery, 6 months after initial stenting procedure. (**h**) Completion DSA image shows satisfactory appearance after additional stenting using 5 mm self-expandable stent-graft (*arrow*) with overlap within the existing stent

Summary

Although peripheral artery disease is prevalent among elderly cancer patients, arterial complications are relatively uncommon in patients undergoing oncologic treatment. Endovascular or surgical revascularization is indicated for critical ischemia and can achieve high rate of limb-salvage in cancer patients. Survival outcome is generally related to the underlying cancer prognosis.

References

1. Levitan N, et al. Rates of initial and recurrent thromboembolic disease among patients with malignancy versus those without malignancy. Risk analysis using Medicare claims data. Medicine (Baltimore). 1999;78(5):285–91.
2. Sorensen HT, et al. Prognosis of cancers associated with venous thromboembolism. N Engl J Med. 2000;343(25):1846–50.
3. Prandoni P, Falanga A, Piccioli A. Cancer and venous thromboembolism. Lancet Oncol. 2005;6(6):401–10.
4. Herrmann J, et al. Vascular toxicities of cancer therapies: the old and the new--an evolving avenue. Circulation. 2016;133(13):1272–89.
5. Lenneman CG, Sawyer DB. Cardio-oncology: an update on cardiotoxicity of cancer-related treatment. Circ Res. 2016;118(6):1008–20.
6. Al-Kindi SG, Oliveira GH. Prevalence of preexisting cardiovascular disease in patients with different types of cancer: the unmet need for onco-cardiology. Mayo Clin Proc. 2016;91(1):81–3.
7. Di Nisio M, et al. Arterial thrombosis in ambulatory cancer patients treated with chemotherapy. Thromb Res. 2011;127(4):382–3.
8. Javid M, Magee TR, Galland RB. Arterial thrombosis associated with malignant disease. Eur J Vasc Endovasc Surg. 2008;35(1):84–7.
9. Bennett KM, et al. Outcomes of surgical revascularization for lower extremity arterial thromboembolism in patients with advanced malignancy. J Vasc Surg. 2014;60(4):987–92.
10. Morris-Stiff G, Lewis MH. Surgical treatment of acute limb ischaemia in the presence of malignancy. Int J Surg. 2010;8(3):233–5.
11. Tsang JS, et al. Acute limb ischemia in cancer patients: should we surgically intervene? Ann Vasc Surg. 2011;25(7):954–60.
12. Mouhayar E, et al. Outcome of acute limb ischemia in cancer patients. Vasc Med. 2014;19(2):112–7.
13. Allison MA, et al. Ethnic-specific prevalence of peripheral arterial disease in the United States. Am J Prev Med. 2007;32(4):328–33.
14. Peripheral Arterial Disease (PAD) Fact Sheet. http://www.cdc.gov/dhdsp/data_statistics/fact_sheets/fs_pad.htm. 2016. 06/16/2016 [cited 2016 9/05/2016].
15. Hirsch AT, et al. Peripheral arterial disease detection, awareness, and treatment in primary care. JAMA. 2001;286(11):1317–24.
16. McDermott MM, et al. Leg symptoms in peripheral arterial disease: associated clinical characteristics and functional impairment. JAMA. 2001;286(13):1599–606.
17. Diehm C, et al. Mortality and vascular morbidity in older adults with asymptomatic versus symptomatic peripheral artery disease. Circulation. 2009;120(21):2053–61.
18. Heart Protection Study Collaborative, G. MRC/BHF Heart Protection Study of cholesterol lowering with simvastatin in 20,536 high-risk individuals: a randomised placebo-controlled trial. Lancet. 2002;360(9326):7–22.
19. Poredos P, Jezovnik MK. Antiplatelet and antithrombotic treatment of patients with peripheral arterial disease. Int Angiol. 2010;29(1):20–6.
20. El Sakka K, et al. Association of malignant disease with critical leg ischaemia. Br J Surg. 2005;92(12):1498–501.
21. Norgren L, et al. Inter-Society Consensus for the Management of Peripheral Arterial Disease (TASC II). J Vasc Surg. 2007;45(Suppl S):S5–67.
22. Fowkes FG, et al. Comparison of global estimates of prevalence and risk factors for peripheral artery disease in 2000 and 2010: a systematic review and analysis. Lancet. 2013;382(9901):1329–40.

23. Fowler B, et al. Improving maximum walking distance in early peripheral arterial disease: randomised controlled trial. Aust J Physiother. 2002;48(4):269–75.
24. Hankey GJ, Norman PE, Eikelboom JW. Medical treatment of peripheral arterial disease. JAMA. 2006;295(5):547–53.
25. Rooke TW, et al. 2011 ACCF/AHA Focused Update of the Guideline for the Management of Patients With Peripheral Artery Disease (updating the 2005 guideline): a report of the American College of Cardiology Foundation/American Heart Association Task Force on Practice Guidelines. J Am Coll Cardiol. 2011;58(19):2020–45.
26. Klinkert P, et al. Vein versus polytetrafluoroethylene in above-knee femoropopliteal bypass grafting: five-year results of a randomized controlled trial. J Vasc Surg. 2003;37(1):149–55.
27. Indes JE, et al. Clinical outcomes of 5358 patients undergoing direct open bypass or endovascular treatment for aortoiliac occlusive disease: a systematic review and meta-analysis. J Endovasc Ther. 2013;20(4):443–55.
28. Conte MS, et al. Results of PREVENT III: a multicenter, randomized trial of edifoligide for the prevention of vein graft failure in lower extremity bypass surgery. J Vasc Surg. 2006;43(4):742–751; discussion 751.
29. Adam DJ, et al. Bypass versus angioplasty in severe ischaemia of the leg (BASIL): multicentre, randomised controlled trial. Lancet. 2005;366(9501):1925–34.
30. Aggarwal V, Waldo SW, Armstrong EJ. Endovascular revascularization for aortoiliac atherosclerotic disease. Vasc Health Risk Manag. 2016;12:117–27.
31. Dake MD, et al. Nitinol stents with polymer-free paclitaxel coating for lesions in the superficial femoral and popliteal arteries above the knee: twelve-month safety and effectiveness results from the Zilver PTX single-arm clinical study. J Endovasc Ther. 2011;18(5):613–23.
32. Tran K, et al. Real-world performance of paclitaxel drug-eluting bare metal stenting (Zilver PTX) for the treatment of femoropopliteal occlusive disease. Ann Vasc Surg. 2017;38:90–8.
33. Candy N, Ng E, Velu R. Paclitaxel-coated balloon reduces target lesion revascularization compared with standard balloon angioplasty. J Vasc Surg. 2017;65(2):558–70. e10
34. Laird JR, et al. Durability of treatment effect using a drug-coated balloon for femoropopliteal lesions: 24-month results of IN.PACT SFA. J Am Coll Cardiol. 2015;66(21):2329–38.
35. Duda SH, et al. Drug-eluting and bare nitinol stents for the treatment of atherosclerotic lesions in the superficial femoral artery: long-term results from the SIROCCO trial. J Endovasc Ther. 2006;13(6):701–10.
36. Hajibandeh S, et al. Covered vs uncovered stents for aortoiliac and femoropopliteal arterial disease: a systematic review and meta-analysis. J Endovasc Ther. 2016;23(3):442–52.
37. Mwipatayi BP, et al. Durability of the balloon-expandable covered versus bare-metal stents in the Covered versus Balloon Expandable Stent Trial (COBEST) for the treatment of aortoiliac occlusive disease. J Vasc Surg. 2016;64(1):83–94. e1
38. McQuade K, et al., Four-year randomized prospective comparison of percutaneous ePTFE/nitinol self-expanding stent graft versus prosthetic femoral-popliteal bypass in the treatment of superficial femoral artery occlusive disease. J Vasc Surg. 2010;52(3):584–90; discussion 590–1, 591 e1–591 e7.
39. Geraghty PJ, et al. Three-year results of the VIBRANT trial of VIABAHN endoprosthesis versus bare nitinol stent implantation for complex superficial femoral artery occlusive disease. J Vasc Surg. 2013;58(2):386–95. e4
40. Modrall JG, Sadjadi J. Early and late presentations of radiation arteritis. Semin Vasc Surg. 2003;16(3):209–14.
41. Baerlocher MO, et al. Primary stenting of bilateral radiation-induced external iliac stenoses. J Vasc Surg. 2004;40(5): 1028–31.
42. Moutardier V, et al. Iliac atherosclerotic occlusive disease complicating radiation therapy for cervix cancer: a case series. Gynecol Oncol. 2002;84(3):456–9.
43. Haddad TC, Greeno EW. Chemotherapy-induced thrombosis. Thromb Res. 2006;118(5):555–68.
44. Fernandes DD, et al. Acute aortic thrombosis in patients receiving cisplatin-based chemotherapy. Curr Oncol. 2011;18(2): e97–100.
45. Schutz FA, et al. Bevacizumab increases the risk of arterial ischemia: a large study in cancer patients with a focus on different subgroup outcomes. Ann Oncol. 2011;22(6):1404–12.
46. Alhawiti N, et al. The tyrosine kinase inhibitor, nilotinib potentiates a prothrombotic state. Thromb Res. 2016;145:54–64.
47. Lang K, et al. Mortality and vascular events among elderly patients with chronic myeloid leukemia: a retrospective analysis of linked SEER-Medicare Data. Clin Lymphoma Myeloma Leuk. 2016;16(5):275–285.e1.

Carotid Artery Disease in Patients with Cancer

10

Tam T.T. Huynh, George T. Pisimisis, Karen C. Broadbent, and Reza J. Mehran

Abstract

Stroke remains the leading cause of permanent disability. Embolic stroke due to severe carotid artery stenosis can be preventable. In this article, we review the management of carotid artery disease with particular focus in cancer patients. Carotid duplex ultrasonography is the screening modality of choice for the detection of cervical carotid artery disease. Surgical carotid endarterectomy remains the gold-standard therapy for all symptomatic patients with severe carotid artery stenosis. Carotid stenting is a minimally invasive alternative treatment for symptomatic patients deemed high-risk for carotid endarterectomy either due to medical or anatomical reasons. Head and neck cancer patients require special considerations due to higher incidence of carotid artery disease, particularly following the radiation treatment.

Keywords

Carotid • Ischemic stroke • Cerebral infarction • Atherosclerosis • Endarterectomy • Stenting • Angioplasty • Cancer • Radiation • Head and neck • Stenosis • Vascular

Introduction

The decline in stroke mortality in the United States over the past decades has been recognized as a major improvement in the medical field. The progress in stroke outcomes results from medical interventions to control cardiovascular risk factors, reduced stroke incidence, and lower case fatality rates [1]. However, stroke remains a leading cause of long-term disability globally. Approximately 70% of stroke survivors require further medical care after sustaining an acute stroke. It is estimated that 87% of all strokes are due to acute ischemic cerebral infarction, 10% to intracranial hemorrhage and 3% to subarachnoid hemorrhage. Severe carotid artery plaque disease accounts for up to 20% of acute ischemic strokes (Fig. 10.1). The incidence of ischemic stroke related to cervical carotid artery plaque disease

T.T.T. Huynh, M.D. (✉) • G.T. Pisimisis, M.D.
Department of Thoracic and Cardiovascular Surgery,
The University of Texas M.D. Anderson Cancer Center,
1515 Holcombe Blvd., Unit 1489, Houston, TX 77030-4009, USA

Department of Interventional Radiology, The University of Texas
M.D. Anderson Cancer Center, Houston, TX, USA
e-mail: tamhuynh@mdanderson.org

K.C. Broadbent, B.S.N., R.N., R.V.T.
Thoracic and Orthopedic Center, The University of Texas
M.D. Anderson Cancer Center, Houston, TX, USA

R.J. Mehran, M.D.
Department of Thoracic and Cardiovascular Surgery,
The University of Texas M.D. Anderson Cancer Center,
1515 Holcombe Blvd., Unit 1489, Houston, TX 77030-4009, USA

S.W. Yusuf, J. Banchs (eds.), *Cancer and Cardiovascular Disease*, https://doi.org/10.1007/978-3-319-62088-6_10

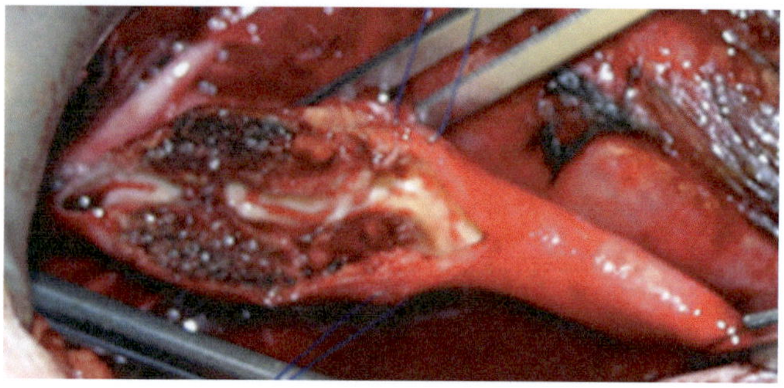

Fig. 10.1 Carotid plaque. Intraoperative photograph of a bisected carotid artery bifurcation, showing the atherosclerotic plaque, intramural thrombus with hemorrhage, and friable debris

will likely continue to rise in the next decade due to the aging of the U.S. baby boomer population. Cardiovascular complications are common in cancer patients. For the cancer patient, the occurrence of an acute stroke will often delay oncologic treatment for that patient until he/she regains adequate functional or performance status. In this article, we review the management of carotid disease with particular focus in cancer patients and provide a consortium of clinical vignettes.

Stroke Risk Factors

Older age, cigarette smoking, hypertension, diabetes, and hyperlipidemia are well-established risk factors for atherosclerotic plaque formation in the cervical carotid arteries, similar to that seen in the coronary and other medium-size arteries. Artery-to-artery atheroembolization from carotid plaque to either a large intracranial branch (e.g. middle cerebral artery) or a smaller cortical branch is recognized as the most common mechanism leading to acute cerebral ischemia (Fig. 10.2). Stroke due to acute carotid artery thrombosis is less common (Fig. 10.3). In general, patients who sustain an acute ischemic stroke due to atheroembolization from carotid artery disease are more likely to experience a recurrent stroke than those with small vessel occlusion or cardioembolism [2]. Lacunar infarcts due to small vessel disease typically result in milder neurologic impairments and are associated with better outcomes when compared to ischemic strokes due to carotid artery atheroembolism. The current management of patients with carotid artery plaque disease is primarily based on the severity of stenosis, and the presence or absence of ipsilateral ischemic neurologic symptoms (symptomatic versus asymptomatic, respectively).

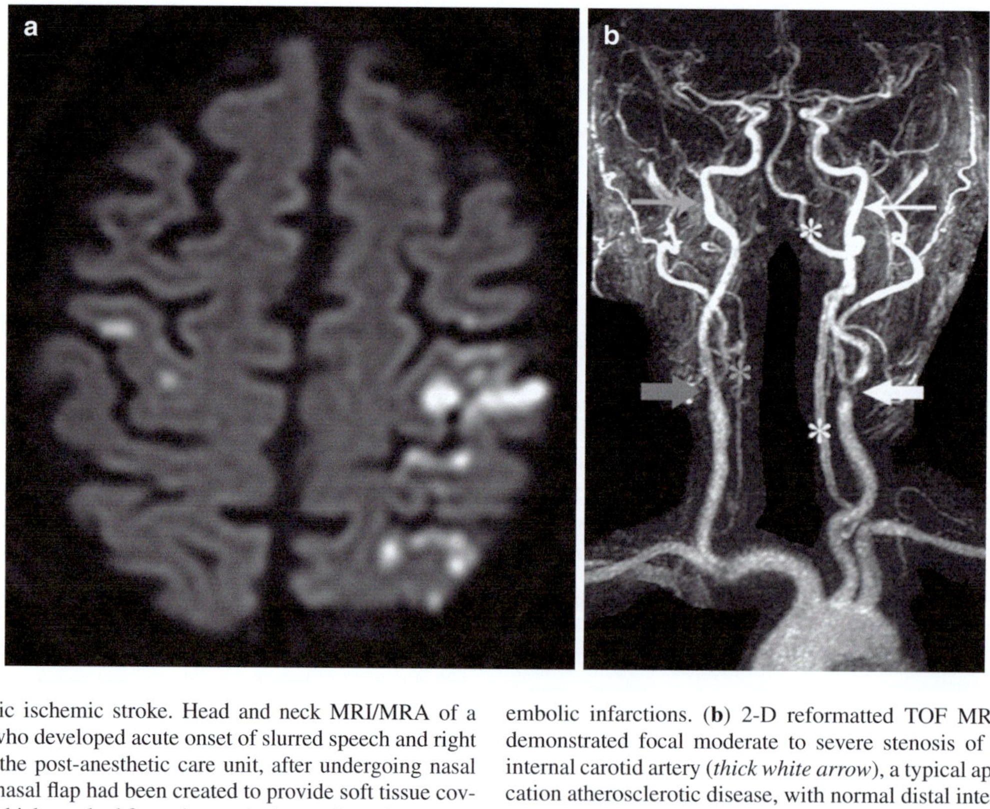

Fig. 10.2 Embolic ischemic stroke. Head and neck MRI/MRA of a 72 year-old man who developed acute onset of slurred speech and right arm weakness in the post-anesthetic care unit, after undergoing nasal flap revision (the nasal flap had been created to provide soft tissue coverage to a defect which resulted from the surgical resection of a cutaneous melanoma lesion 3 weeks prior). (**a**) Axial MRI image showed multiple scattered foci of restricted diffusion (bright signals on DWI) concentrated in the left frontal and parietal lobes, and in the left occipital and right posterior frontal lobes, consistent with multiple acute embolic infarctions. (**b**) 2-D reformatted TOF MRA coronal image demonstrated focal moderate to severe stenosis of the left proximal internal carotid artery (*thick white arrow*), a typical appearance of bifurcation atherosclerotic disease, with normal distal internal carotid artery (*thin white arrow*). The left vertebral artery is normal and dominant (*white asterisks*). The right carotid bifurcation has mild disease (*thick grey arrow*) and distal right internal carotid artery is normal (*thin grey arrow*). The right vertebral artery is hypoplastic (*grey asterisk*). The patient also had paroxysmal atrial fibrillation

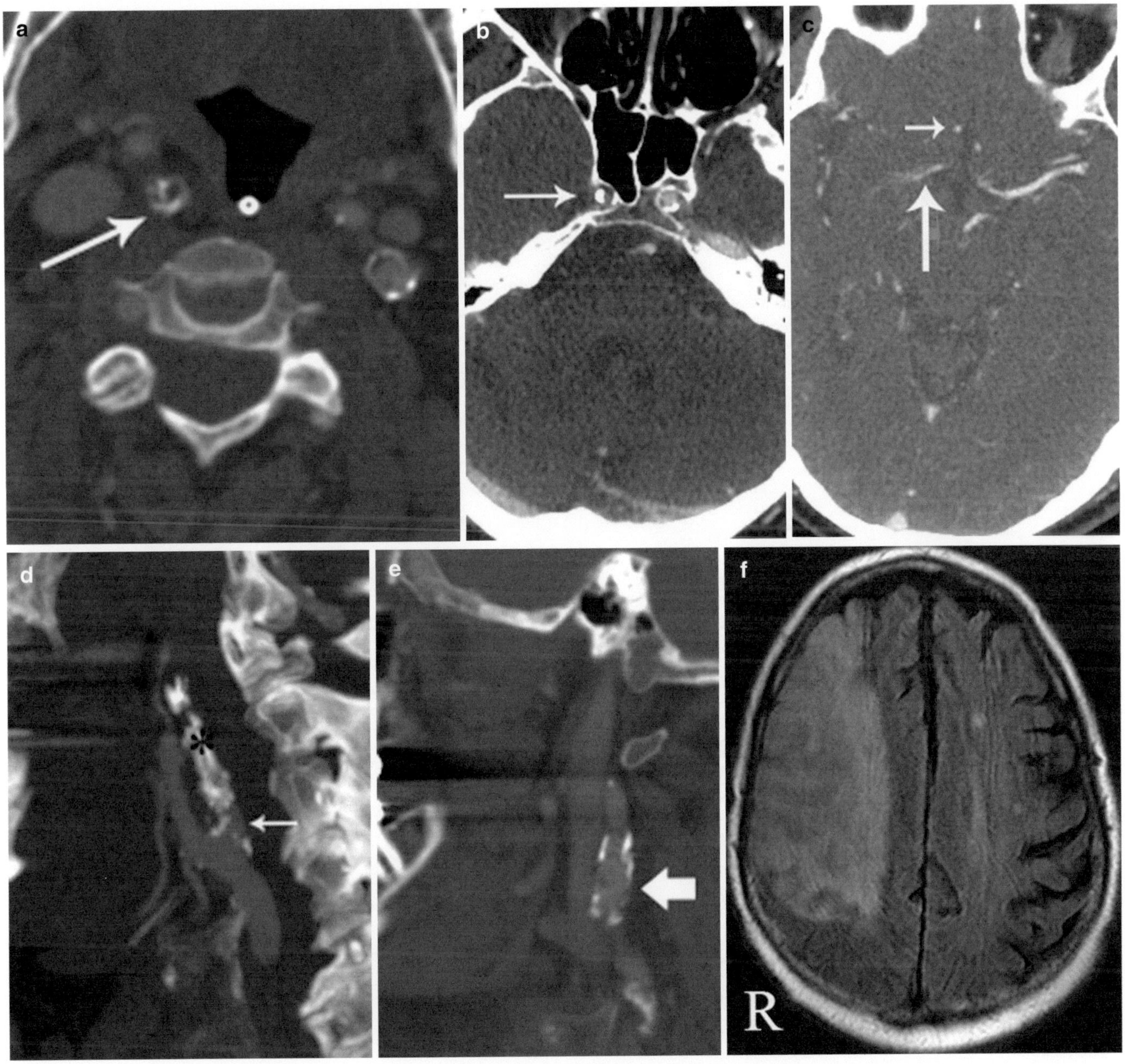

Fig. 10.3 Acute internal carotid artery thrombosis. A 70 year-old man sustained acute middle cerebral artery territory large ischemic stroke due to acute right internal carotid artery thrombosis, following repair of a femoral artery pseudoaneurysm, which occurred after extensive common femoral endarterectomy and patch angioplasty reconstruction. CT angiogram axial images revealed (**a**) acute thrombosis of the proximal right internal carotid artery (*arrow*), extending into the (**b**) clinoid segment of the vessel (*arrow*), which is also heavily calcified, and (**c**) reconstitution of flow in the right middle (*large arrow*) cerebral and anterior (*small arrow*) cerebral arteries via collaterals. On sagittal views, (**d**) extensive calcified complex plaque disease (*asterisk*) is seen with interruption of contrast flow just above the carotid bifurcation in the right cervical internal carotid artery (*arrow*), and (**e**) moderate stenosis of the left proximal internal carotid artery is shown (*arrow*). (**f**) Brain MRI axial T2 flair image (11 days after the acute stroke event) showed the large acute/subacute infarction involving the right middle cerebral artery territory, and smaller acute embolic infarcts in the left middle cerebral territory. The patient had received immunotherapy (nivolumab trial) for metastatic urothelial cancer for approximately 3 years without progression of cancer disease and had remote history of coronary artery bypass

Diagnostic Imaging

Carotid duplex ultrasound examination is the initial imaging modality of choice to evaluate the cervical carotid artery bifurcation for the presence of plaque disease and stenosis (Fig. 10.4). Duplex ultrasound is a non-invasive test with high sensitivity and specificity. Characterization of the carotid bifurcation plaque on gray-scale imaging provides useful information about its morphology and composition. Certain characteristics such as soft plaque (homogenous and

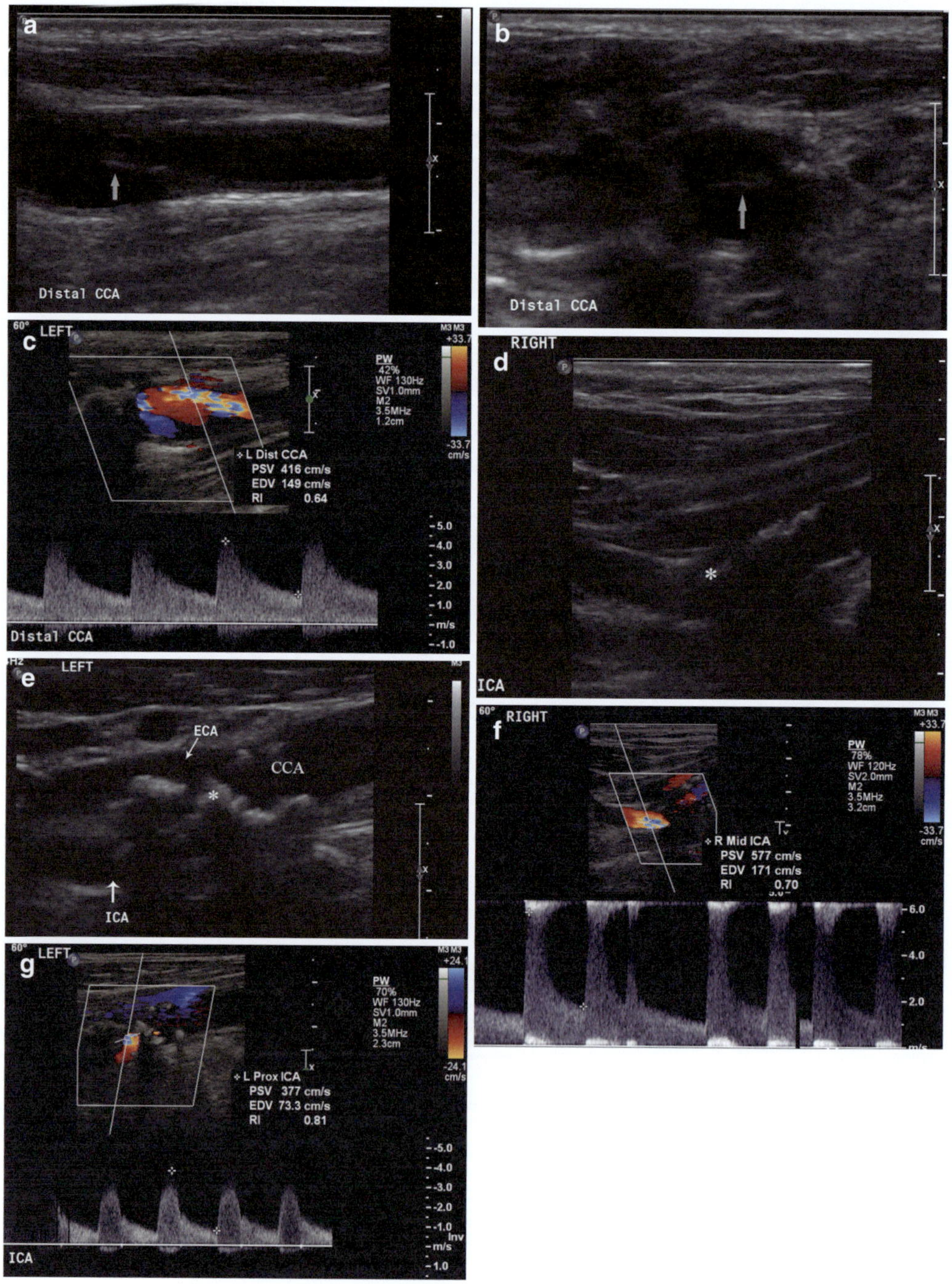

Fig. 10.4 Carotid Duplex ultrasound. (**a–c**) Duplex carotid ultrasound of an asymptomatic 75 year-old man, 30 years after surgical neck dissection, muscle flap reconstruction and external beam radiation for oropharyngeal squamous cell cancer. Gray scale ultrasound shows a focal dissection intimal flap (*arrow*) in the distal common carotid artery (CCA) on (**a**) longitudinal and (**b**) axial views; the intimal flap is likely chronic and related to the remote surgery. (**c**) Doppler interrogation demonstrates markedly increased peak systolic velocity indicating greater than 50% stenosis of the distal common carotid artery. (**d–g**) Duplex carotid ultrasound of a 72 year old-man with right small glottic cancer and asymptomatic severe bilateral carotid artery stenosis. Gray scale longitudinal ultrasound images show complex plaque (*asterisk*) disease in the (**d**) right and (**e**) left carotid internal carotid arteries (ICA). Doppler interrogation suggests high-grade stenosis in both (**f**) mid right internal carotid artery and (**g**) proximal left internal carotid artery. The patient had 75 pack-years smoking tobacco and hypertension. Clopidogrel and atorvastatin therapy was initiated and the patient had successful definitive intensity-modulated radiation therapy (IMRT) for the glottic cancer. Patient sustained a minor myocardial infarction 2 years after radiation treatment, but has had no ischemic neurologic events

echolucent), intraplaque hemorrhage and plaque ulceration have been associated with higher incidence of distal embolization compared to heterogenous and calcified plaques. However, the severity of luminal stenosis is still the strongest predictor of stroke risk. By convention, the determination of carotid artery stenosis is provided in ranges based on the Doppler derived flow velocities, and not by diameter measurement. The criteria recommended by the Ultrasound Consensus Panel remains the most commonly used to determine the severity of stenosis of the cervical internal carotid artery [3].

Carotid duplex scanning in the head and neck cancer patient is often challenging. Preoperatively, a large tumor mass in the neck can displace, compress or encase the cervical carotid vessels (Fig. 10.5). Soft tissue changes secondary to surgery and/or radiation treatment can limit visualization. Irradiated tissue becomes fibrotic over time, hampering transmission of the ultrasound beam and causes acoustic shadowing that can obscure segment of the carotid arteries. Removal of the sternocleidomastoid muscle with radical neck dissection eliminates an important acoustic window for a posterior approach to the already superficial location of the carotid arteries. The presence of a tracheostomy further narrows the scanning window, and in particular, view of the common carotid artery, which is often very close to the stoma, can be suboptimal.

The finding of a severe carotid artery stenosis (70–99%) detected on duplex ultrasound performed in an accredited vascular laboratory is generally deemed sufficient evidence for determining therapy or intervention [4]. However, further evaluation with either magnetic resonance angiography (MRA) or computed tomographic angiography (CTA) is warranted to confirm the severity of stenosis, and to assess for presence of proximal vessel disease, or tandem intracranial stenosis. Imaging technology and post-processing methods of MRA and CTA are constantly evolving. In our institution, CTA is more commonly used than MRA to evaluate patients with suspected carotid disease, in part due to the local expertise (Fig. 10.6). The multi-slice helical CT scanner provides higher spatial resolution than MR imaging. One additional advantage of CTA over MRA is better characterization of calcification. However, the diagnostic value of conventional CTA (single-energy source CT) is limited when there is extensive calcification in the carotid bifurcation, and the severity of stenosis can be either over- or under-estimated. The recent introduction of dual-energy source CT systems

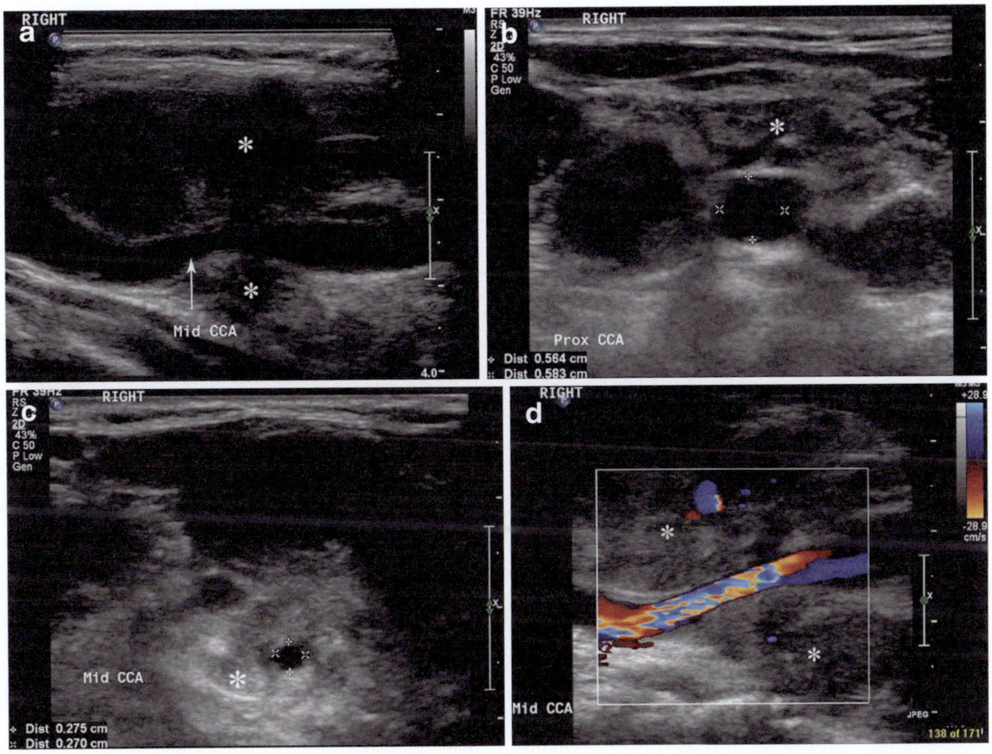

Fig. 10.5 Thyroid tumor encasing carotid artery bifurcation. (**a–e**) Ultrasound images of a large papillary thyroid cancer mass (*asterisk*) encasing and narrowing the right mid-common carotid artery (CCA) in a 52 year-old woman: (**a**) gray scale long view of mid-CCA encased by tumor; transverse views showing (**b**) normal diameter of proximal CCA and (**c**) reduced diameter of mid CCA; (**d**) disturbed colorflow seen in mid CCA associated with (**e**) increased Doppler peak systolic velocities, indicating luminal stenosis (due to external compression by the encasing tumor). The vessel wall including intima is otherwise normal and free of plaque disease.

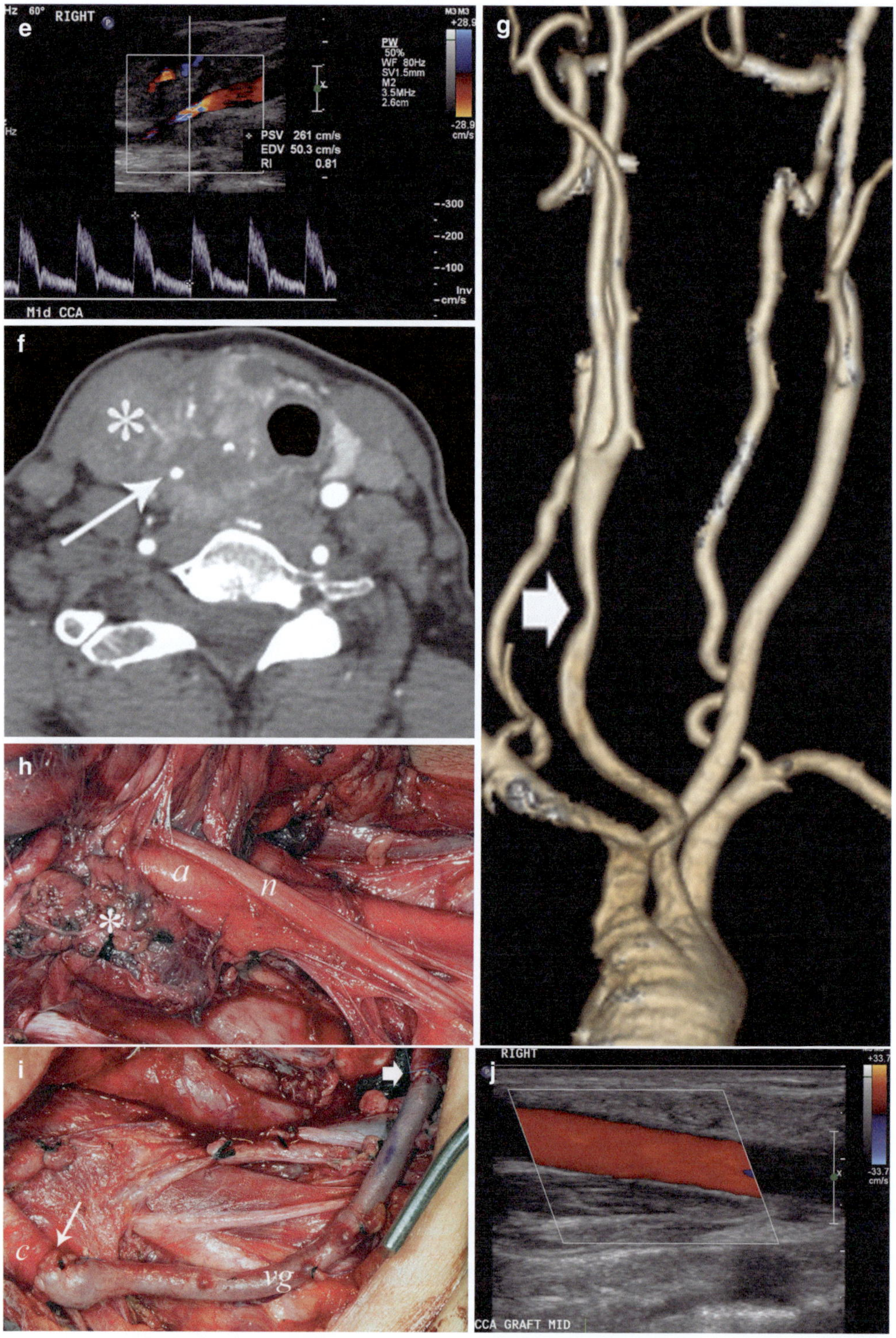

Fig. 10.5 (continued) (**f**) Axial CT neck shows the large papillary thyroid cancer mass (*asterisk*) with extensive locoregional disease, encasing the right mid-common carotid artery (*arrow*). (**g**) Reformatted 3-D CT angiogram depicts focal narrowing (*arrow*) of the right common carotid artery caused by tumor encasement. (**h**) Intra-operative photograph shows tumor (*asterisk*) encasing the right common carotid artery (*a*) and right vagus nerve (*n*). (**i**) Following en-bloc tumor and carotid artery resection, reconstruction of the right common carotid artery (*c*) using reversed saphenous vein graft (*vg*) is shown on photograph; proximal (*short arrow*) and distal (*long arrow*) anastomoses are depicted. (**j**) Colorflow ultrasound image of the reconstructed right common carotid artery (vein graft) at 6 months following surgery and post-operative external radiation

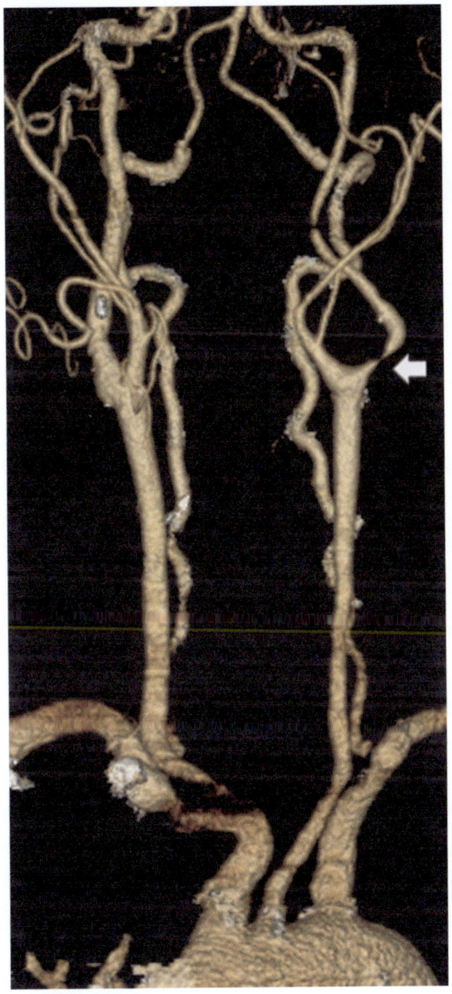

Fig. 10.6 3-D reformatted CT angiogram. A sixty-three year-old man who had left tonsillar HPV-related squamous cell cancer intensity modulated radiotherapy to 66 Gy in 2009. CT surveillance showed no evidence of cancer recurrence but revealed an incidental asymptomatic severe stenosis of the proximal left internal carotid artery in 2015. Reformatted 3-D image depicts the focal high-grade stenosis (*arrow*) of the proximal left internal carotid artery with small caliber vessel distal to the stenosis. The patient subsequently had successful carotid endarterectomy

may potentially overcome this limitation. Analysis of tube voltage-dependent attenuation differences between iodine and calcium enables rapid and fully automated subtraction of calcification from CTA datasets by dedicated post-processing software tools. Preliminary data suggests that dual-energy CTA may become the preferred imaging modality of choice for assessing patients with severely calcified carotid artery bifurcation disease [5]. Surveillance contrast-enhanced CT of the neck soft tissue is routinely obtained in head and neck cancer survivors in the first 5 years after completion of treatment and periodically thereafter. The presence of carotid artery disease can be noted on these CT, but it is often not assessed or reported because it is not the primary reason for the test. Indeed more attention should be paid to the carotid arteries in contrast-enhanced neck CT surveillance done for head and neck cancer patients, as the incidental finding of significant carotid stenosis is not infrequent. In our institution, we are working with our neuroradiologists towards standardizing reports on contrast-enhanced CT of neck soft tissue to include a comment on the carotid arteries.

MRA imaging incurs no radiation risk and does not require the use of intravenous iodinated contrast. Contrast-enhanced MRA with intravenous injection of gadolinium can provide accurate assessment of the plaque, residual lumen and degree of stenosis (Fig. 10.2b) [6]. However, in patients with renal insufficiency, TOF-MRA can provide adequate evaluation of the carotid artery bifurcation without need for contrast, avoiding the risk of nephrogenic systemic fibrosis. Invasive intra-arterial carotid angiography (selective digital subtraction angiography) was the historical gold standard test for evaluating carotid artery disease. However, with the improved diagnostic accuracy of the non-invasive carotid duplex ultrasound, MRA and CTA imaging, invasive carotid angiography is currently reserved for therapeutic intervention such as carotid stenting or when there is discordance in the findings of the non-invasive imaging tests.

Medical Therapy in Stroke Prevention

There is large body of evidence to support the routine use of aspirin and statin to prevent stroke in patients who either have symptomatic atherosclerotic cardiovascular disease, or are considered high-risk [7]. Aspirin (75–325 mg daily) has been shown to be effective in preventing stroke in patients at increased risk of for cardiovascular events, including those who sustain an acute myocardial infarction or ischemic stroke, unstable or stable angina, or those with prior history of myocardial infarction, stroke, and peripheral arterial disease [8, 9]. However, in patients without known cardiovascular disease or risk factors for atherosclerosis, the benefit of aspirin therapy remains uncertain. Large clinical trials have shown significant reduction in first and recurrent incidence of stroke in high-risk patients taking statin [10, 11]. Moreover, high-risk patients with established cardiovascular disease can benefit from statin regardless of their cholesterol level. In a prospective cohort of 68 asymptomatic patients with greater than 50% carotid artery stenosis, the use of statin therapy was associated with reduced rate of carotid plaque progression on MRI [12]. The beneficial effects of statin is not directly related to lipid-lowering, but rather can be linked to pleiotropic effects which are still not well understood [13].

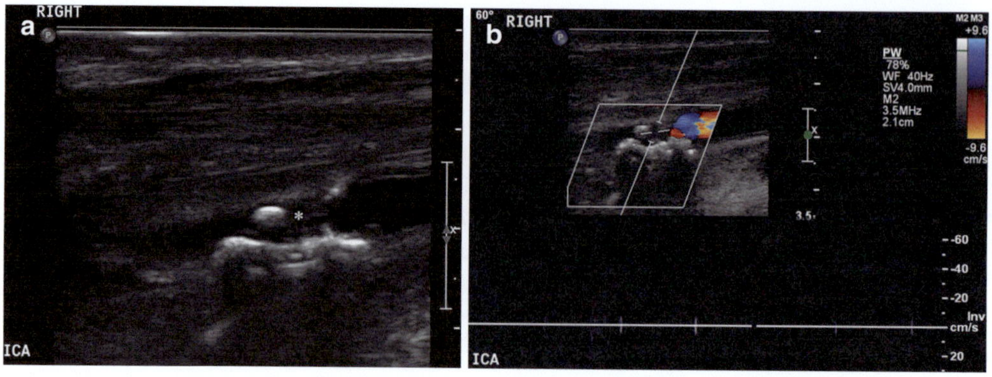

Fig. 10.7 Acute ischemic stroke during induction chemotherapy. A sixty-two year-old man, heavy smoker with prior history of myocardial infarction and coronary stenting, sustained right hemispheric stroke while undergoing induction chemotherapy (docetaxel and carboplatin) for synchronous squamous cell cancer in floor of the mouth and oropharynx. Although the patient had been on clopidogrel, it was halted for lymph node biopsy and not resumed until he developed an acute ischemic stroke. Duplex carotid ultrasound showed (**a**) calcified occlusive plaque (*asterisk*) in the right carotid bulb and (**b**) no Doppler colorflow, consistent with complete occlusion of the internal carotid artery. Fortunately, the patient recovered full neurologic function, and went on to receive successful definitive chemoradiation therapy within a month after the stroke. The patient remained on clopidogrel and atorvastatin during oncologic treatment and has had no recurrent ischemic neurologic events for 2 years since the incident stroke

In oncologic patients, there can often be competing treatment goals. Antiplatelet therapy is frequently put on hold during chemotherapy regimens that are known to cause bone marrow suppression and thrombocytopenia. However, patients with prior history of coronary artery or carotid disease (with or without stenting), myocardial events, or ischemic stroke should be reminded to remain on antiplatelet therapy throughout their oncologic treatment to reduce risk of cardiovascular events unless they develop major bleeding complications. The mere bleeding potential risk related to the combination of platelet inhibition and thrombocytopenia is not a valid contra-indication to interrupt antiplatelet therapy during oncologic treatment (Fig. 10.7). On occasions, patients may be temporarily unable to take their regular medications due to side effects of the oncologic treatment. When these side effects subside, patients with the above listed cardiovascular conditions should resume their cardiovascular drugs, including statin therapy as soon as possible while completing their cancer treatment.

Surgical Carotid Endarterectomy

Surgical carotid endarterectomy (CEA) remains the gold-standard treatment for stroke prevention in patients with severe cervical carotid artery stenosis. The benefit of CEA over medical therapy alone in stroke prevention is well established for symptomatic patients with severe carotid artery disease (70–99% stenosis). The North American Symptomatic Carotid Endarterectomy Trial (NASCET) reported a cumulative stroke rate of approximately 9% for patients with severe carotid artery stenosis randomized to CEA versus 26% for patients in the medical therapy group [14]. CEA was also shown to benefit patients with moderate carotid artery stenosis (50–69%); the 5-year fatal or nonfatal ipsilateral stroke rate was 16% in the surgically treated group versus 22% in the medically treated group [15]. The European Carotid Surgery Trial (ECST) demonstrated similar findings of the efficacy of CEA in reducing recurrent stroke rate for symptomatic patients with moderate to severe carotid artery stenosis [16]. However, CEA does not reduce risk of recurrent stroke in symptomatic patients with less than 50% carotid stenosis compared to medical therapy alone [15].

The surgical techniques of carotid endarterectomy continue to be refined. There are variations in the conduct of the procedure with regard to anesthesia, neurologic monitoring, type of skin incision, endarterectomy approach, artery closure, and carotid shunting. We describe our technique briefly as follows (Fig. 10.8). We prefer general anesthesia for most patients. A dedicated neurophysiology team monitors the patient's intra-operative electroencephalography (EEG) and somatosensory evoked potentials (SSEP). Using a portable duplex ultrasound, we visualize the carotid bifurcation to be treated and we mark its level and side. We make a curvilinear transverse incision along a skin fold centered on the diseased carotid artery bifurcation. Superior and inferior subplatysmal myocutanous flaps are created. We open the carotid fascia and mobilize the common carotid and internal carotid arteries circumferentially, proximally from below the bifurcation to as high as possible distally. Not infrequently, we divide the inferior belly of the omohyoid muscle to get adequate exposure of the lower part of the common carotid

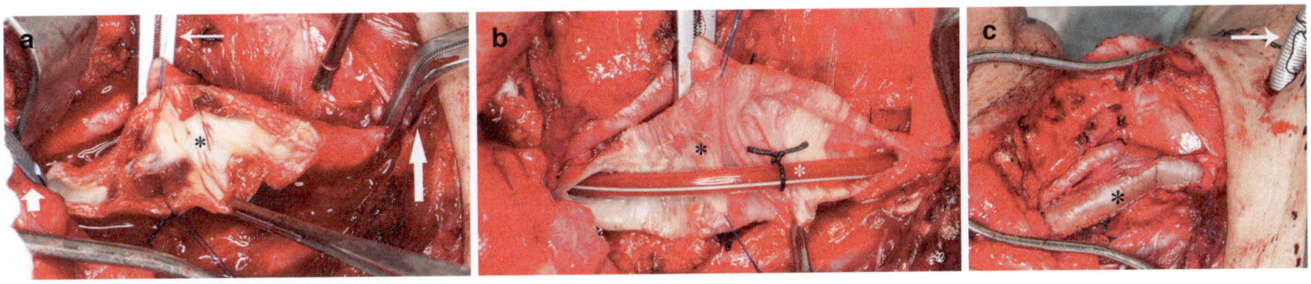

Fig. 10.8 Surgical carotid endarterectomy (CEA). A fifty-five year-old man had right partial glossectomy, neck dissection and postoperative external beam radiation to total dose of 60 Gy to the right tongue and 50 Gy to the right neck in 1997. The patient developed new primary cancer of the left lateral tongue at the end of year 2013 and underwent left partial glossectomy and neck dissection. Patient received additional postoperative radiation using IMRT to total of 60 Gy. The patient subsequently developed bilateral osteoradionecrosis of mandibles and worsening asymptomatic severe stenosis of the cervical right internal carotid artery in 2016. The patient underwent combined mandibulectomy, reconstruction using left fibula osteocutanous free flap, and right carotid endarterectomy. Base of the neck is to right in photographs. (**a**) Standard exposure of the right carotid artery bifurcation is shown. Clamps are placed across the proximal common (*large arrow*), external (*thin arrow*) and distal internal (*short arrow*) carotid arteries. Through the longitudinal arteriotomy, the diseased ulcerated plaque (*asterisk*) is seen. (**b**) The endarterectomized surface (*black asterisk*) is shown after plaque excision, with the temporary shunt (white asterisk) inside the artery. (**c**) Image depicts the patch angioplasty closure (*asterisk*) and prophylactic tracheostomy (*arrow*). The patient recovered well without neurologic or other postoperative complications. Patient's tracheotomy tube was removed and patient was discharged home on post-operative day 8

artery in the neck. This is particularly desirable when intra-arterial shunting is used. Distally, the posterior belly of the digastric muscle can be divided to expose the distal internal carotid artery. The common facial vein is commonly divided as it crosses anterior to the carotid artery. The hypoglossal and vagus nerves are always preserved. We administer heparin (1 mg/kg) intravenously prior to carotid cross-clamping. The external, internal, and common carotid arteries are sequentially clamped. A longitudinal arteriotomy is made to open the common carotid artery from below the bifurcation to distally beyond the diseased plaque onto the mid-distal internal carotid artery**.** We perform the endarterectomy by gently finding the normal plane within the thickened wall of the carotid plaque, removing the occlusive plaque, and leaving the outer layer (adventitia) of the vessel wall intact. Tacking sutures are placed distally using 6-0 or 7-0 Polypropylene sutures when necessary to appose the intima (and prevent an intimal flap). We carefully flush out and remove any loose debris from the endarterectomized surface. To optimize distal cerebral flow, we routinely use an intra-arterial shunt and aim to keep the systolic blood pressure 90–120 mmHg during the period when the carotid artery is opened. We typically close the longitudinal arteriotomy by sewing a commercially available pericardial bovine patch (or autologous saphenous vein patch). The temporary shunt is removed just before completion of the patch angioplasty. Flow is restored to the external carotid artery first then to the internal carotid artery. Protamine sulfate is administered to reverse effect of heparin (1:1) before wound closure. Antiplatelet therapy is resumed immediately after surgery. Patients are typically discharged home 1–2 days after carotid endarterectomy.

Carotid Artery Stenting

The introduction of carotid artery stenting (CAS) provided a minimally invasive alternative treatment for patients with severe carotid stenosis. Endovascular techniques for CAS and the use of temporary embolic protection have continued to evolve over the last decade. There have been numerous clinical studies examining the role of CAS in carotid revascularization. SAPPHIRE (Stenting and Angioplasty with Protection in Patients at High-Risk for Endarterectomy) was the first large clinical trial that showed results of carotid stenting comparable (non-inferior) to endarterectomy [17]. However, the initial enthusiasm for CAS was hampered by subsequent publication of the French multicenter randomized controlled Endarterectomy Versus Angioplasty (EVA-3S) trial showing higher rate of disabling stroke or death with CAS than with CEA in patients with symptomatic severe carotid artery stenosis (incidence of disabling stroke or death at 30-day was 1.5% after CEA and 3.4% after CAS) [18]. Furthermore, the findings of this study suggested that the use of temporary cerebral protection devices during CAS may reduce periprocedural strokes by approximately threefold [19]. Subsequently, the long awaited results of the North American randomized Carotid Revascularization Endarterectomy versus Stenting Trial (CREST) comparing CEA versus CAS were published in 2011 [20]. CREST demonstrated that both CEA and CAS are good options for carotid revascularization because the overall complication rates for both procedures are within the range of current treatment guidelines. However, peri-procedural risk of stroke and death was significantly higher in CAS versus CEA for the subgroup of symptomatic patients (6% vs. 3.2%).

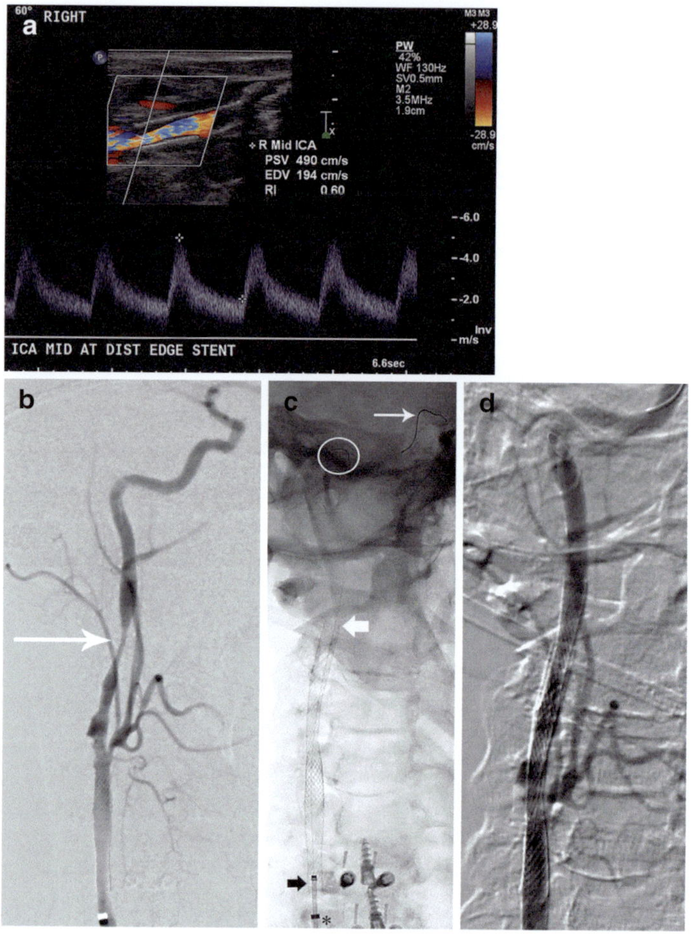

Fig. 10.9 Carotid artery stenting (CAS). A seventy year-old man with history of supraglottic squamous cell cancer had definitive chemoradiation in 2009. Patient developed a recurrence in 2012 in a left retropharyngeal lymph node and received additional 66 Gy proton therapy. Patient subsequently developed severe right internal carotid artery stenosis with neurologic symptoms and had carotid artery stenting in 2015. (**a**) At 1-year follow-up, duplex ultrasound surveillance showed severe in-stent restenosis of the right internal carotid artery with recurrent neurologic symptoms. The patient underwent successful repeat carotid stenting without complications. (**b**) Selective carotid arteriogram confirmed severe stenosis at the distal edge of the previous stent in the right internal carotid artery. (**c**) Spot fluoroscopic image depicts the tip of the sheath (*asterisk*), top of the new stent (still constrained within the delivery catheter; *small black arrow*), existing overlapping stents in the carotid artery (*large white arrow* denotes distal edge), and the temporary filter wire (nitinol loop-*white circle*; *thin white arrow points* to distal tip of wire). (**d**) Completion arteriogram after new stent deployment and post-stent balloon angioplasty demonstrates satisfactory result

Many carotid stents and distal embolic protection devices have become commercially available since the Federal Drug Administration first approved CAS in 2004. Transfemoral approach remains the standard conventional technique (Fig. 10.9). In brief, CAS is typically performed under conscious sedation. During the procedure, the patient's neurologic status is assessed periodically. Intra-procedure transcranial Doppler monitoring can detect intra-operative cerebral embolization and flow disturbances. Following standard arch aortogram, the external carotid artery is cannulated and a 6F or 7F sheath is advanced into the common carotid artery. Bivalirudin, a bivalent direct thrombin inhibitor, is administered intravenously as an initial bolus (0.75 mg/kg) then continued as a continuous infusion at a rate of 1.75 mg/kg/h. Distal embolic protection device (filter) is navigated carefully across the diseased plaque and deployed in the normal distal internal carotid artery. Various stent diameters and lengths are available. The self-expandable carotid stent is deployed across the target lesion. Post-stent balloon angioplasty is inflated gently and briefly. Intravenous atropine is frequently required to treat severe bradycardia or asystole, which can occur during stent deployment or balloon angioplasty. Following satisfactory completion angiogram, the temporary filter is removed, completing the procedure. Peri-procedural embolic stroke risk, in part related to crossing of the aortic arch, remains the Achilles heel of transfemoral CAS. More recently, transcarotid stenting using a novel neuroprotection device (flow reversal) has produced promising results with lower perioperative stroke risk [21]. We recommend long-term clopidogrel therapy following carotid stenting.

Asymptomatic Carotid Artery Stenosis

In 2012, 90,800 CEA and 16,300 CAS procedures were performed in the United States. Approximately 70–80% of carotid interventions (CEA and CAS) are done for asymptomatic carotid stenosis. Controversy remains in the treatment of asymptomatic carotid artery stenosis for primary stroke prevention [22]. Two large multicenter randomized clinical trials have shown significant reduction in stroke risk for patients with severe asymptomatic carotid artery stenosis treated by CEA versus medical therapy. The North American Asymptomatic Carotid Arteriosclerosis Study (ACAS) was published in 1998 and showed that the 5-year risk for any perioperative stroke or death was 5.1% for CEA patients and 11.0% for patients treated medically [23]. Subsequently, the European Asymptomatic Carotid Surgery Trial (ACST) showed similar results [24]. The first report of this trial showed 5-year risk for all strokes to be 6.4% in the surgical arm compared to 11.8% in the medical arm. This risk reduction was maintained in long-term follow up study for patients younger than 75 years of age, with 10-year stroke risk reduction observed to be 13.4% for CEA patients versus 17.9% for medically treated patients [25]. Critics of these older trials contend that medical therapy has improved greatly, and the current best medical therapy, particularly, the prevalent use of lipid-lowering drugs and the ameliorated control of hypertension, would void the potential benefits of CEA.

Results of more recent trials have emerged comparing CEA versus CAS for severe asymptomatic carotid stenosis in patients on contemporary medical therapy. There were 1181 asymptomatic patients with high-grade carotid artery stenosis randomized to CAS or CEA in the CREST trial, the periprocedural stroke and death rate was similar in both groups (2.5% in CAS versus 1.4% CEA) [20]. Most recently, results of the ACT randomized trial were published in February 2016, comparing CAS vs. CEA in patients with severe asymptomatic carotid artery stenosis [26]. The investigators showed that CAS was non-inferior to CEA for patients with severe asymptomatic carotid artery stenosis with 30-day rate of stroke or death of 2.9% in CAS group and 1.7% for CEA group, and cumulative 5-year rate of stroke-free survival of 93.1% in CAS and 94.7% in CEA groups, respectively. Three current multicenter randomized trials in Europe and North America, Stent-Protected Angioplasty versus Carotid Endarterectomy, Carotid Revascularization Endarterectomy versus Stenting Trial, and European Carotid Surgery Trial (SPACE-2, CREST-2, and ECST-2, respectively) are currently enrolling patients to address the important question: does intervention by either CAS or CEA offer additional benefit over contemporary best medical therapy alone in patients with severe asymptomatic carotid artery stenosis.

Special Considerations for Patients with Head and Neck Cancer

The development of carotid artery stenosis is a well-recognized late complication in patients receiving high-dose external beam radiation for head and neck cancers. It has been estimated that the relative risk of ischemic stroke is at least double following head and neck radiotherapy [27]. A review of a Medicare-cohort of 6862 patients with head and neck cancer (Surveillance Epidemiology and End-Results—SEER) between 1992 and 2012 found a 10-year incidence of cerebrovascular events of 34% in patients undergoing definitive radiotherapy, compared with 25% in patients with surgery plus post-operative radiotherapy, and 26% in patients treated with surgery alone [28]. Although this report did not differentiate the location or cause of stroke, it suggests an association between high radiation dose and an overall increased risk of stroke. The factors leading to radiation-induced vasculopathy and accelerated atherosclerosis have not yet been clearly defined, but are thought to be in part due to combined radiation effects on the vascular endothelium and the vasa vasorum of the adventitia [29]. Although most carotid lesions in radiated field have similar appearance compared to typical atherosclerotic bifurcation disease (Figs. 10.1 and 10.6), the former can be more extensive, involving the proximal common carotid, and/or mid to distal internal carotid artery not infrequently (Fig. 10.10). Several investigators have recommended routine screening and surveillance for carotid occlusive disease in all patients following external beam high dose radiation for head and neck [30–33]. However, evidence-based guidelines for the treatment of asymptomatic patients with radiation-induced carotid disease are still lacking, and optimal medical treatment has not yet been defined. Unfortunately, most of the past and current large carotid multicenter randomized trials, described in the prior sections, have excluded patients with history of neck radiation, neck dissection and active/recent cancer.

Carotid endarterectomy in radiated field can be done safely, but can be associated with increased risk of surgical complications including up to approximately 25% incidence of cranial nerve injury [34, 35]. Carotid stenting provides an alternative less-invasive treatment for affected patients with radiation induced severe carotid artery stenosis. However, carotid stenting for radiation induced carotid artery stenosis have resulted in higher rate of in-stent restenosis (Fig. 10.9) [35, 36]. A recent three-center retrospective review showed no significant differences in the peri-operative complications and restenosis in patients having carotid artery stenting with or without prior neck radiation therapy [37]. At our institution, the management of patients with radiation induced carotid stenosis follows the same principles as that for non-radiated patients. Carotid intervention, either stenting or endarterectomy is recommended for symptomatic patients with moderate to severe carotid artery stenosis. Currently, our group offers surgical carotid endarterectomy as the first option to symptomatic patients considered good operative candidates. Surgical dissection in irradiated tissue can be more difficult because of presence of scar tissues with obliteration of the normal tissue planes. We have found sharp tissue dissection to be particularly useful in redo and irradiated neck to avoid inadvertent injuries. Admittedly, carotid endarterectomy in patients who had prior neck dissection or high dose radiation is more tedious than surgery in a neck without prior such treatment, but it can be done successfully in experienced hands. However, in patients with extensive soft tissue deformity in the neck, chronic tracheostomy, or high medical risks, we favor carotid stenting for symptomatic severe carotid artery stenosis.

On rare occasions, patients can present with neck wound complications after extensive neck dissection and radiation that can lead to contained carotid artery pseudoaneurysm or catastrophic carotid blow-out (Fig. 10.11). Emergency endo-

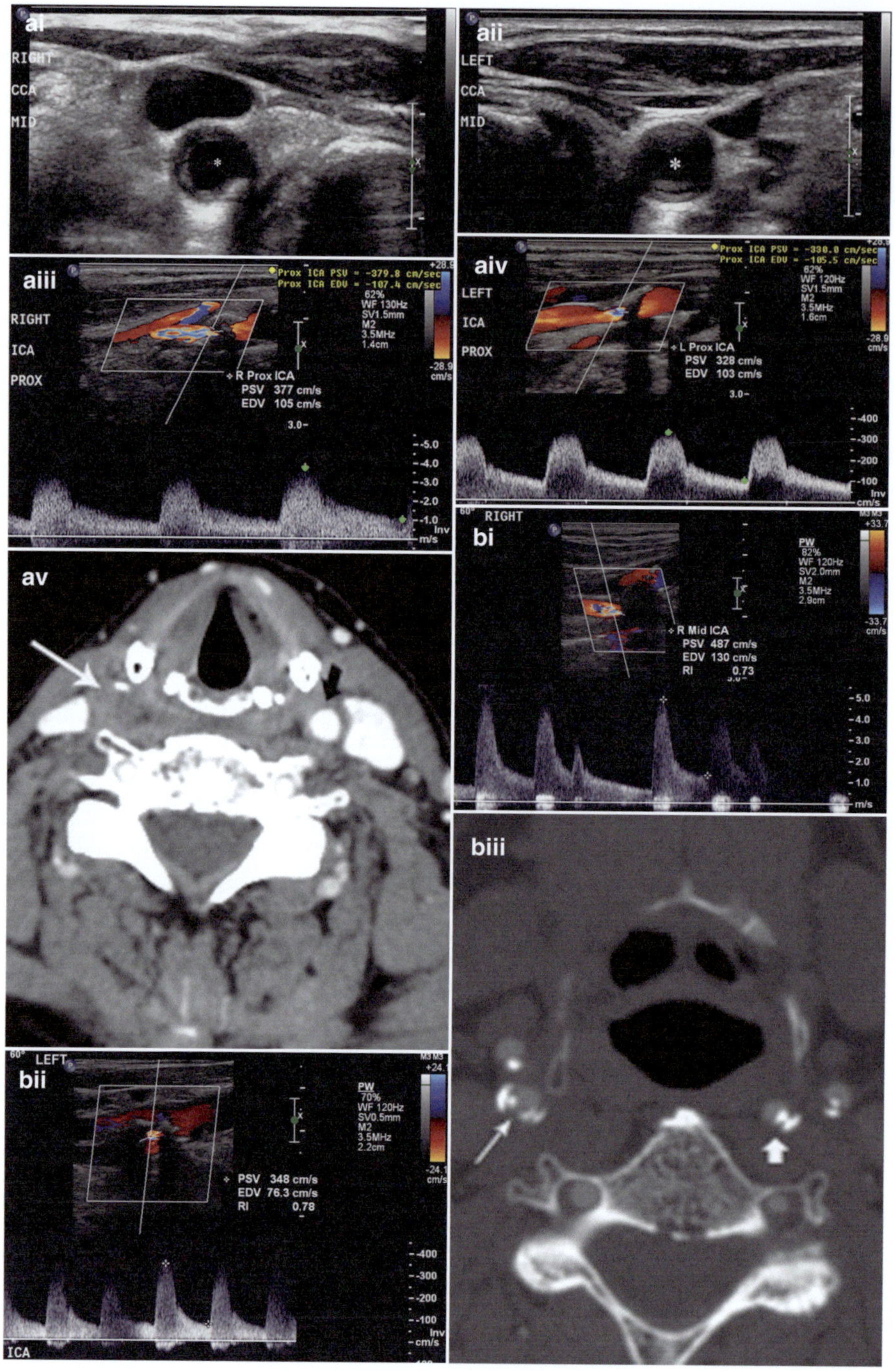

Fig. 10.10 Radiation-induced carotid artery vasculopathy. Carotid plaque formation in patients after external radiation can lead to accelerated atherosclerosis of the carotid bifurcation, similar to the typical atherosclerotic process. However, radiation-induced vasculopathy can also produce more extensive plaque formation, involving the common carotid and/or the internal carotid artery beyond the bulb. Below we describe the progression of carotid disease in two patients who had neck radiation for nasopharyngeal and laryngeal cancer. (**a**) A sixty-three year-old woman presented with local cancer recurrence involving the left maxilla. Twelve years prior, the patient had surgical resection of squamous cell cancer of the right hard palate and alveolar ridge, and postoperative external beam radiation therapy (65 Gy to the operative bed and retropharyngeal nodes and 50 Gy to the right hemineck). The patient continued to smoke tobacco and was on chronic warfarin therapy for history of DVT. Carotid duplex ultrasound showed wall thickening of (i) right and (ii) left common carotid arteries (*asterisk*) and moderate to severe stenosis of (iii) right and (iv) left proximal internal carotid arteries (worse on the right). We recommended continuing medical therapy for her carotid disease. The patient then underwent partial resection of the left maxilla to remove the local recurrence without complications. (v) The patient subsequently developed asymptomatic interval occlusion of the right common (*white arrow*) and internal carotid arteries on CT imaging at 7 months postoperatively; black arrow points to a patent left common carotid artery. (**b**) A seventy-two year-old man smoker with known asymptomatic bilateral carotid artery stenosis was referred for laryngeal squamous cell cancer in 2014. Patient received IMRT to 63 Gy to the vocal cord without complications. The patient has since quit tobacco and remains on clopidogrel and statin. At 2-year follow-up, carotid duplex images show (i) moderate to severe stenosis of the right mid-internal carotid artery and (ii) moderate stenosis of the left mid-internal carotid artery; and (iii) axial CT image depicts significant calcification of bilateral carotid bifurcation. The patient has remained asymptomatic on medical therapy

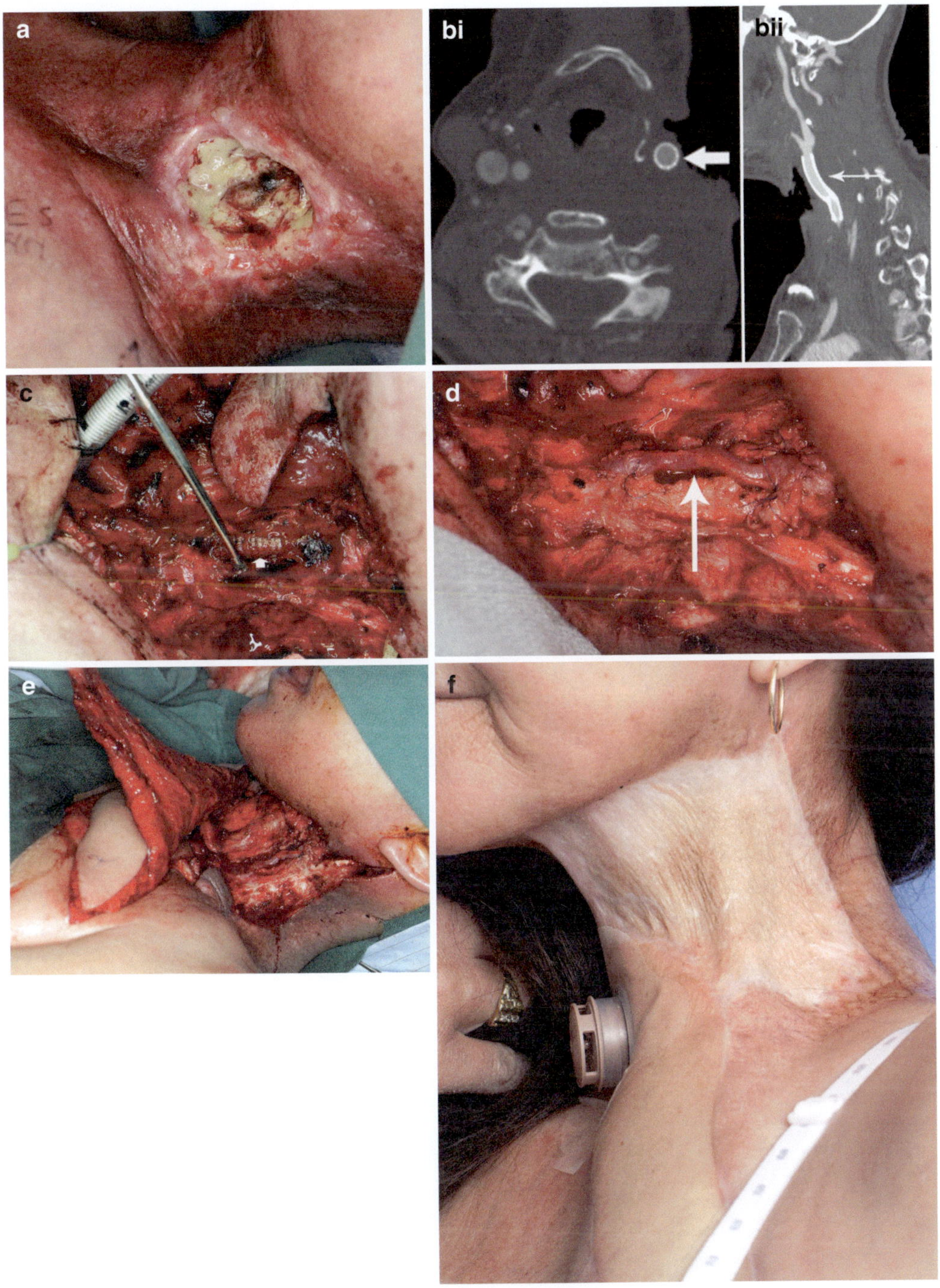

Fig. 10.11 Neck wound complication and muscle flap coverage. A fifty-eight year-old woman was referred to our center for management of chronic non-healing neck wound. The patient had initially received definitive external radiation therapy for laryngeal cancer in 1999. She subsequently developed a recurrence in 2004 and underwent left neck dissection and had postoperative chemoradiation therapy. In 2010, the patient acquired a wound in her left neck, which progressed despite local wound care and hyperbaric treatment. The patient developed bleeding in the left neck wound associated with presence of a left common carotid artery pseudoaneurysm. Stenting of the pseudoaneurysm using covered stent temporarily stopped the bleeding. The patient was then transferred to our center for definitive treatment. Intra-operative photographs are provided courtesy of Dr. Peirong (Ron) Yu, Plastic Reconstructive Surgery, University of Texas MD Anderson Cancer Center. (**a**) Photograph of left neck wound (base of neck to right). (**b**) CT images show patent left common carotid artery stent (*arrow*) on (i) axial and (ii) sagittal views. (**c**) Intra-operative photograph showing covered stent (*arrow*; base of neck to right). (**d**) Reconstruction of the left common carotid artery using reversed saphenous vein graft (*arrow*) after extensive neck wound debridement; base of neck to the right. (**e**) Transposition of pedicle left latissimus dorsi myocutaneous flap to cover large wound defect. (**f**) Photograph of patient's neck at 1-year follow up

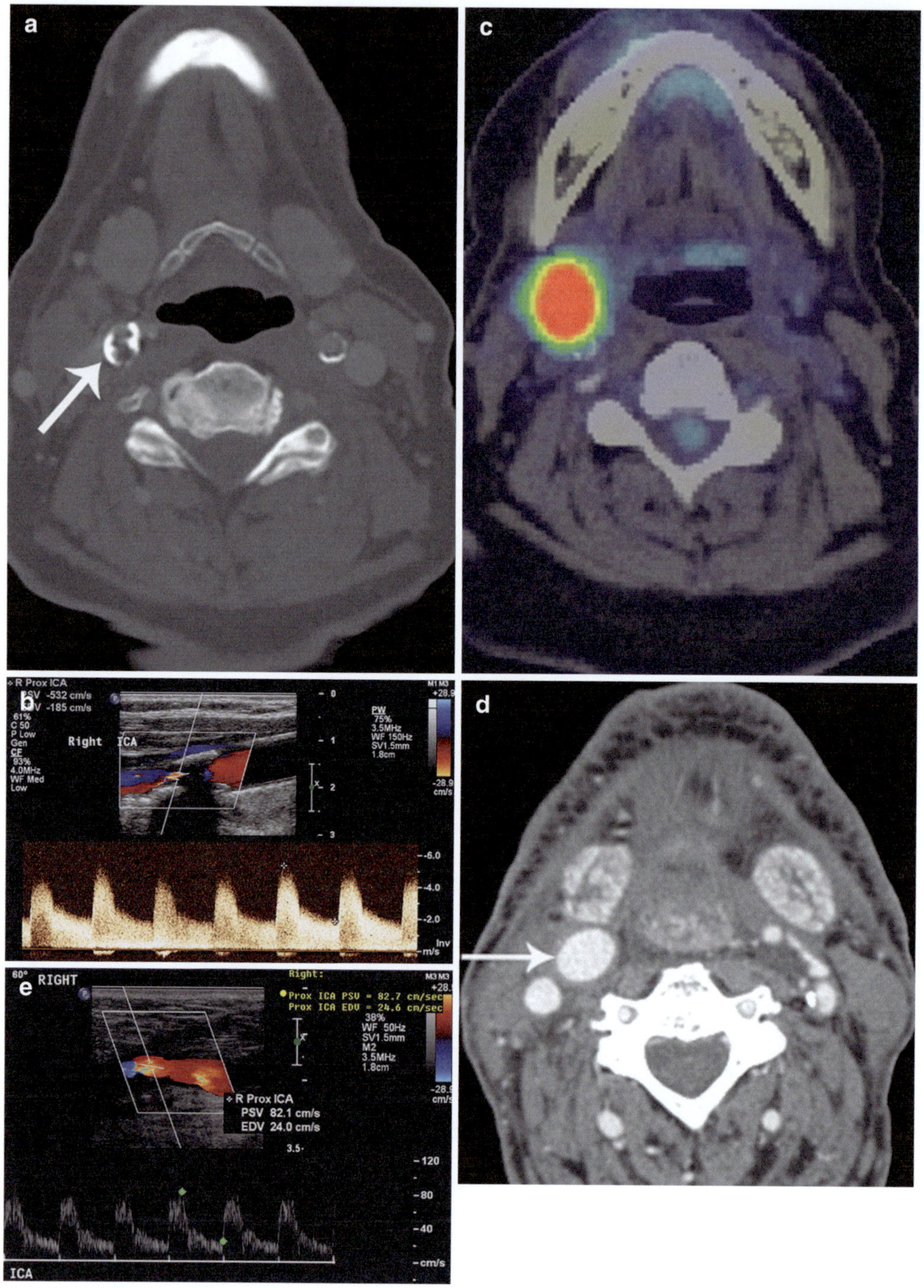

Fig. 10.12 Concomitant oncologic neck dissection and CEA. A sixty-five year-old woman was found to have right tonsillar squamous cell cancer with nodal metastatic disease and severe right proximal internal carotid artery stenosis while undergoing work-up for right eye amaurosis fugax in 2011. Patient underwent concomitant tonsillectomy, right neck dissection, and right carotid endarterectomy. The patient received postoperative chemotherapy (cetuximab) and external neck radiation to the tumor bed (total dose of 66 Gy). At 5 years post-treatment, the patient is without evidence of cancer 5 years and has had no recurrent ischemic neurologic events. Pre-operative (**a**) CT image showed bulky calcified plaque causing near occlusion of the proximal right internal carotid artery (*arrow*), (**b**) ultrasound image demonstrated markedly elevated velocities consistent with greater than 80% stenosis of the proximal right internal carotid artery, and (**c**) PET/CT revealed large FGD-avid right neck lymph node. At 5 year post-treatment, (**d**) CT showed no evidence of recurrent cancer and satisfactory appearance of the right internal carotid artery patch angioplasty (*arrow*), and (**e**) normal flow velocities in the right internal carotid artery on Doppler ultrasound

vascular intervention to repair carotid artery rupture using covered stent can be a life-saving measure. Muscle flap reconstruction is often required to provide adequate soft tissue coverage of the carotid artery and soft tissue defect in irradiated neck wound (Fig. 10.11).

The incidence perioperative stroke risk after neck dissection for head and neck cancer patients remains debatable with reports ranging from 0.2% to as high as 4.8% [38, 39]. We currently screened patients with newly diagnosed oropharyngeal or nasopharyngeal cancers for carotid artery disease if they have underlying risk factors for atherosclerotic disease such as tobacco smoking, older age, diabetes, hypertension, or hyperlipidemia. Screened patients are initiated on antiplatelet and statin therapy if found to have greater than 50% stenosis of the internal carotid artery. On rare occasions, we have successfully performed concomitant oncologic neck surgery such as nodal dissection, thyroidectomy, tracheal and esophageal resection combined with carotid endarterectomy in patients also found to have severe carotid artery stenosis (>80% stenosis) (Fig. 10.12). For cancer survivors who develop asymptomatic carotid artery stenosis following neck radiation, more studies are needed to determine whether any carotid intervention is indicated over best medical therapy. Currently, we reserved carotid intervention in asymptomatic patients only for truly high-grade (>80% stenosis). It is conceivable that early medical intervention can alter or halt the progression of radiation induced carotid plaque formation, but the role of routine screening for carotid disease in head and neck cancer patients remains to be determined in future longitudinal prospective studies. This is particularly important as we consider the changing demographics of patients diagnosed with oropharyngeal cancer. The new emerging data show that affected patients are of younger age and predominantly male (without cardiovascular risk factors), and have higher prevalence of human papilloma virus (HPV) infection and better long-term survival than in the past [40].

Peri-operative Stroke Prevention

Routine preoperative carotid screening for cancer patients prior to oncologic surgical resection is generally not recommended. Carotid intervention for unilateral asymptomatic carotid stenosis is not warranted as the perioperative stroke risk is low in non-cardiac and non-vascular surgery [41]. However, some patients with bilateral high-grade carotid artery stenosis (or unilateral high grade carotid stenosis with contralateral carotid occlusion) may benefit from carotid revascularization before elective oncologic surgery. We have favored offering surgical carotid endarterectomy for these patients unless they are deemed to have high medical or anatomical risks. The rationale for carotid endarterectomy rather than carotid stenting is in part because of the need for at least 4–6 weeks of uninterrupted clopidogrel treatment after stenting, which would increase the perioperative risk of bleeding or delay oncologic surgery significantly. Typically, patients recover quickly after carotid endarterectomy and are ready for major oncologic surgery within 1–2 weeks, requiring only maintenance aspirin therapy peri-operatively.

The optimal level of blood pressure during surgery to prevent stroke is still controversial. For patients with occlusive cerebrovascular disease including carotid disease, we recommend keeping the peri-operative mean arterial systolic blood pressure at a level similar to preoperative baseline, or at 80–100 mmHg (permissive hypertension) to keep relatively higher cerebral perfusion pressure. In patients with known cardiovascular diseases, early resumption (or initiation) of aspirin and statin has been shown to reduce cardiovascular events [41]. Two particular subtypes of solid tumors, lung cancer and urothelial (urinary bladder) are particularly associated with tobacco smoking. Expectedly, there is a higher incidence of carotid disease and cardiovascular complications in these two subgroups of patients undergoing oncologic surgery. Cardiovascular screening and optimal medical therapy is strongly recommended in these patients with cardiovascular risk factors.

Carotid Body Tumor

Carotid body tumor (CBT) is the most common head and neck paraganglioma, a rare neuroendocrine tumor. CBT typically presents sporadically in the third or fourth decade as a slow-growing unilateral painless neck mass that is located in the carotid artery bifurcation. CBT is benign in >95% of cases with small risk of malignancy. Surgical resection is the treatment of choice for CBT. Pre-operative embolization for CBT >5 cm can be done prior to surgical excision and may help reduce intra-operative blood loss, although a recent meta-analysis did not show any benefit [42]. CBT has a very typical appearance on imaging (ultrasound, CT or MR). It is seen as a hypervascular mass, getting its blood supply from branches of the external carotid artery (most commonly the ascending pharyngeal branch), splaying the carotid artery bifurcation. Approximately 90% of CBTs can be resected without carotid artery reconstruction and only 10% require some form of carotid reconstruction such as graft interposition, patch angioplasty or primary repair [43]. The incidence of cranial nerve injury is slightly higher in patients with large tumor size (>5 cm). Surgical treatment is curative. Patients with heritable head and neck paragangliomas are more likely to present at a younger age, and have bilateral CBTs and multiple paragangliomas [44]. Management of a large CBT is shown in Fig. 10.13.

Recommendations Regarding Carotid Screening

Many professional societies and associations, including the Society for Vascular Surgery, the American Heart Association, American Stroke Association, and the American College of Cardiology, have put forth guidelines and recommendations regarding the management of extra-cranial carotid disease, individually or part of consensus statement [4, 7]. We have adopted these recommendations in part and put forth the following guidelines for carotid screening [45]:

1. Carotid duplex ultrasound in an accredited vascular laboratory is the initial diagnostic imaging of choice for screening and evaluating the severity of stenosis in asymptomatic and symptomatic patients.
2. Asymptomatic patients should be screened only if they have one or more of the following associated conditions:
   (a) Symptomatic peripheral arterial disease
   (b) Coronary artery disease

(c) Risk factors for atherosclerosis including tobacco smoking, hypertension, hyperlipidemia, or family history in a first-degree relative of atherosclerosis manifested before age 60 years.

3. Routine carotid duplex ultrasound screening is *not* indicated to detect clinically asymptomatic carotid stenosis in patients without associated risk factors of atherosclerosis (including patients with incidental neck bruits). The principal rationale against screening for carotid stenosis in these patients is that the potential for overall benefit is limited by low prevalence and possible harms of intervention.

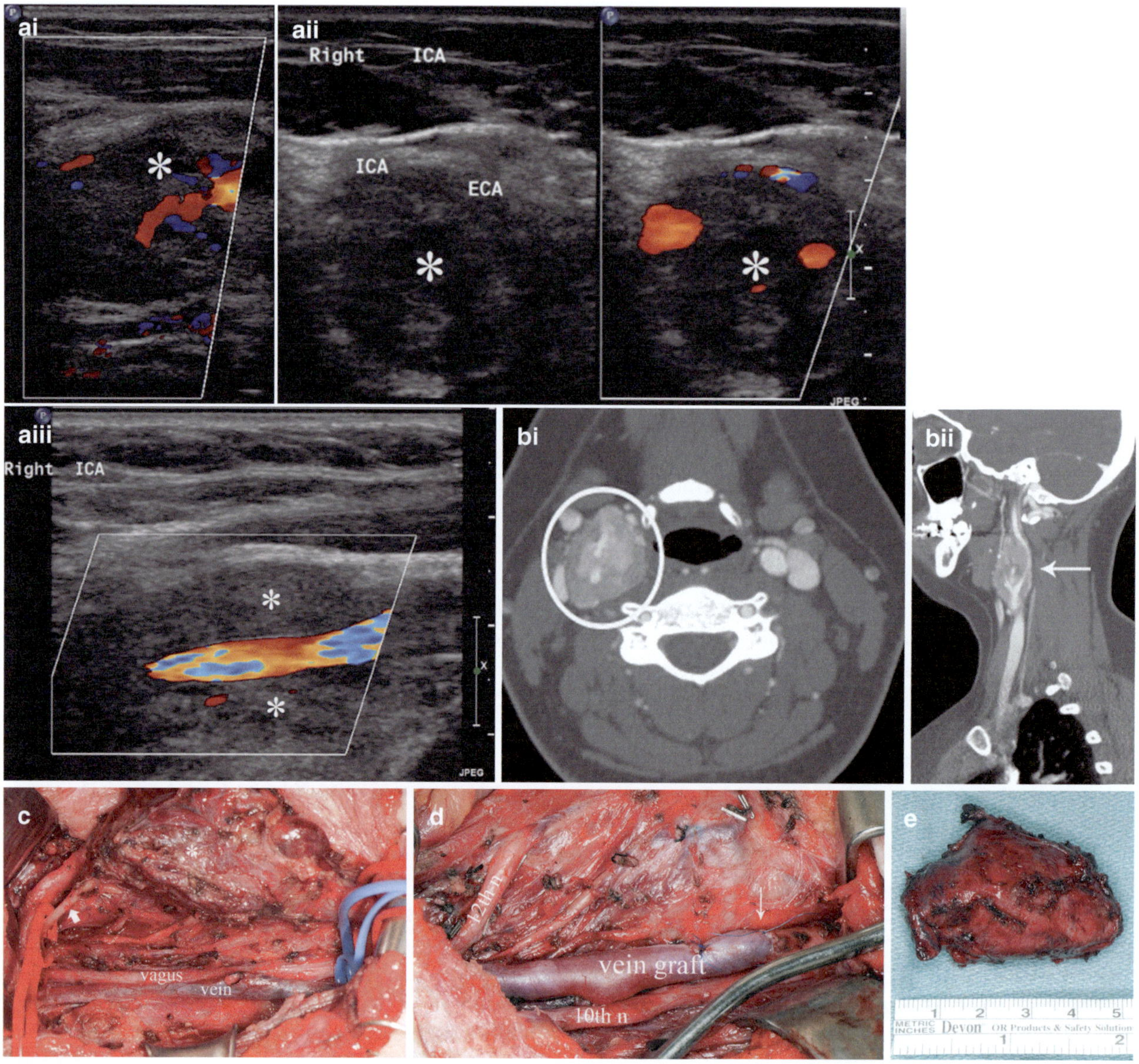

Fig. 10.13 Carotid body tumor (Paraganglioma). The majority of carotid body tumors can be resected without requiring carotid artery reconstruction. We report a relatively rare case of a 17 year-old girl who presented with a large right carotid body tumor (5 cm) encasing the carotid artery bifurcation. The ascending pharyngeal branch of the right external carotid artery, the main blood supply to the tumor, was embolized using Onyx liquid polymer the day prior to surgical resection. (**a**) Pre-operative ultrasound images show (i) the large hypervascular tumor (*asterisk*), (ii) tumor encasing the internal and external carotid arteries on axial views; longitudinal view (iii) depicts normal flow in the encased internal carotid artery. (**b**) Pre-operative CT images demonstrates the large carotid body tumor encasing the carotid artery bifurcation on axial view (i), and sagittal view (ii). (**c**) Intra-operative photograph depicts the carotid body tumor (*asterisk*) encasing the carotid artery bifurcation (mobilized medially); other structures shown include the vagus nerve (vagus), hypoglossal nerve (*arrow*), an internal jugular vein (vein). Base of the neck to the right. (**d**) Intraoperative photograph of the reconstructed carotid artery with non-reversed ipsilateral jugular vein graft (after en-bloc resection of the carotid body tumor including the carotid artery bifurcation). *Arrow* points to the proximal end-to-end anastomosis of the vein graft to the proximal common carotid artery. Base of neck to the left. (**e**) Photograph of the excised specimen.

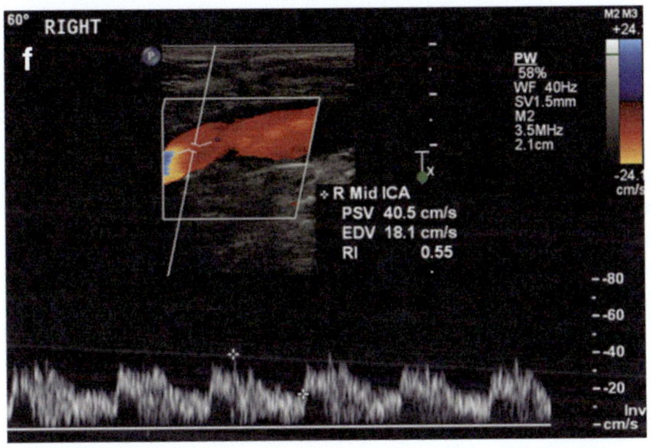

Fig. 10.13 (continued) (**f**) Duplex ultrasound surveillance of right carotid artery demonstrates satisfactory appearance of the vein graft at 22 months post-operatively

4. Post-intervention carotid duplex ultrasound surveillance is recommended within 30 days after carotid endarterectomy or stenting to assess the site of intervention. Further follow-up carotid duplex evaluation of the endarterectomy or stented carotid artery can be considered at intervals after intervention. Carotid duplex ultrasound evaluation of the contralateral carotid artery is also indicated if found to be greater than 50% stenosis.
5. We caution the use of routine screening in asymptomatic patients after neck irradiation therapy until more studies can show its benefit.

Summary

In summary, carotid endarterectomy remains the gold-standard treatment for symptomatic patients with moderate to severe carotid artery stenosis. Carotid stenting is a comparable alternative treatment in symptomatic patients deemed high-risk for carotid endarterectomy either due to medical or anatomical reasons. For asymptomatic patients with severe carotid artery stenosis, carotid endarterectomy is warranted albeit with a narrow benefit margin over best medical therapy. Head and neck cancer patients are at increased risks for radiation-induced injury. The current management of carotid disease in head and neck cancer patients follows the same principles as that for non-cancer patients. While receiving oncologic treatment patients with known cardiovascular risk factors and carotid artery stenosis should be on concurrent antiplatelet agent and statin to minimize risk of stroke. We continue to refine our diagnostic imaging, medical therapy, surgical and endovascular techniques. The results of the ongoing clinical trials will hopefully resolve the controversy as to whether either method of carotid intervention (carotid endarterectomy or stenting) is superior to best medical therapy for asymptomatic patients with severe carotid artery stenosis.

References

1. Mozaffarian D, Benjamin EJ, Go AS, Arnett DK, Blaha MJ, et al. Heart Disease and Stroke Statistics-2016 update: a report from the American Heart Association. Circulation. 2016;133(4):e38–60.
2. Petty GW, Brown RD Jr, Whisnant JP, Sicks JD, O'Fallon WM, Wiebers DO. Ischemic stroke subtypes : a population-based study of functional outcome, survival, and recurrence. Stroke. 2000;31(5):1062–8.
3. Grant EG, Benson CB, Moneta GL, Alexandrov AV, Baker JD, Bluth EI, et al. Carotid artery stenosis: gray-scale and Doppler US diagnosis–Society of Radiologists in Ultrasound Consensus Conference. Radiology. 2003;229(2):340–6.
4. Ricotta JJ, Aburahma A, Ascher E, Eskandari M, Faries P, Lal BK. Updated Society for Vascular Surgery guidelines for management of extracranial carotid disease: executive summary. J Vasc Surg. 2011;54(3):832–6.
5. Korn A, Bender B, Brodoefel H, Hauser TK, Danz S, Ernemann U, et al. Grading of carotid artery stenosis in the presence of extensive calcifications: dual-energy CT angiography in comparison with contrast-enhanced MR angiography. Clin Neuroradiol. 2013;25:33–40.
6. Etesami M, Hoi Y, Steinman DA, Gujar SK, Nidecker AE, Astor BC, et al. Comparison of carotid plaque ulcer detection using contrast-enhanced and time-of-flight MRA techniques. AJNR Am J Neuroradiol. 2013;34(1):177–84.
7. Brott TG, Halperin JL, Abbara S, Bacharach JM, Barr JD, Bush RL, et al. ASA/ACCF/AHA/AANN/AANS/ACR/ASNR/CNS/SAIP/SCAI/SIR/SNIS/SVM/SVS guideline on the management of patients with extracranial carotid and vertebral artery disease: executive summary. A report of the American College of Cardiology Foundation/American Heart Association Task Force on Practice Guidelines, and the American Stroke Association, American Association of Neuroscience Nurses, American Association of Neurological Surgeons, American College of Radiology, American Society of Neuroradiology, Congress of Neurological Surgeons, Society of Atherosclerosis Imaging and Prevention, Society for Cardiovascular Angiography and Interventions, Society of Interventional Radiology, Society of NeuroInterventional Surgery, Society for Vascular Medicine, and Society for Vascular Surgery. Circulation. 2011;124(4):489–532.
8. Collaborative meta-analysis of randomised trials of antiplatelet therapy for prevention of death, myocardial infarction, and stroke in high risk patients. BMJ. 2002;324(7329):71–86.
9. Baigent C, Blackwell L, Collins R, Emberson J, Godwin J, Peto R, et al. Aspirin in the primary and secondary prevention of vascular disease: collaborative meta-analysis of individual participant data from randomised trials. Lancet. 2009;373(9678):1849–60.
10. Plehn JF, Davis BR, Sacks FM, Rouleau JL, Pfeffer MA, Bernstein V, et al. Reduction of stroke incidence after myocardial infarction with pravastatin: the Cholesterol and Recurrent Events (CARE) study. The Care Investigators. Circulation. 1999;99(2):216–23.
11. MRC/BHF Heart Protection Study of cholesterol lowering with simvastatin in 20,536 high-risk individuals: a randomised placebo-controlled trial. Lancet. 2002;360(9326):7–22.
12. Saam T, Yuan C, Chu B, Takaya N, Underhill H, Cai J, et al. Predictors of carotid atherosclerotic plaque progression as measured by noninvasive magnetic resonance imaging. Atherosclerosis. 2007;194(2):e34–42.
13. Paciaroni M, Bogousslavsky J. Primary and secondary prevention of ischemic stroke. Eur Neurol. 2010;63(5):267–78.
14. North American Symptomatic Carotid Endarterectomy Trial Collaborators. Beneficial effect of carotid endarterectomy in symptomatic patients with high-grade carotid stenosis. N Engl J Med. 1991;325(7):445–53.

15. Barnett HJ, Taylor DW, Eliasziw M, Fox AJ, Ferguson GG, Haynes RB, et al. Benefit of carotid endarterectomy in patients with symptomatic moderate or severe stenosis. North American Symptomatic Carotid Endarterectomy Trial Collaborators. N Engl J Med. 1998;339(20):1415–25.
16. Randomised trial of endarterectomy for recently symptomatic carotid stenosis: final results of the MRC European Carotid Surgery Trial (ECST). Lancet. 1998;351(9113):1379–87.
17. Yadav JS, Wholey MH, Kuntz RE, Fayad P, Katzen BT, Mishkel GJ, et al. Protected carotid-artery stenting versus endarterectomy in high-risk patients. N Engl J Med. 2004;351(15):1493–501.
18. Mas JL, Chatellier G, Beyssen B, Branchereau A, Moulin T, Becquemin JP, et al. Endarterectomy versus stenting in patients with symptomatic severe carotid stenosis. N Engl J Med. 2006;355(16):1660–71.
19. Mas JL, Chatellier G, Beyssen B. Carotid angioplasty and stenting with and without cerebral protection: clinical alert from the Endarterectomy Versus Angioplasty in Patients With Symptomatic Severe Carotid Stenosis (EVA-3S) trial. Stroke. 2004;35(1):e18–20.
20. Silver FL, Mackey A, Clark WM, Brooks W, Timaran CH, Chiu D, et al. Safety of stenting and endarterectomy by symptomatic status in the Cartotid Revascularization Endarterectomy Versus Stenting Trial (CREST). Stroke. 2011;42(3):675–80.
21. Kwolek CJ, Jaff MR, Leal JI, Hopkins LN, Shah RM, Hanover TM, et al. Results of the ROADSTER multicenter trial of transcarotid stenting with dynamic flow reversal. J Vasc Surg. 2015;62(5):1227–34.
22. Kakisis JD, Avgerinos ED, Antonopoulos CN, Giannakopoulos TG, Moulakakis K, Liapis CD. The European Society for Vascular Surgery guidelines for carotid intervention: an updated independent assessment and literature review. Eur J Vasc Endovasc Surg. 2012;44(3):238–43.
23. Endarterectomy for asymptomatic carotid artery stenosis. Executive Committee for the Asymptomatic Carotid Atherosclerosis Study. JAMA 1995;273(18):1421–8.
24. Halliday A, Mansfield A, Marro J, Peto C, Peto R, Potter J, et al. Prevention of disabling and fatal strokes by successful carotid endarterectomy in patients without recent neurological symptoms: randomised controlled trial. Lancet. 2004;363(9420):1491–502.
25. Halliday A, Harrison M, Hayter E, Kong X, Mansfield A, Marro J, et al. 10-year stroke prevention after successful carotid endarterectomy for asymptomatic stenosis (ACST-1): a multicentre randomised trial. Lancet. 2010;376(9746):1074–84.
26. Rosenfield K, Matsumura JS, Chaturvedi S, Riles T, Ansel GM, Metzger DC, et al. Randomized trial of stent versus surgery for asymptomatic carotid stenosis. N Engl J Med. 2016;374(11):1011–20.
27. Plummer C, Henderson RD, O'Sullivan JD, Read SJ. Ischemic stroke and transient ischemic attack after head and neck radiotherapy: a review. Stroke. 2011;42(9):2410–8.
28. Smith GL, Smith BD, Buchholz TA, Giordano SH, Garden AS, Woodward WA, et al. Cerebrovascular disease risk in older head and neck cancer patients after radiotherapy. J Clin Oncol. 2008;26(31):5119–25.
29. Abayomi OK. Neck irradiation, carotid injury and its consequences. Oral Oncol. 2004;40(9):872–8.
30. Cheng SW, Wu LL, Ting AC, Lau H, Lam LK, Wei WI. Irradiation-induced extracranial carotid stenosis in patients with head and neck malignancies. Am J Surg. 1999;178(4):323–8.
31. Carmody BJ, Arora S, Avena R, Curry KM, Simpkins J, Cosby K, et al. Accelerated carotid artery disease after high-dose head and neck radiotherapy: is there a role for routine carotid duplex surveillance? J Vasc Surg. 1999;30(6):1045–51.
32. Cheng SW, Ting AC, Ho P, Wu LL. Accelerated progression of carotid stenosis in patients with previous external neck irradiation. J Vasc Surg. 2004;39(2):409–15.
33. Ikawa H, Sato K, Tonogi M, Yamane GY, Kimura M, Tatsuno S, et al. Head and neck contrast-enhanced CT for identification of internal carotid artery stenosis progression on the affected side after treatment for oral squamous cell carcinoma. Oral Radiol. 2013;29(1):1–5.
34. Kashyap VS, Moore WS, Quinones-Baldrich WJ. Carotid artery repair for radiation-associated atherosclerosis is a safe and durable procedure. J Vasc Surg. 1999;29(1):90–6, discussion 97–9
35. Tallarita T, Oderich GS, Lanzino G, Cloft H, Kallmes D, Bower TC, et al. Outcomes of carotid artery stenting versus historical surgical controls for radiation-induced carotid stenosis. J Vasc Surg. 2011;53(3):629–36.e1–5.
36. Favre JP, Nourissat A, Duprey A, Nourissat G, Albertini JN, Becquemin JP. Endovascular treatment for carotid artery stenosis after neck irradiation. J Vasc Surg. 2008;48(4):852–8.
37. Ravin RA, Gottlieb A, Pasternac K, Cayne N, Schneider D, Krishnan P, et al. Carotid artery stenting may be performed safely in patients with radiation therapy-associated carotid stenosis without increased restenosis or target lesion revascularization. J Vasc Surg. 2015;62(3):624–30.
38. Thompson SK, Southern DA, McKinnon JG, Dort JC, Ghali WA. Incidence of perioperative stroke after neck dissection for head and neck cancer: a regional outcome analysis. Ann Surg. 2004;239(3):428–31.
39. Macellari F, Paciaroni M, Agnelli G, Caso V. Perioperative stroke risk in nonvascular surgery. Cerebrovasc Dis. 2012;34(3):175–81.
40. Pytynia KB, Dahlstrom KR, Sturgis EM. Epidemiology of HPV-associated oropharyngeal cancer. Oral Oncol. 2014;50(5):380–6.
41. Selim M. Perioperative stroke. N Engl J Med. 2007;356(7):706–13.
42. Abu-Ghanem S, Yehuda M, Carmel NN, Abergel A, Fliss DM. Impact of preoperative embolization on the outcomes of carotid body tumor surgery: a meta-analysis and review of the literature. Head Neck. 2016;38(Suppl 1):E2386–94.
43. Power AH, Bower TC, Kasperbauer J, Link MJ, Oderich G, Cloft H, et al. Impact of preoperative embolization on outcomes of carotid body tumor resections. J Vasc Surg. 2012;56(4):979–89.
44. Sridhara SK, Yener M, Hanna EY, Rich T, Jimenez C, Kupferman ME. Genetic testing in head and neck paraganglioma: who, what, and why? J Neurol Surg B Skull Base. 2013;74(4):236–40.
45. Huynh TT, Broadbent KC, Jacob AD, James S, Erasmus JJ. Screening for carotid artery stenosis. Semin Roentgenol. 2015;50(2):127–38.

Venous Diseases in Malignancy

11

Rohit Ram and Joshua Kuban

Abstract

Malignancy is known to induce a hypercoagulable state and literature evidence has long supported that a significant proportion of morbidity and mortality in patients with a known malignancy is attributable to thromboembolic events. A high incidence of venous and, to a lesser extent, arterial thrombosis is observed and in several instances a thromboembolic event such as deep venous thrombosis or pulmonary embolism may be the presenting event that leads to unmasking an underlying malignancy. This dates back to Trousseau's astute description in 1860s of migratory thrombophlebitis harboring an occult malignancy [1].

Keywords

Venous disease • Malignancy

Malignancy is known to induce a hypercoagulable state and literature evidence has long supported that a significant proportion of morbidity and mortality in patients with a known malignancy is attributable to thromboembolic events. A high incidence of venous and, to a lesser extent, arterial thrombosis is observed and in several instances a thromboembolic event such as deep venous thrombosis or pulmonary embolism may be the presenting event that leads to unmasking an underlying malignancy. This dates back to Trousseau's astute description in 1860s of migratory thrombophlebitis harboring an occult malignancy [1].

The primary mechanism by which a prothrombotic state is induced is complex, and fundamentally involves increase in expression of hemostatic proteins (tumor factor), inflammatory cytokines (tumor necrosis factor-alpha, interleukin-1), angiogenic factors (vascular endothelial growth factor) and adhesion molecules [2]. Recent evidence demonstrates that alteration in host response and hemostatic mechanisms also promotes tumor progression, and certain types of malignancies specifically activate clotting and upregulate procoagulant molecules as part of the neoplastic transformation [2]. Independent host risk factors associated with increased thrombosis such as advanced age, sex, obesity, immobilization and treatment related risk factors of hypercoagulability, both surgical and medical, add to the increased incidence of thromboembolic events in patients with a malignancy. The clinical presentation of a patient in a procoagulant state is not always predictable and the spectrum ranges from subclinical thrombophilia sometimes evidenced only by laboratory abnormalities in coagulation studies, or present with fatal pulmonary embolism or stroke. Clinicians have advocated the use of risk assessment models to stratify patients for better screening and prompt institution of treatment. In this chapter, we present a variety of primary venous thromboembolic (VTE) manifestations of malignancy, the diagnosis and management of complications related to such events.

Deep Venous Thrombosis

Venous thromboembolic disease can be broadly categorized into deep venous thrombosis (DVT) and pulmonary embolism (PE) and is thought to represent 1% of hospital admissions in the US. In the general public, there are approximately 900,000 cases of VTE per year resulting in up to 300,000 deaths [3], and is now the third most common cause of life-threatening cardiovascular disease in the United States. Although DVT and PE are categorized separately, the underlying pathophysiology is identical and represents two entities in the spectrum of VTE.

R. Ram, M.D. • J. Kuban, M.D. (✉)
University of Texas MD Anderson Cancer Center, Baylor College of Medicine, Houston, TX, USA
e-mail: jdkuban@mdanderson.org

S.W. Yusuf, J. Banchs (eds.), *Cancer and Cardiovascular Disease*, https://doi.org/10.1007/978-3-319-62088-6_11

Over the years, there has been an increase in overall reports of VTE in cancer patients and can be attributed to an increased awareness of risk and more patients undergoing cancer treatments [4]. Population based studies have assessed risk factors for development of DVT and demonstrated malignancy as an independent risk factor in 18–34% of cases [3, 5]. In fact, depending on the type of malignancy and presence of metastases, the risk of acquiring a first time venous thrombosis rises up to seven fold (odds ratio 6.7; 95% confidence interval, 5.2–8.6) [6]. When combined with additional risk factors such as surgery, hospitalization, immobility, and chemotherapy, the risk of DVT rises substantially. This has been validated both in the US and Europe. A cohort study from the UK estimated that incidence of venous thrombosis for all types of cancer was 13.9 per 1000 person-years (95% CI: 13.4–14.4) and up to 68 per 1000 person-years (95% CI: 48–96) among cancer patients with high-grade or metastatic disease or those treated with therapeutic strategies that increased thromboembolic risk [4, 7]. In another study by Blom et al., patients with metastatic disease were 20 times more likely to have a VTE than those with local disease, and 50 times more likely to have an event than controls without cancer [6, 8].

Primary factors that contribute to development of thrombosis can be attributed to Virchow's triad of hypercoagulability, stasis and endothelial injury. In a healthy adult, small thrombi form in the deep veins, however, an intact thrombolytic system is able to prevent progression to a larger thrombus. When the thrombolytic system is overwhelmed or impaired, this dynamic process is interrupted and leads to larger thrombus formation that eventually may lead to clinical symptoms.

Classification

Diagnosis of DVT is most commonly confirmed by ultrasound examination of the extremities, which demonstrates echogenic intraluminal thrombus, which may be non-compressible or partially compressible, with or without blood flow (Fig. 11.1). Findings vary depending on the severity and duration of occlusion. In the lower extremity, DVT can be further subcategorized based on location—proximal DVT such as those affecting the iliofemoral and popliteal veins (*see Iliofemoral*) and distal DVT that are primarily below the popliteal trifurcation affecting the calf and distal veins. In the past, distal (below the knee) DVTs were thought to be clinically insignificant and were not screened for in an asymptomatic patient. However, the rate of proximal extension of distal DVTs has been debated, and there is evidence from smaller studies to suggest that, in the short term, patients harboring a malignancy with distal DVTs are still at high risk for PE and recurrent VTE [9–12].

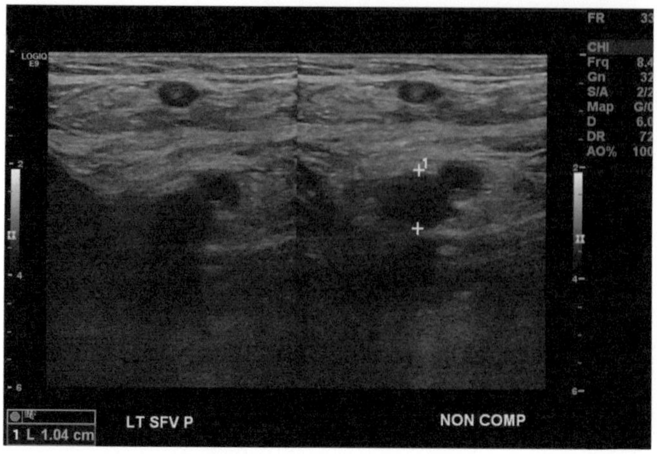

Fig. 11.1 Grayscale images demonstrating echogenic, non-compressible clot within the left femoral vein and peroneal veins

Iliofemoral

Acute iliofemoral DVT is defined as complete or partial occlusion of the iliac vein and/or the common femoral vein that has been present for less than 14 days [13]. The commonly described scenario involves compression of the left iliac vein between the right iliac artery and a lumbar vertebral body (May Thurner Syndrome, Fig. 11.2). The distinction between iliofemoral and a more distal DVT (e.g. infrapopliteal) is important, as the latter group is more amenable to endogenous recanalization and development of collateral circulation. An occluded iliac or proximal femoral vein rarely recanalizes and leads to chronic venous outflow obstruction [14]. Increased incidences of post-thrombotic syndrome (discussed below), valve incompetency leading to venous reflux and claudication, poor physical functioning and worsening quality of life have all been reported [15]. Due to serious long-term complications, identification of this particular entity is important as management varies from a popliteal DVT (discussed under treatment).

Complications

Although pulmonary embolism is the most feared complication of DVT, long-term complications such as post-thrombotic syndrome (PTS) and to a lesser extent chronic pulmonary hypertension are also debilitating. PTS is reported in 20–50% of patients even with appropriate treatment [16, 17] and is a constellation of findings wherein patients present with chronic limb pain, swelling, cramping, heaviness, edema and in extreme cases, venous ulcers. Recurrent DVT is an additional complication of VTE with an approximately 30% 10 year recurrence rate, with the highest recurrence occurring within the first 6 months [18]. A population cohort study of residents in Olmsted County, MN by Heit et al. evaluated effectiveness of anticoagulation and reported that active cancer was the

Fig. 11.2 Eighteen year old female who originally presented with left lower extremity swelling and suspicion for May Thurner syndrome presents again with worsening swelling. Digital subtraction angiography images of the left common iliac vein (LCIV) demonstrate complete occlusion of the LCIV at the confluence (*black arrow*) and no flow of contrast in the inferior vena cava. There are multiple lumbar collaterals (*white arrows*) that drain centrally

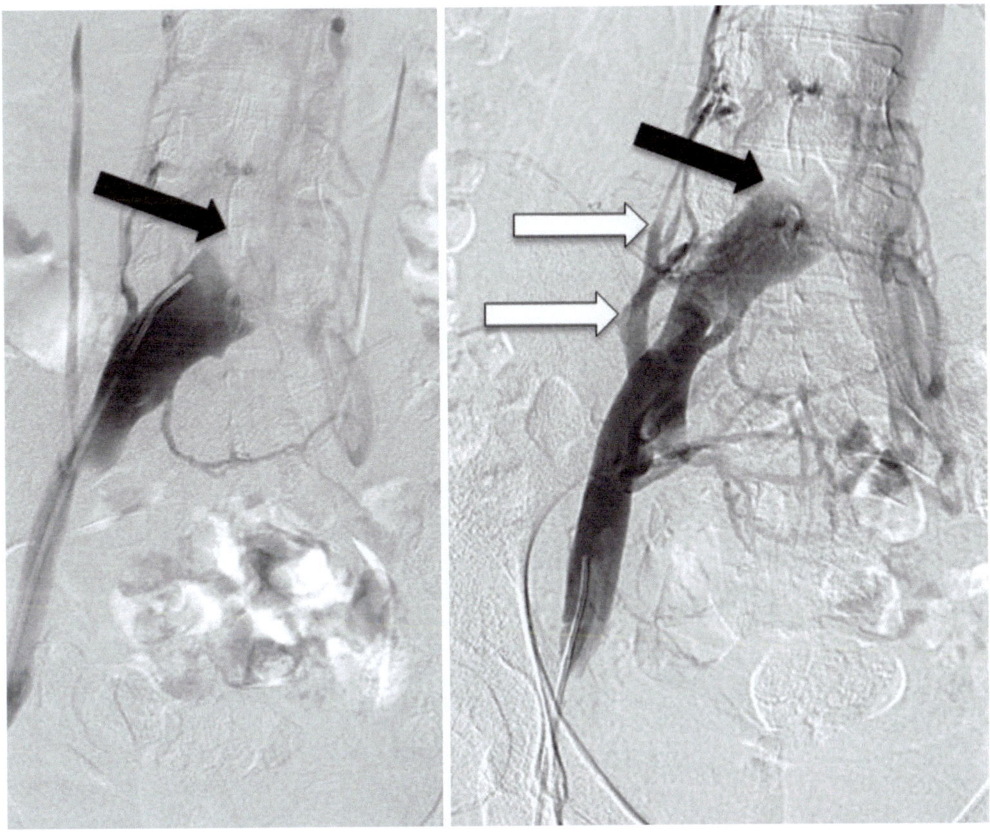

only independent predictor of early VTE recurrence, with about a three-fold increased hazard rate [19]. Another study, utilizing the same cohort of patients, showed that malignant neoplasms accounts for almost one fifth of all cases of VTE in the community [20]. About 16% of active cancer patients develop recurrence within 6 months compared to 4% of patients with idiopathic VTE [18].

Presentation

The clinical presentation of DVT varies depending on the site of thrombosis but classically, patients present with swelling, pain and erythema of the involved extremity (Fig. 11.3). There is significant overlap in presentation with other conditions and differential considerations include cellulitis, musculoskeletal strain or injury, superficial thrombophlebitis, lymphatic obstruction and chronic venous insufficiency [21]. While patients with cancer are at highest risk for developing DVTs, finding a DVT in an otherwise "normal" patient should not lead to a malignancy workup [22]. In the setting of malignancy, however, patients are at highest risk for developing DVTs within the first few months of diagnosis [6].

For patients with large iliofemoral clot burden, acute phlegmasia may be a rare but potentially fatal presentation with evidence of arterial insufficiency due to severe venous outflow obstruction. There is evidence of marked swelling

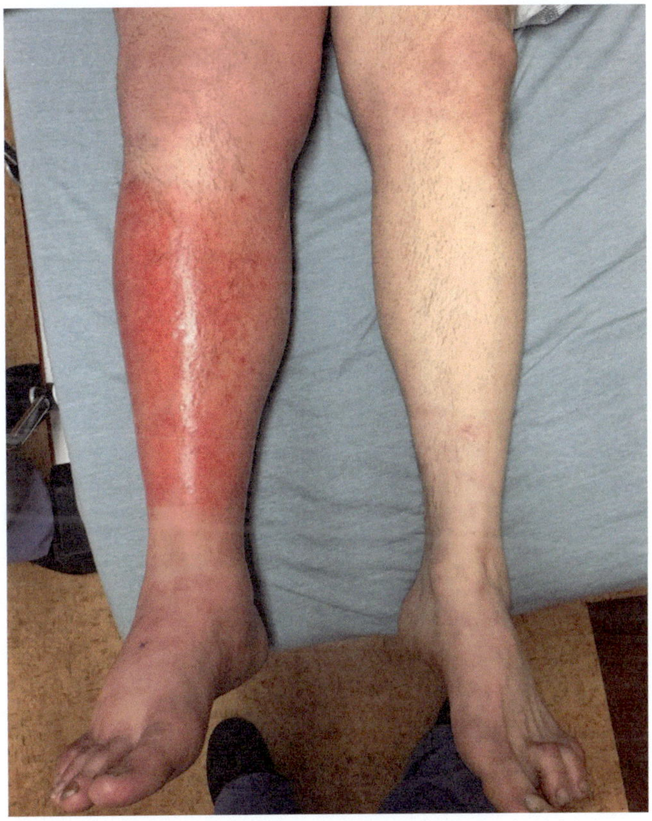

Fig. 11.3 Right lower extremity acute DVT. Note swelling, erythema and skin changes

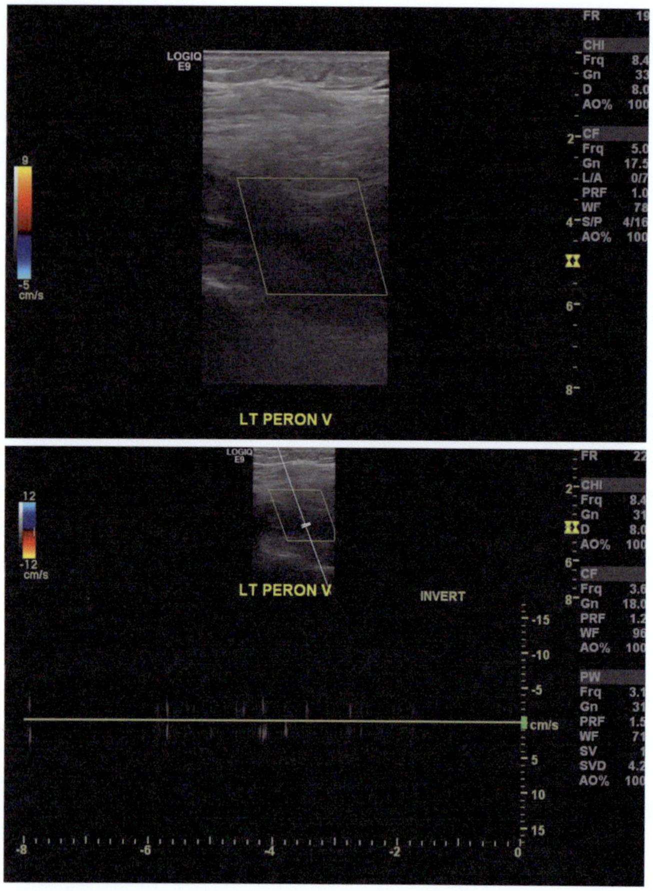

Fig. 11.4 Color Doppler images of the peroneal vein ("distal DVT") demonstrating no color flow (*top image*). Spectral Doppler tracing reveals no waveforms compatible with occlusive thrombus

and discoloration, which eventually leads to compartment syndrome, arterial compromise and venous gangrene. Malignancy is the most common risk factor in patients presenting with phlegmasia cerulea dolens [23].

Diagnosis

Diagnosis of DVT should initially start with a clinical probability assessment such as the Wells score [24] or the Geneva score [25]. D-dimer is a degradation product of a cross-linked fibrin clot frequently used an adjunct laboratory marker and in combination with a low pre-test probability, has a high negative predictive value for isolated DVT [11]. For peripheral extremity DVT, venous ultrasound with compression has remained the mainstay of noninvasive imaging and has largely replaced venography (Figs. 11.4, 11.5, and 11.6). For the deep pelvic veins, however, ultrasound is limited by poor acoustic windows and in these scenarios CT, or less commonly MR venography offers a more sensitive evaluation (Fig. 11.7). Catheter-based diagnostic venography is rarely used, though this technique was the historical gold standard for diagnosis (Fig. 11.8). Catheter venography is still used in preparation for catheter based intervention.

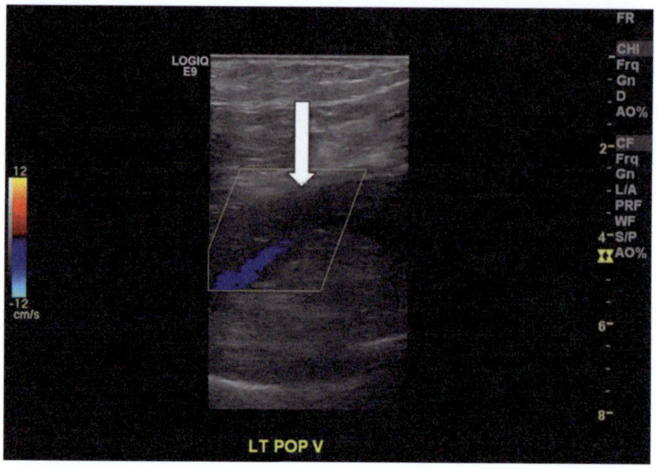

Fig. 11.5 Color Doppler image of the popliteal vein demonstrates echogenic thrombus within the vein (*arrow*). Color flow is demonstrated in the adjacent popliteal artery

Treatment

The treatment algorithm of venous thromboembolic disease is aimed at preventing pulmonary embolism, to decrease the risk of clot propagation, DVT recurrence and post-thrombotic syndrome. Treatment can be broadly categorized as medical, surgical or catheter directed. Surgical thrombectomy is reserved for very few scenarios (see iliofemoral).

Medical

Pharmacologic approach classically has involved initiation of IV heparin such as unfractionated heparin (UFH), a mixture of sulphated glucosaminoglycans that binds to antithrombin (AT), and inactivates several clotting factors (Xa, IXa, XIa, XIIa) including thrombin (factor IIa). In the unfractionated form, UFH contains polymers of several lengths and weights that are not fractioned with non-specific binding affinities to endothelial cells and platelets. This contributes to its unpredictable pharmacokinetics and increased incidence of side effects. Low molecular weight heparin (LMWH) on the other hand is the fractionated form that is derived from UFH by depolymerization, with a more predictable dose-response and fewer side effects. Although UFH had been used for several decades, the improved and desired safety profile and equal effectiveness of LMWH has mostly replaced UFH. Vitamin K antagonist (VKA), mainly warfarin, is the most common anticoagulant used for prevention and long-term treatment of VTE. The main disadvantages include slow onset of action, various interactions with food and other drugs, narrow therapeutic window and need for close monitoring. Patients can easily under treat or over treat and adverse effects can be fatal if compliance is not strict, both by providers and patients.

Newer generation of anticoagulants have been developed to increase the safety and efficacy of systemic therapy, and target specific factors in the coagulation cascade. Fondaparinux

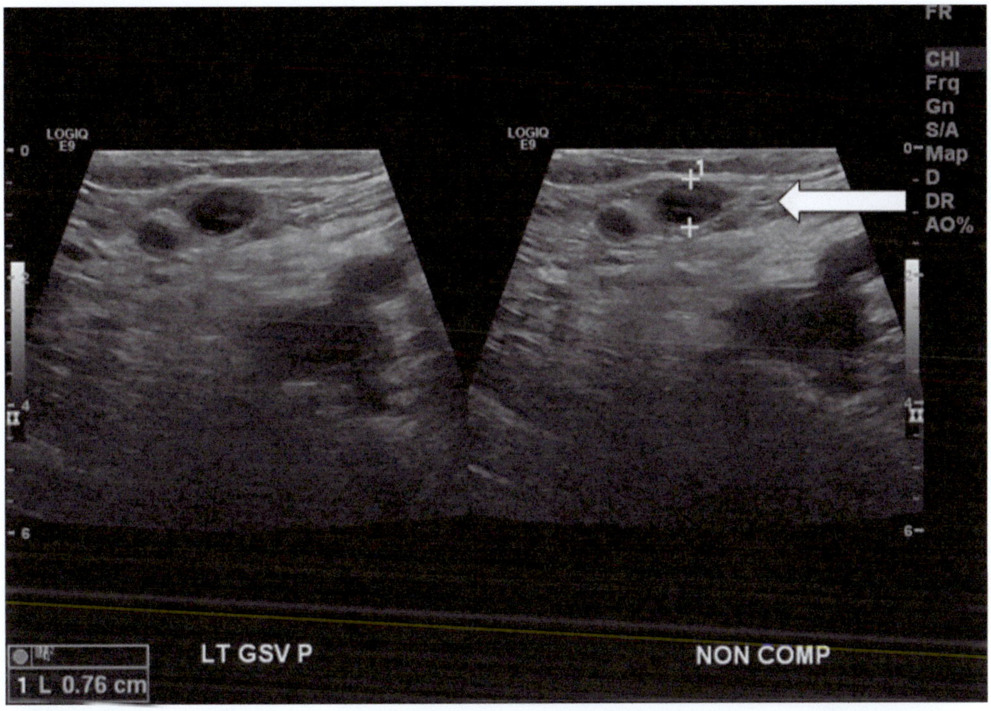

Fig. 11.6 Non-compressible and echogenic intraluminal thrombus in the left greater saphenous vein (GSV). Although the GSV is considered a superficial vein, there should be a thorough investigation as there is a high incidence of concomitant DVT, especially in those patients harboring a malignancy

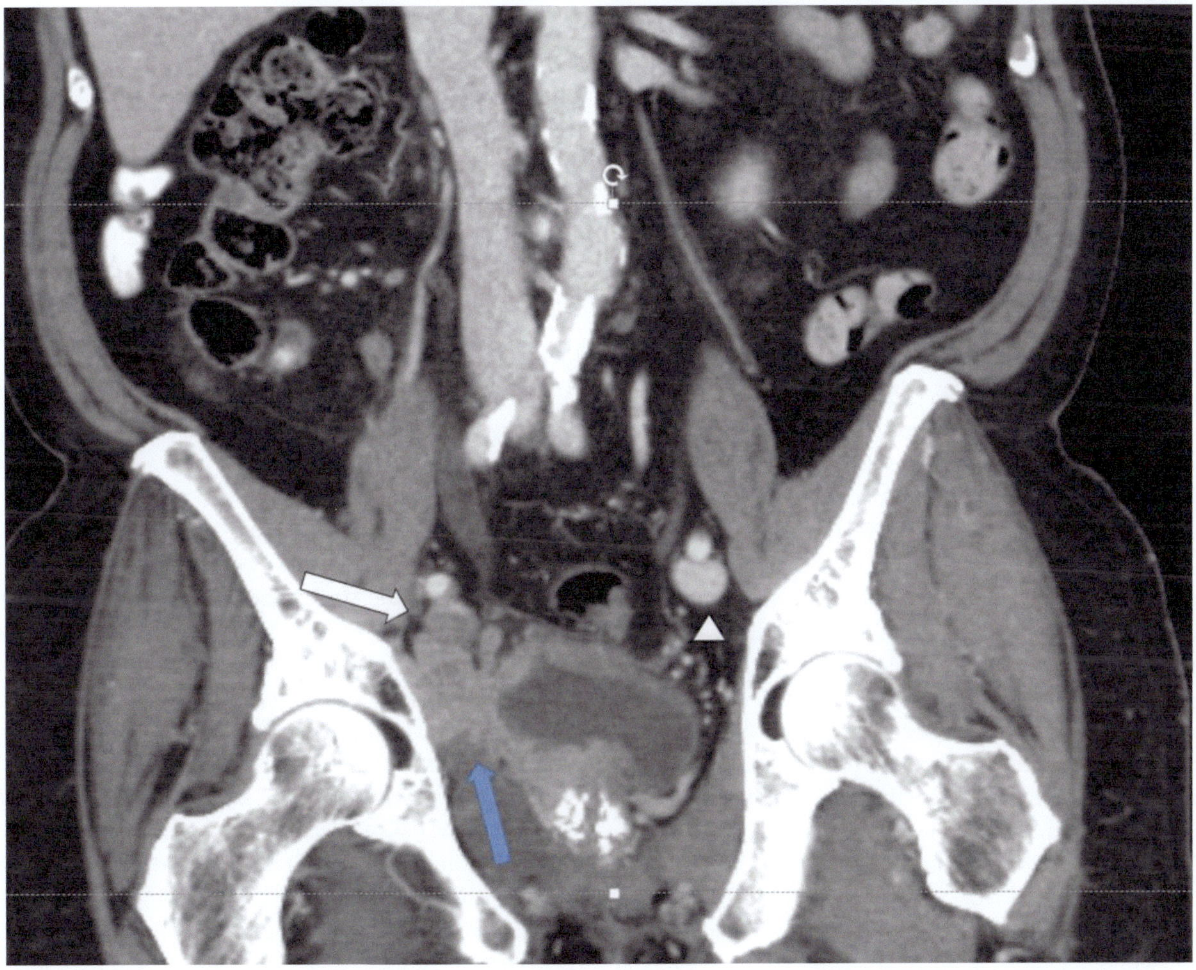

Fig. 11.7 Acute right iliac deep venous thrombosis on CT venogram. Intraluminal filling defect in the right iliac vein (*white arrow*) compared with appearance of normal iliac vein appearance on the left side (*arrowhead*). More distally, the right external ilia vein was compressed by exophytic bladder mass (*blue arrow*)

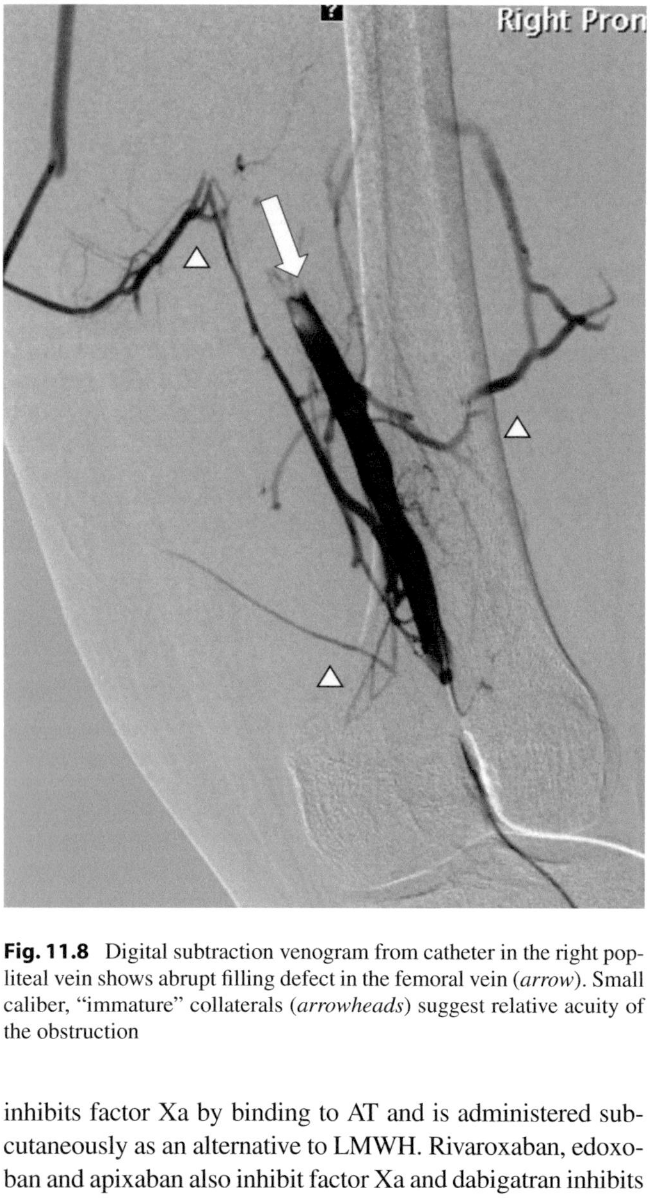

Fig. 11.8 Digital subtraction venogram from catheter in the right popliteal vein shows abrupt filling defect in the femoral vein (*arrow*). Small caliber, "immature" collaterals (*arrowheads*) suggest relative acuity of the obstruction

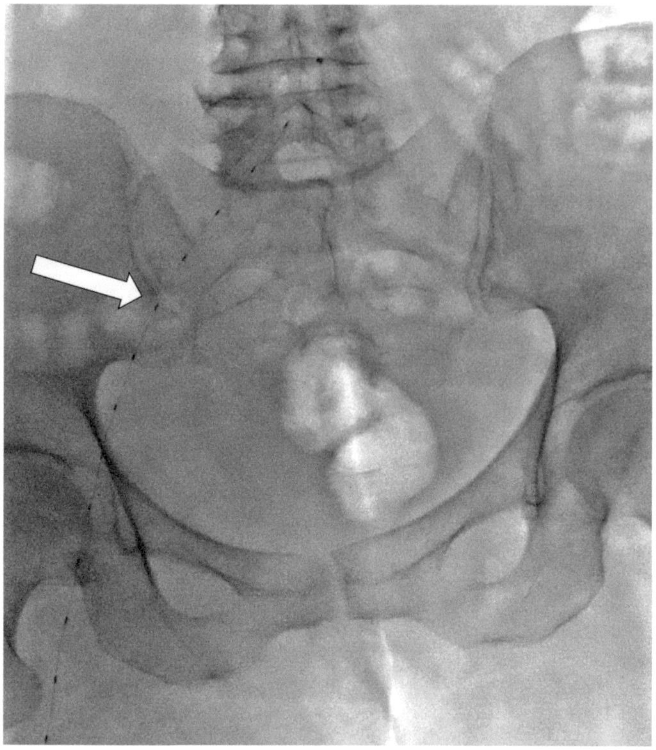

Fig. 11.9 Fluoroscopic spot image of the pelvis demonstrates an EKOS infusion catheter placed in the left femoral, external and common iliac veins for catheter directed thrombolysis

inhibits factor Xa by binding to AT and is administered subcutaneously as an alternative to LMWH. Rivaroxaban, edoxoban and apixaban also inhibit factor Xa and dabigatran inhibits thrombin and are all administered orally and referred to as non-vitamin K oral anticoagulants (NOACs). There is now enough evidence (RE-COVER, RE-COVER II, EINSTEIN DVT, EINSTEIN PE, AMPLIFY, Holusai-VTE trials) [26–31] that the newer oral anticoagulants are safer and equally effective, that in the most recent AT10 guidelines, ACCP now recommends NOACs over VKA therapy for patients with DVT of the leg or PE and without cancer [32]. For patients with cancer, LMWH is still preferred over VKA and the NOACs [32].

Acute therapy should be aimed at prevention extension of thrombus or PE, and should continue for a transient period until the thrombus has recanalized or organized, or the "activated" inflammatory state has resolved [18]. ACCP has specific recommendations for various clinical scenarios, but generally, medical therapy is continued for 3 months for patients without cancer. In patients with DVT or PE and active cancer (cancer-associated thrombosis), who do not have high bleeding risk the recommendation is for extended anticoagulant therapy (no scheduled stop date) over 3 months of therapy (Grade 1B) [32]. For cancer associated thrombosis, LMWH is preferred over oral anticoagulants [32]. In the setting of cancer-associated thrombosis, treatment for longer than 3 months is recommended even for those patients with high bleeding risk (Grade 2B), however, with periodic reassessment [32, 33]. For extended therapy, there should generally be no need to change the choice of anticoagulant after the first 3 months unless patient's circumstances change [32, 33].

Catheter Directed Therapy

Catheter directed therapy can be divided into pharmacological, mechanical and pharmacomechanical techniques. Pharmacologic catheter directed therapy involves gaining catheter access to the thrombosed vessel and administering thrombolytic medications directly into the clot, usually alteplase (tPA). The advantage of local delivery is the ability to achieve high concentrations of tPA within the clot without high systemic concentrations, thereby minimizing the risk of systemic bleeding complications. Catheter directed thrombolysis (CDT) is usually administered via a multiside hole infusion catheter (Fig. 11.9).

Mechanical catheter techniques include clot disruption, rheolytic aspiration, suction thrombectomy and stent-assisted thrombectomy. Pharmacomechanical thrombolysis refers to a combination of catheter directed thrombolysis in

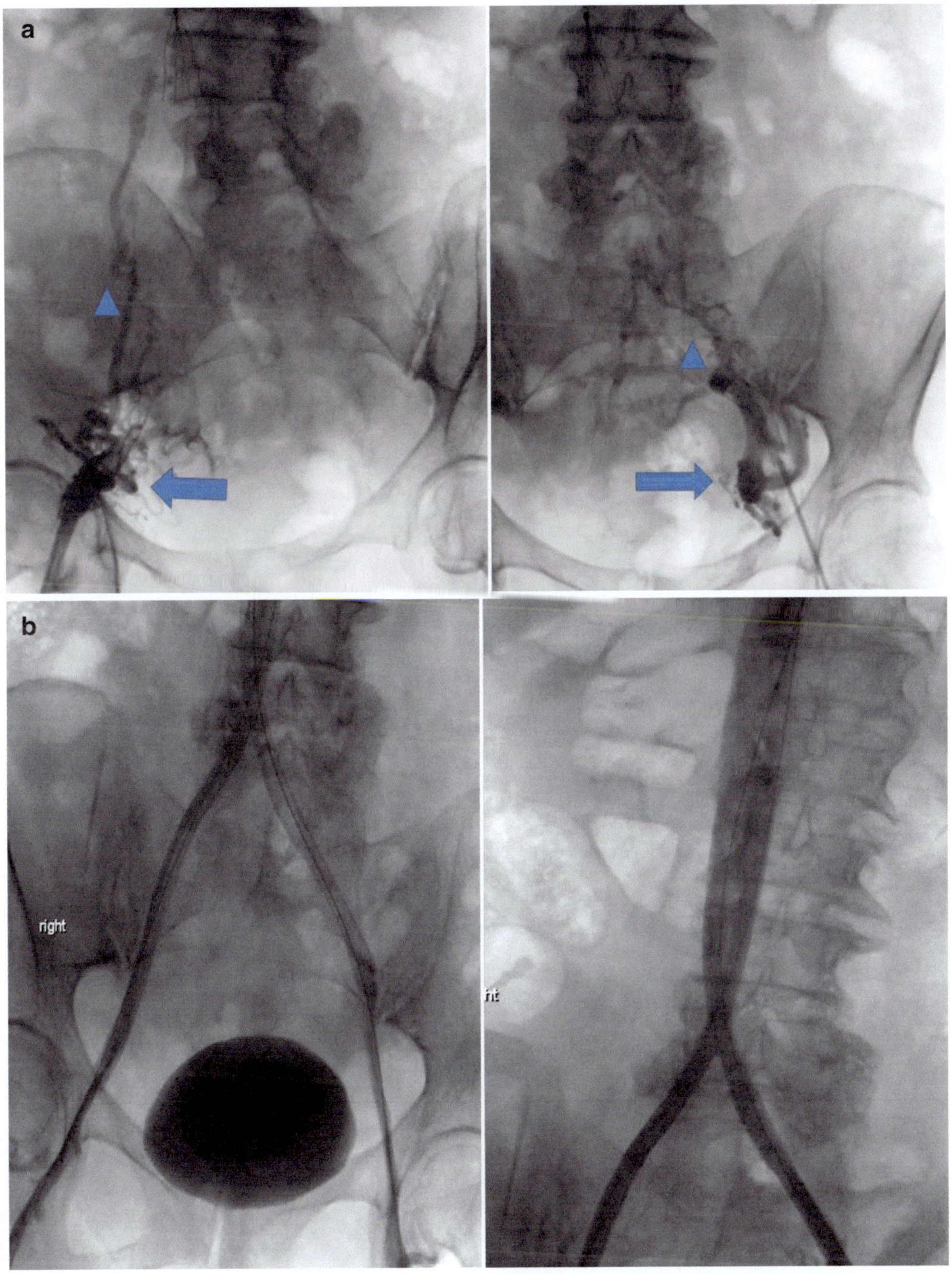

Fig. 11.10 (**a**) 71F with bilateral leg swelling and pain. Bilateral iliac venograms from catheters in the common femoral veins show chronic total occlusion of both external iliac veins (*arrows*). Collateral veins (*arrowheads*) have formed in an attempt to circumvent the occlusions. (**b**) Bilateral venograms after bilateral iliac stent placement and angioplasty show restored venous flow without filling of collaterals. Note the IVC filter has been removed

conjunction with mechanical disruption or thrombectomy. Result in experimental model indicates that ultrasound exposure causes reversible disaggregation of the uncrossed linked fibers into smaller fibers, which may alter flow resistance and improve fibrinolytic therapy [34]. A subtype of pharmacomechanical thrombolysis is ultrasound-assisted thrombolysis (UAST). In this technique, a catheter (Ekos catheter, Ekos, Bothell, WA) is placed across the thrombosed vessel that both infuses thrombolytic medications and delivers high frequency, low power sound waves to loosen clot and expose plasminogen receptor sites [35]. Once the acute thrombus is removed, any underlying cause of obstruction can be treated with angioplasty or stent placement (Fig. 11.10).

The main complications of CDT are related to major bleeding risks such as intracranial hemorrhage and those extra-cranial bleeds that are significant to require transfusions, cessation of therapy, or cause death. In a pooled analysis the cumulative major bleeding rate for CDT was reported to be 8% [35–37]. However, with lower doses of tPA gaining favor, rates of major bleeding complications have been decreasing.

For patients with acute iliofemoral or proximal DVT, ACCP recommends systemic anticoagulation as first line therapy [32, 33]. However, due to long-term morbidity associated with PTS, catheter directed thrombolysis techniques are supported by the Society of Interventional Radiology (SIR) for those patients who have acute iliofemoral DVT for

<14 days, good functional status, and low risk of bleeding, and in rare cases limb threatening venous compromise [32, 33, 37]. Both the SIR and AACP recognize the limitations of published studies and available evidence. Therefore, an individualized approach to stratify patients that may benefit from CDT is recommended until further evidence is established [32, 33, 37].

Pulmonary Embolism

Acute pulmonary embolism (PE) is the most feared complication of deep venous thrombosis. As mentioned earlier (see DVT), most thrombi form in the deep veins of the calf, and propagate proximally. PE is thought to be the sequela of treated or untreated thrombi commonly in the proximal lower extremity veins. Once thrombus is in the popliteal or femoral veins, approximately 50% patients are at risk for acute symptomatic pulmonary embolism [38]. A systemic review demonstrated that up to 95% of PE are caused by thrombus in the deep veins of the lower limbs [39]. Diagnosis of PE is most commonly done with CT angiography of the pulmonary artery (CTPA) (Fig. 11.11). In patients unable to have a CT scan, a nuclear medicine ventilation/perfusion scan (VQ) is most commonly used (Fig. 11.12). Catheter-based pulmonary arteriography is no longer used as a diagnostic modality but is performed as part of any catheter based intervention (see treatment below).

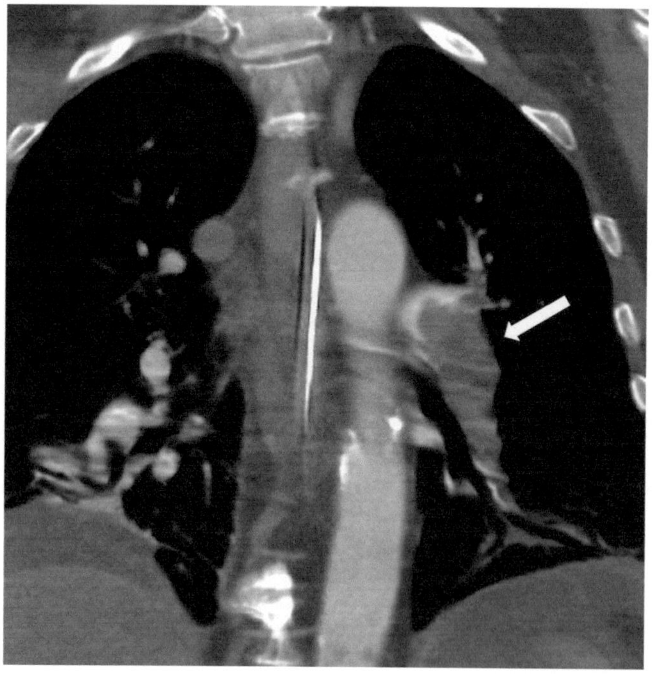

Fig. 11.11 Coronal projection from CT angiogram of the pulmonary artery shows large filing defect (*arrow*) in the left main and lower lobe pulmonary arteries

A risk-based classification taking into account patient presentation and morbidity stratifies PE as non-massive or low-risk, submassive and massive.

Massive or high risk PE is defined as acute PE with sustained hypotension (systolic blood pressure <90 mmHg for at least 15 min or requiring inotropic support), not due to a cause other than PE (i.e. arrhythmia, hypovolemia, sepsis, or left ventricular dysfunction), pulselessness, or persistent profound bradycardia (heart rate < 40 bpm with signs or symptoms of shock) [40]. Submassive PE is defined as acute PE without systemic hypotension (systolic blood pressure ≥ 90 mmHg) but with either right ventricular (RV) dysfunction (RV dilation, brain natriuretic peptide elevation, echocardiographic changes) or myocardial necrosis (elevated troponin I or troponin T) [40]. The ratio of diameters of the right ventricle to the left ventricle (RV:LV ratio) on CT is the most commonly used metric for imaging evidence of right heart dysfunction owing to its availability (Fig. 11.13). An RV:LV ratio greater than 1 is a significant predictor of persistent pulmonary symptoms and mortality at 3 months post PE. Echocardiography can be used to further investigate right heart function. Low-risk PE is defined as acute PE and the absence of the clinical markers of adverse prognosis that define massive or submassive PE [40]. The distinction is important not only for risk stratification and morbidity but also for management as discussed below.

Treatment

Systemic pharmacologic treatment for acute PE is dictated by classification. Patients with low-risk acute PE are treated with systemic anticoagulation alone. There is no role for systemic lytic treatment in this group.

For patients in the massive or high risk PE group, prompt aggressive therapy is warranted given an estimated 30% mortality for patients with acute PE and hypotension [41]. All patients in this group should be started on weight based heparin infusion with bolus dose, except where absolutely contraindicated. Current ACCP guidelines recommend administration of systemic thrombolytic therapy if no contraindication exists [32, 33]. Current guidelines are based on multiple randomized trials [42, 43], as well as analysis showing thrombolysis improves pulmonary arterial pressures, oxygenation, and pulmonary perfusion [44].

A meta-analysis by Wan et al. analyzed 11 randomized trials comparing heparin alone to heparin and systemic

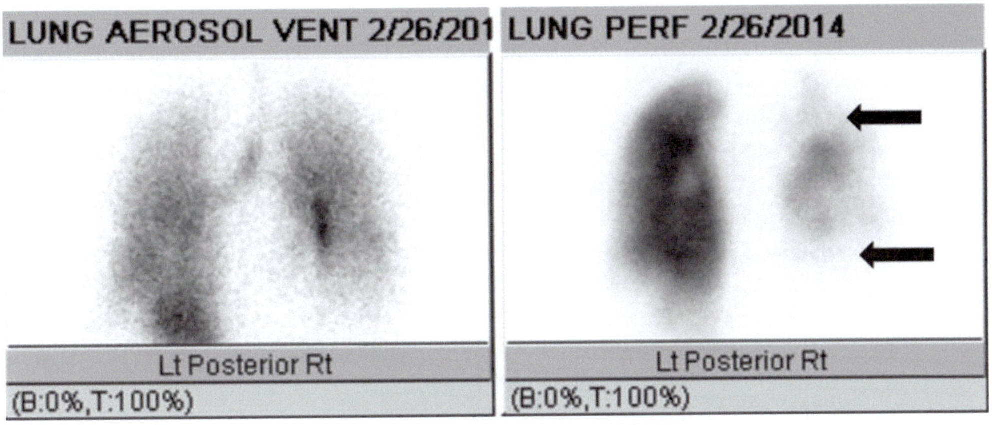

Fig. 11.12 Posterior projections of a high risk ventilation perfusion scan. The *right* images shows physiologic disruption of ventilator tracer. Image on the *left* shows multiple peripheral areas of decreased lung perfusion (*arrows*) indicating pulmonary embolism

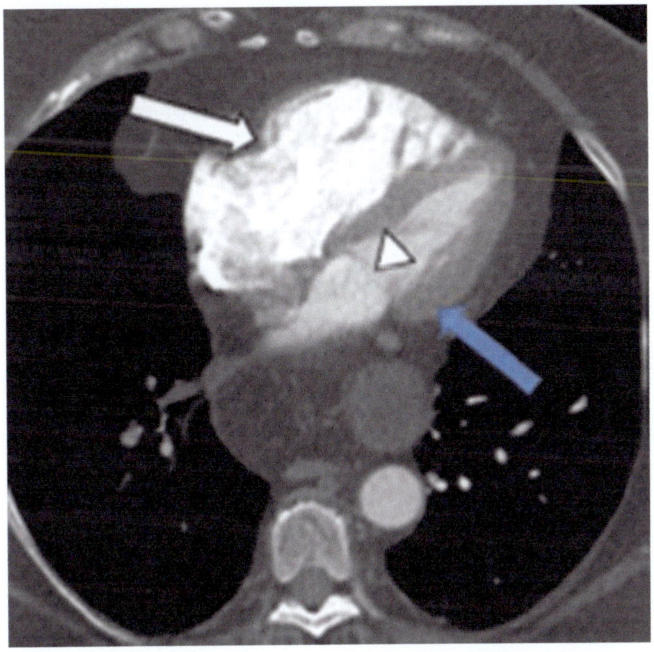

Fig. 11.13 Axial image from CT of the chest and abdomen in a patient with acute pulmonary embolism. The right ventricle (*white arrow*) is dilated and is larger in diameter than the left ventricle (*blue arrow*). The RV:LV ratio is 2.1, indicating severe right heart strain. The normally convex intraventricular septum (with respect to the ventricle) is flattened and slightly bowed toward the left ventricle (*arrowhead*)

thrombolysis, involving 748 patients with acute PE [45]. There were no significant differences in recurrent PE/death or major bleeding complications in an unselected population. However, in trials that enrolled patients with high-risk PE, patients treated with systemic thrombolysis and heparin had a significantly less recurrent PE or death compared to patients treated with heparin alone (9.4% vs. 19%, OR 0.45 95% CI 0.22–0.92). In most centers, administration of systemic thrombolytic therapy for acute high-risk PE is standard of care, except where contraindicated. Contraindications to systemic thrombolysis are the same as those encountered for acute ischemic stroke and ST segment elevation MI. Of particular note is that cancer itself does not present a contraindication to systemic thrombolysis.

For patients in the sub-massive or intermediate-risk group, current ACCP guidelines (2016) do not recommend treatment with systemic thrombolysis for most patients with intermediate-risk PE [33]. However, more recent trials addressing this issue have been completed and are worth consideration. The PEITHO trial, conducted by Meyer et al., was a randomized double-blind trial comparing treatment with heparin alone vs. heparin plus systemic thrombolysis for 1006 patients with intermediate-risk PE, specifically defined in this trial as RV dysfunction on imaging AND evidence of myonecrosis via a positive troponin test [46]. Patients treated with systemic thrombolysis had a significantly decreased incidence of the composite endpoint death/hemodynamic collapse compared with heparin alone (2.6% vs. 5.6%, $p = 0.015$). It is worth noting that there was no significant difference in mortality alone. Patients treated with systemic thrombolysis did have increased incidence of major bleeding compared with the patients treated with heparin alone (11.5% vs. 2.4%, $p < 0.0001$), including a 2.0% rate of hemorrhagic stroke in the thrombolysis group. A recent meta-analysis by Goa et al. analyzed prospective randomized controlled trials of patients with intermediate-risk PE treated with systemic thrombolysis, including PEITHO and seven additional trials encompassing 1755 patients [47]. Patients treated with systemic thrombolysis and heparin had significantly lower mortality than patients treated with heparin alone (1.39% vs. 2.92%, RR 0.52; 95% CI 0.28–0.97). However, as shown in the PEITHO trial, this decrease in mortality was at the expense of increased major bleeding events in the group treated with systemic thrombolysis (7.8% vs. 2.28% RR 3.35; 95% CI 2.03–5.54). It is worth noting that one of the randomized trials included in the study (MOPETT trial, Sharifi et al.), showed that compared with heparin alone, patients treated with low-dose systemic tPA (50 mg rather than 100 mg) and heparin had decreased incidence of recurrent PE, pulmonary hypertension, and length of hospital stay without a significant increase in major bleeding complications [48].

Further studies are needed to evaluate the impact on mortality of low dose systemic tPA as well as to identify predictive factors for subgroups of patients with submassive PE who will benefit most from systemic thrombolysis.

Catheter Directed Therapy

Catheter directed therapy (CDT) includes catheter based thrombolysis, pharmacomechanical thrombectomy and mechanical thrombectomy (Fig. 11.14). CDT has proven to be useful in patients with acute PE and systemic hypotension (massive or high-risk PE), particularly when there is a relative or absolute contraindication to systemic thrombolysis. In a systematic review by Kuo et al., six prospective and 29 retrospective uncontrolled studies were identified in which catheter directed therapy was used to treat 594 patients with acute high-risk PE [49]. Clinical success, defined as stabilization of hemodynamics, resolution of hypoxia and survival from massive PE, was achieved in 86.5% of patients, with 2.4% of patients experiencing major complications. It is worth noting that 96% of patients in this analysis did not receive systemic thrombolysis, while 66% of patients received thrombolytic during catheter directed therapy, presumably at a low dose. Although uncontrolled, the results of this analysis are favorable when compared with historical rates of survival (77%) and major hemorrhage (22%) following systemic thrombolysis and to overall mortality from acute high risk PE (30%) [41]. Therefore, catheter directed therapy for acute high-risk PE should be considered in cases where there is a relative or absolute contraindication to systemic thrombolysis or in the case of ineffective systemic thrombolysis.

Multiple recent prospective, randomized clinical trials have shown that treatment of patients with intermediate-risk (submassive) PE with systemic thrombolysis and heparin significantly improves patient mortality, RV function, risk of recurrent PE and hemodynamic collapse compared with patients treated with heparin alone [46–48]. However, this benefit comes at the expense of a significant increase in major bleeding complications, including >2% risk of hemorrhagic stroke. It has been postulated that catheter directed therapy, specifically catheter directed ultrasound assisted thrombolysis (USAT), can achieve the same benefit

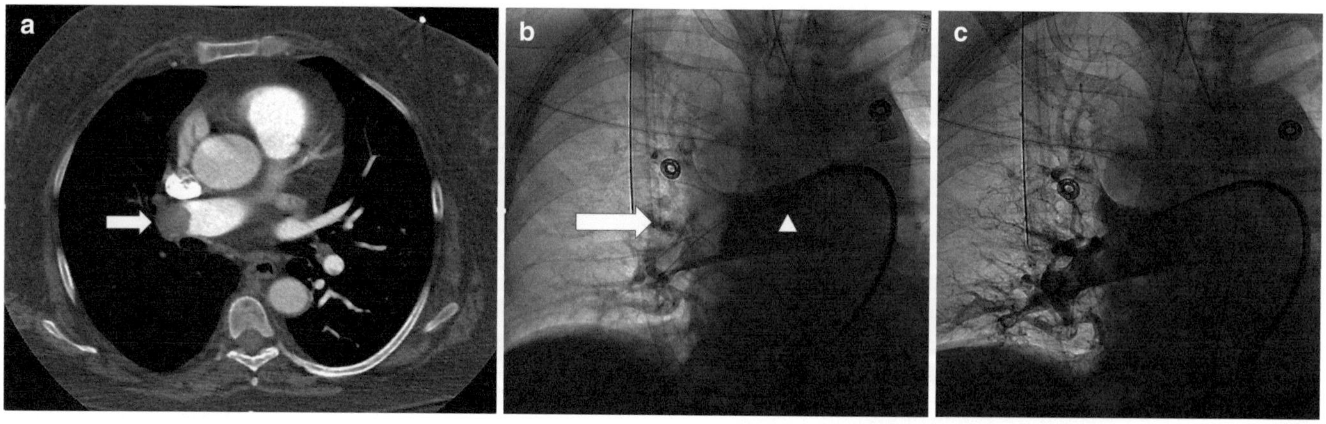

Fig. 11.14 (**a**) 53F with history of colon cancer presents with hypoxia and hypotension. Axial CT angiogram of the pulmonary artery shows thombus in the right main pulmonary artery (*arrow*). (**b**) Pulmonary angiogram showing corresponding filling defect in the right pulmonary artery (*arrow*) causing total absence of flow to the right lung and increased right ventricular afterload. Note the enlargement of the contrast-opacified main pulmonary artery (*arrowhead*). (**c**) After mechanical clot disruption, there is restored flow to the right lung. This caused an immediate reduction in pulmonary resistance and prevented acute right heart failure. Multiple filling defects remain, particularly in the right upper lobe. These were further treated with catheter directed thrombolysis

in these patients with lower systemic doses and bleeding complications. The SEATTLE II trial by Piazza et al. was a prospective non-controlled study of UAST in patients with high-risk and intermediate-risk PE [50] where a total of 24 mg of tPA was administered via the Ekos catheter in 150 patients. This study found significant decreases in RV strain, pulmonary pressure and pulmonary artery obstruction compared with baseline. Importantly, there were no intracranial hemorrhages and a 10% rate of major hemorrhage. Multiple additional non-controlled studies have found efficacy of catheter directed therapy for intermediate-risk PE with low rates of bleeding [51–53]. In the only prospective controlled randomized trial (Ultima trial), Kucher et al. randomized 59 patients with intermediate-risk PE to heparin alone vs. heparin with USAT (10–20 mg tPA). Significant improvements in right heart strain, as measured by RV/LV ratio, were seen in the USAT group compared with heparin alone (1.28–0.99 vs. 1.20–1.17, $p < 0.001$). Significantly, there were no major bleeding events or deaths in the USAT group [54]. Although not currently recommended for most patients with submassive or intermediate risk PE [32], these more recent studies support the claim that catheter directed therapy can deliver similar cardiovascular benefit as systemic thrombolysis with significantly fewer bleeding complications. As such, catheter directed therapy should be considered in the treatment algorithm for patients with intermediate risk PE.

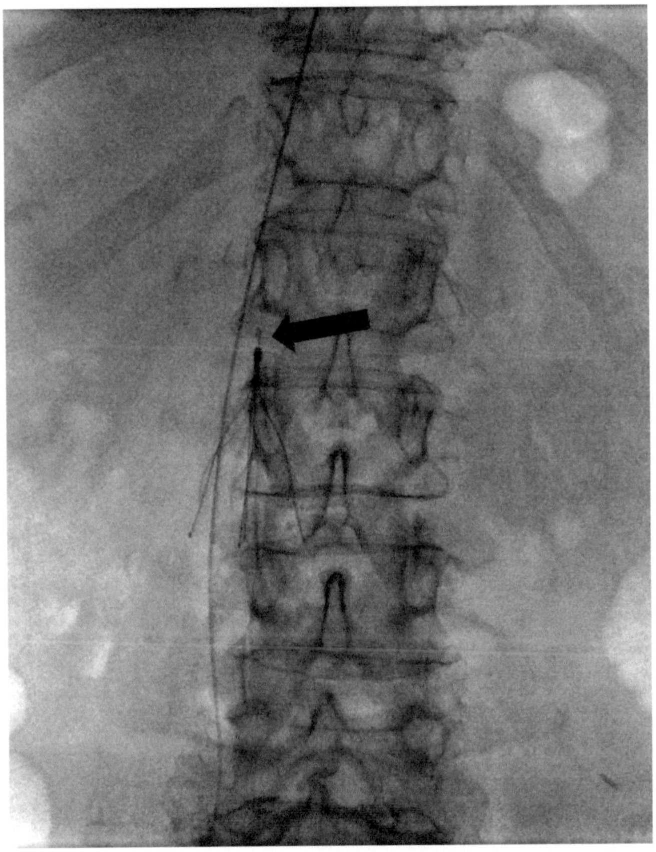

Fig. 11.15 Retreivable infrarenal IVC filter. Note the hook on the superior tip of the filter (*arrow*) to facilitate endovascular retreival

IVC Filter

IVC filters have been placed for over 40 years since the Greenfield filter was first introduced in 1973. The original filter was conical in shape, which helped trap clot within its central seams while still providing enough caval blood flow [55, 56]. There have been several filters that have adopted a similar design and several others that are entirely different in shape (Figs. 11.15 and 11.16). However, all filters are designed to primarily prevent significant PE by trapping venous emboli originating from the deep veins of the lower extremity.

The PREPIC trial was the first randomized control trial to evaluate the effectiveness of IVC filters [55, 57], which demonstrated a statistically significant 78% reduction in the risk of an acute pulmonary embolic event [57]. A follow up study 8 years after filter placement revealed a statistically significant 6.2% reduction in symptomatic PEs, however, with a 35% increased risk of symptomatic DVT in the filter group [57]. More recently, PREPIC 2 randomized trial found that even in high risk patients who are anti-coagulated systemically, placement of an IVC filter for 3 months actually did not reduce recurrent PE, including fatal PE [32, 58]. In the Olmsted cohort study, IVC filter placement increased the risk of VTE recurrence by almost 50%, and one third of early recurrences were related to PE [19]. In light of DVT complications, placement of IVC filters has been controversial and highly debated topic.

There have been no randomized controlled trials that have demonstrated superiority of a particular filter. However, modern filters have evolved to be less thrombogenic, less prone to breakage, and are MRI compatible [56]. There are two broad groups of IVC filters: retrievable and permanent. Permanent filters have been available for several years and are placed in patients who have lifelong risk of PE [55, 56]. Complications related to long-term filters and need for short-term prophylaxis, has resulted in a rise in placement of retrievable filters [55]. Subgroup of retrievable filters includes temporary filters (*must* be retrieved) that are tethered to the skin by a wire/catheter, and optionally retrievable filters that can be left in situ as a permanent device [55]. More recently, there has been a dramatic shift towards placement of retrievable/optional filters as they offer flexibility of retrieval if clinically indicated [59]. The ideal time frame for filter retrieval is within the first 3 months. However, it is possible to remove filters that have been in for much longer time periods, in some cases up to 10 years. Chronic indwelling filters, or filters with significant tilting of the tip, usually require retrieval with endovascular forceps (Fig. 11.17) or laser assisted.

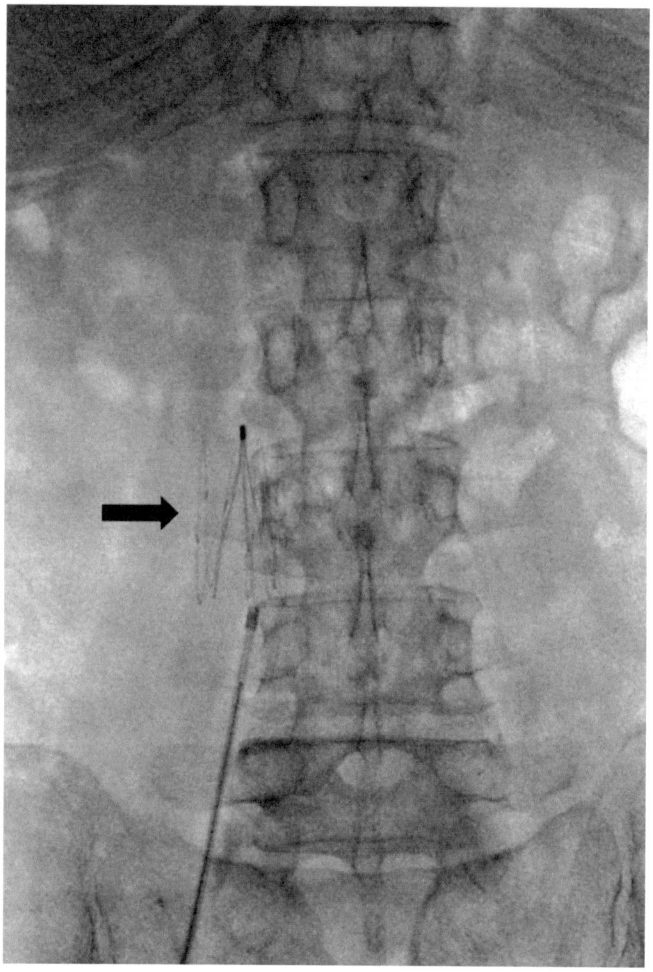

Fig. 11.16 Permanent infrarenal IVC filter. In addition to conical shape, permanat filters do not have a retreiveal hook and have more contact with the caval wall

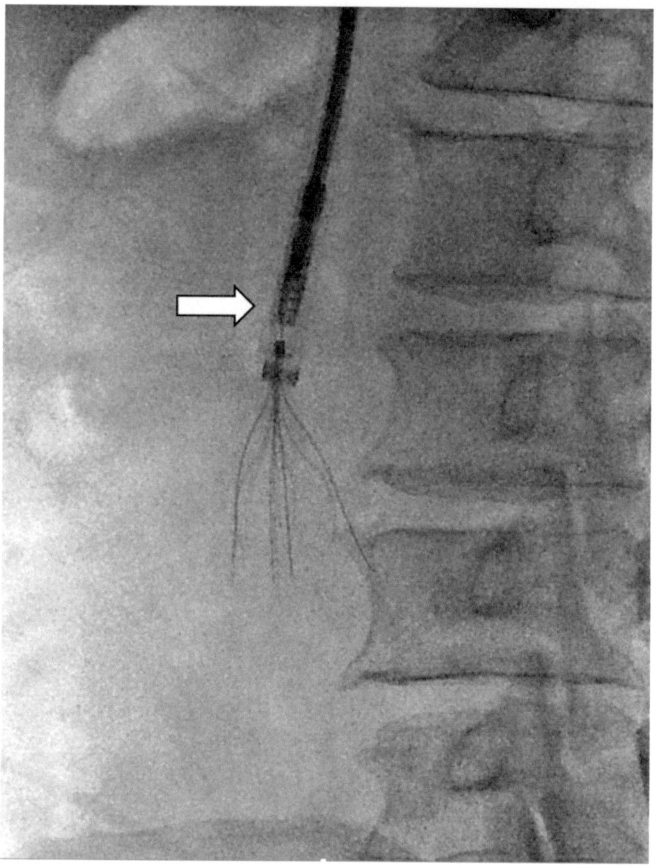

Fig. 11.17 Endobronchial forceps (*white arrow*) used to grasp a retrievable filter that had been indwelling for 3 years. The forceps are used to stabilize the filter as vascular sheath is advanced over the forceps and filter to collapse the filter legs and ultimately free the filter from the caval wall. Note this is an off-label use of endobronchial forceps

Majority of IVC filters for lower extremity DVTs are placed in an infra renal location. Suprarenal IVC filters are also placed, however, should be performed judiciously in select patients with specific indications due to a shorter length of the suprarenal IVC, and theoretical risk of filter induced renal vein thrombosis and subsequent renal failure. Recent retrospective evidence however, supports the original finding from Greenfield that suprarenal filters are equally effective in preventing PE without added risk of complications compared to infra-renal filters [60, 61]. Filters have also been placed for upper extremity DVTs that occur in the axillary, subclavian, brachiocephalic veins or SVC (Fig. 11.18). Although upper extremity DVTs are rare and are less likely to result in PE, if indicated, filters can be placed in the SVC just distal to the confluence of brachiocephalic veins, albeit with a slightly higher rate of complications such as caval perforation (4% in the SVC compared to 0.5% in the IVC) [62].

Indications for placement of both therapeutic and prophylactic IVC filters have been formulated by the American College of Radiology ACR/Society of Interventional Radiology (SIR) and are similar to those recommended by the American College of Chest Physicians (ACCP). The 10th edition of Antithrombotic guidelines (AT 10) from the ACCP however, recommended against placement of an IVC filter as primary prophylaxis for any patient or for VTE treated with anticoagulants [33]. Although filters have been around for several years, lack of significant level I evidence for IVC filter placement and research questions remain to be addressed. Nevertheless, there are several circumstances such as pregnancy, and trauma where a filter has shown significant benefit. In the setting of malignancy, however, the evidence is mixed. Filters still offer protection for PE related mortality, however, the stage of disease and type of cancer also questions the validity of placement in patients with advanced disease who succumb to the cancer earlier [63]. In one study that included 116 patients with malignancy, 46% of patients with stage IV disease who had a filter placed died of cancer within 6 weeks, and only 14% of patients were still alive after 1 year [64]. However, another study at a major cancer center examined 308 patients

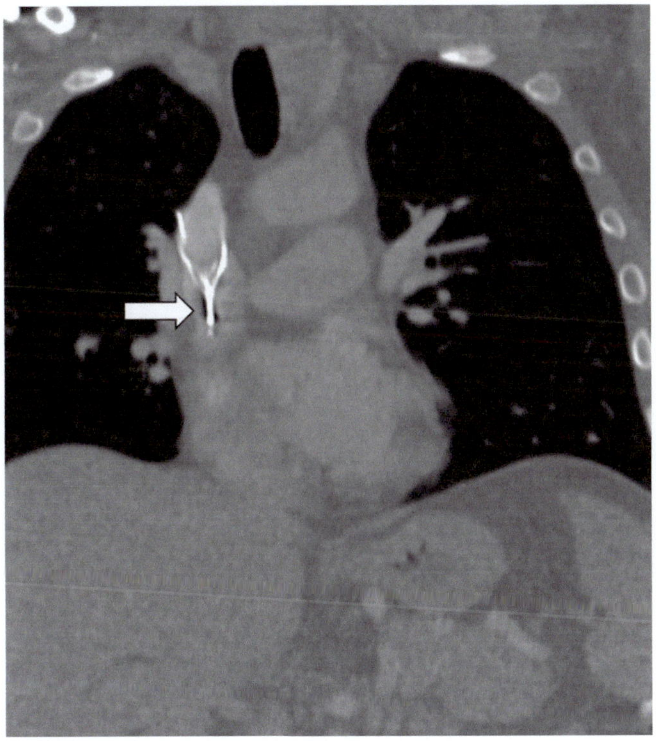

Fig. 11.18 Superior vena cava filter

with cancer and VTE, and found substantial mortality benefit for those patients with IVC filters in preventing PE-related deaths [65]. Given the controversy and lack of significant level 1 evidence, an individualized approach taking into account the stage and prognosis will likely offer the most benefit.

Additional filter complications include filter tilt, fracture, migration, embolization, caval wall perforation, IVC stenosis/occlusion and in some cases PTS (Figs. 11.19, 11.20, and 11.21). In response to growing complications, in 2010 the FDA issued a medical device Alert and Notice titled "Removing Retrievable Inferior Vena Cava Filters: Initial Communication," in which it cited concerns that retrievable filters are not retrieved after the patients' risk profile for PE has diminished, resulting in increased complications. The FDA recommended all physicians carefully evaluate patients for filter retrieval at regular intervals and prudent decision-making is imperative for any patient who receives a filter.

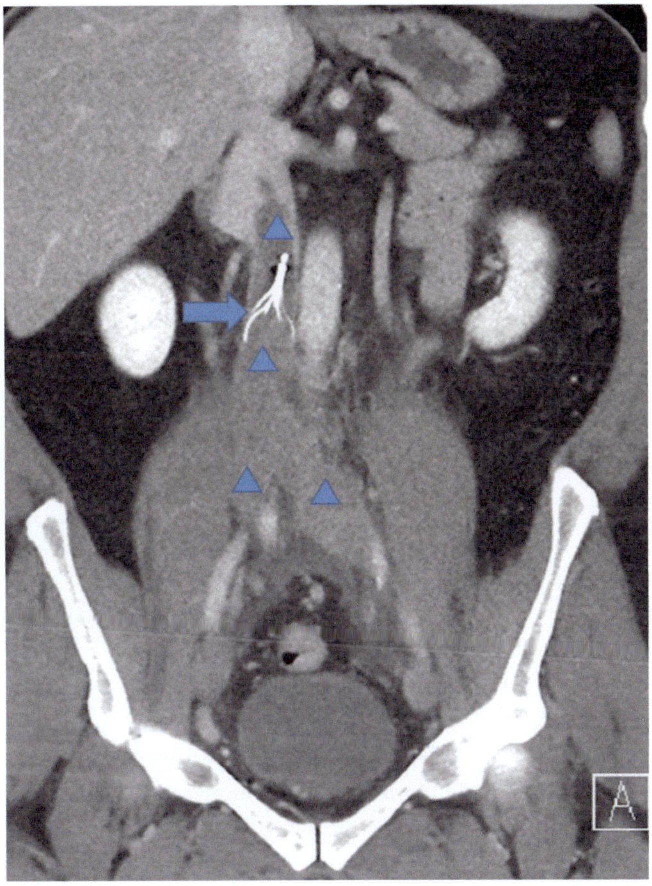

Fig. 11.19 Coronal CECT showing indwelling IVC filter (*arrow*) with filter associated IVC and iliac thrombosis (*arrowheads*)

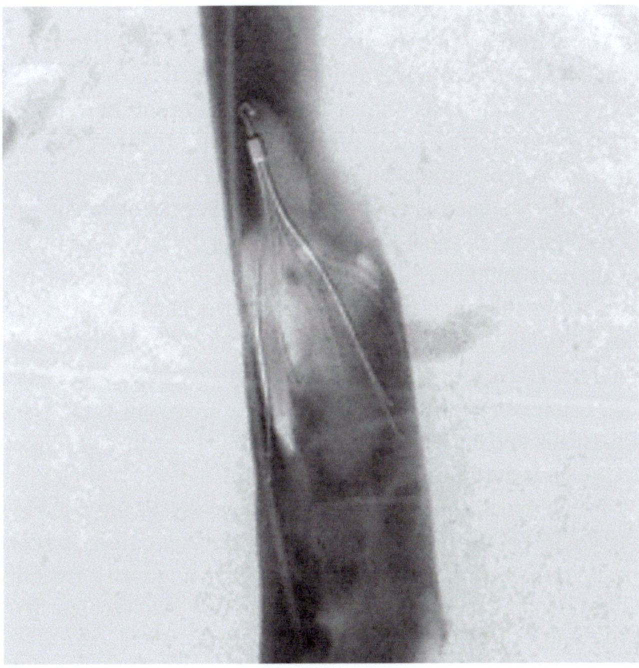

Fig. 11.20 Digital subtraction cavogram demonstrating intraluminal thrombus in and around the IVC filter

Superior Vena Cava Syndrome

Superior vena cava (SVC) syndrome was first described by William Hunter in 1757 and is a clinical manifestation of compression of the SVC, originally described in a patient with a syphilitic aortic aneurysm [66]. Compression may be extrinsic of the SVC itself, or of the greater veins emptying into the SVC. Although infectious causes accounted for a majority of the cases when originally described, over the last

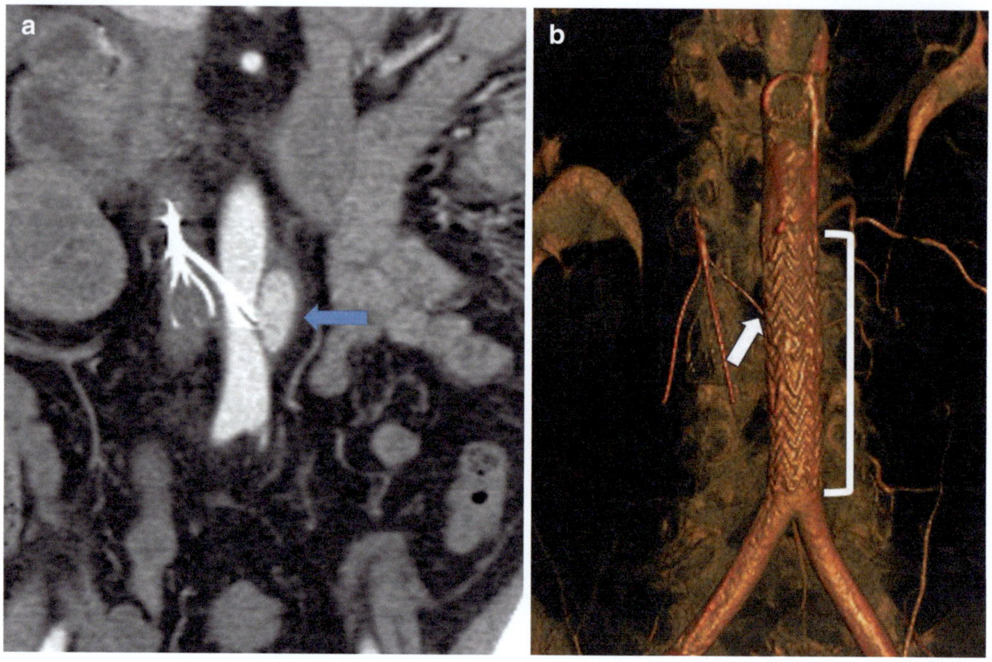

Fig. 11.21 (**a**) Coronal CECT showing perforation of the IVC by filter strut. The strut extends into the aorta and results in aortic pseudoaneurysm (*arrow*). (**b**): 3D reconstruction of aortogram after placement of aortic stent graft (*bracket*) with successful exclusion of the pseudoaneurysm. Filter, with perforated strut (*arrow*) was then successful removed

few decades SVC syndrome is most often a result of a malignant process in the thorax, most commonly lung cancer [67] and up to 35% of cases are due to non-malignant causes mostly secondary to use of intravascular devices resulting in thrombotic occlusion [68]. Once the SVC is occluded, venous return is impaired and alternate pathways mainly the azygous venous system, internal mammary/epigastric system, and superficial subcutaneous venous system act as collateral pathways (Fig. 11.22).

Early recognition of presentation of SVC syndrome is crucial since cerebral edema can be fatal if not treated promptly. Diagnosis is most often apparent by clinical assessment; however, CT of the chest with contrast offers a more sensitive evaluation of the etiology and in some cases MRI may be used if contrast medium is not tolerated. The constellation of signs and symptoms include edema of the head, neck and upper extremities, distention of subcutaneous vessels in the upper thorax, head and neck, laryngeal and nasal edema, and rarely cerebral edema [67]. Unless absolutely emergent, diagnosis of the underlying cause should be first established with tissue sampling or cytological analysis. Prognosis and survival in these patients are primarily related to the underlying cause of obstruction.

Management of SVC syndrome depends on the underlying cause of obstruction and acuity of presentation. A scoring system has been developed in order to stratify patients based on symptom severity and help guide management [69, 70] (Table 11.1).

Radiation therapy has been used since the 1970s used for emergent, palliative or definitive therapy. Emergency radiotherapy is started without histologic diagnosis when patients present acutely with severe symptoms [71]. In some cases of malignant obstruction from lymphoma or lung cancer, fractionated radiotherapy has shown to improve clinical symptoms with relief noted as early as 3–4 days in some patients [72]. In other cases, chemotherapy may be preferable if there is prior histologic diagnosis and the tumor is chemosensitive (e.g. small cell lung cancer, non-Hodgkin's lymphoma, germ cell tumors). However, more recently percutaneous stent placement, if feasible, has become the first line of treatment especially for those patients with malignant obstruction and results in immediate symptomatic relief when compared to emergent radiation. Radiation therapy and/or chemotherapy generally follows stent placement in the emergent setting, however, in the non-emergent setting may precede stent placement. Stent placement was introduced in the 1980s and has been refined over the years to reduce complications related to stent migration [73]. A prospective study by Gwon et al. reported a 94% patency rate for covered stents vs. 48% patency for non-covered stents over a 12-month period [74]. Despite this, non-covered stents are most often used owing to anatomic considerations when covered stents may cover collateral pathways or contralateral venous drainage. Although no randomized control trials exist to prove superiority of stenting compared to alternative therapies, there are several smaller case reports and studies that have established long

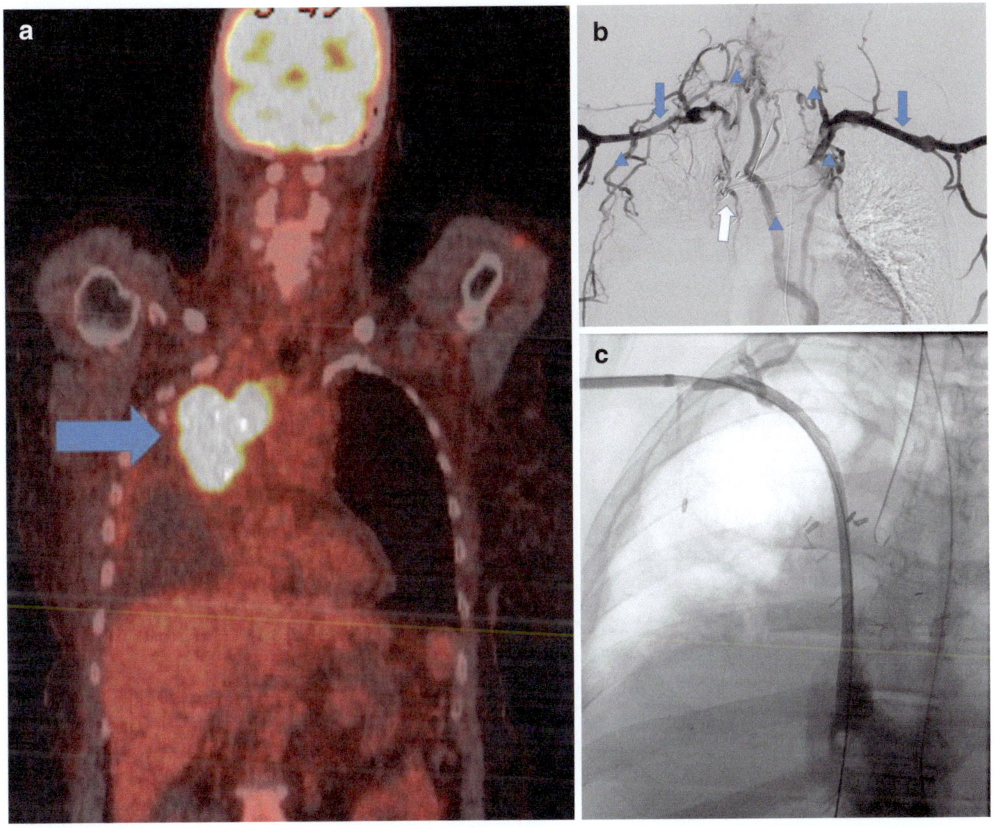

Fig. 11.22 (**a**) 61F with PET avid non-small cell lung carcinoma in the right upper lobe. (**b**) Patient developed face/arm swelling and shortness of breath while laying down 6 months after right upper and middle lobectomy. She was found to have mediastinal recurrence. Digital subtraction angiogram from both arms show patent subclavian veins (*blue arrows*). There is no flow into the superior vena (*white arrow*). There is filling of multiple collateral venous pathways (*blue arrowheads*). (**c**) Restoration of antegrade flow from the right subclavian vein to the heart after placement of 22 mm wallstent. Patient's symptoms resolved

Table 11.1 Superior vena cava (SVC) syndrome

Grade	Category	Estimated incidence (%)	Definition[a]
0	Asymptomatic	10	Radiographic superior vena cava obstruction in the absence of symptoms
1	Mild	25	Edema in head or neck (vascular distention), cyanosis, plethora
2	Moderate	50	Edema in head or neck with functional impairment (mild dysphagia, cough, mild or moderate impairment of head, jaw or eyelid movements, visual disturbances caused by ocular edema)
3	Severe	10	Mild or moderate cerebral edema (headache, dizziness) or mild/moderate laryngeal edema or diminished cardiac reserve (syncope after bending)
4	Life-threatening	5	Significant cerebral edema (confusion, obtundation) or significant laryngeal edema (stridor) or significant hemodynamic compromise (syncope without precipitating factor, hypotension, renal insufficiency)
5	Fatal	<1	Death

[a]Adopted from Yu et al. [70]

term success with minimal complication rate. Major complications include stent migration, bleeding, pericardial tamponade, pulmonary edema and pulmonary embolism [75].

Although stenting has changed management over the last few decades, not every patient is a candidate. Until further evidence is established, stent placement should be reserved for patients who have significant, life style altering symptoms that are either too great to wait for chemotherapy or radiation or who do not respond to these modalities. In general stenting should be avoided or used as a last resort in patients with a good chance of recovery and longer life expectancy, to prevent long-term complications such as stent occlusion [75]. In these patients, primary angioplasty with local catheter directed thrombolytic therapy and early institution of systemic anticoagulation is generally preferred [75]. Adjunct therapies to alleviate symptoms include head elevation, supplemental oxygen, diuretics and corticosteroids to decrease laryngeal and cerebral edema [73]. As with most interventions, approach to patient selection for the appropriate mode of therapy is vital in improving overall outcomes.

Splanchnic Vein Thrombosis and Stenosis

Splanchnic venous thrombosis (SVT) is an uncommon yet potentially fatal manifestation of VTE. The splanchnic system encompasses the hepatic veins, and the portal circulation. Primary presentations of SVT are Budd-Chiari syndrome, portal vein thrombosis (PVT) and mesenteric vein thrombosis (MVT) with the PVT and MVT constituting the majority of cases.

Risk factors of SVT include cirrhosis, and abdominal malignancies (mainly gastrointestinal, pancreatic or hepatobiliary system) present in 34% and 31% of PVT patients, respectively [76, 77]. In the last few decades, myeloproliferative neoplasm has accounted for a majority of SVT cases [76]. A gain-of-function mutation of the tyrosin-kinase JAK2 (JAK2V617F), has also been strongly associated with development of both myeloproliferative neoplasm and SVT [76, 78–80]. A recent meta-analysis found a prevalence of JAK2 mutation of 32.7% (95% CI, 25.5–35.9%) in patients with known SVT, and also reported a strong association between JAK2 mutation and the development of SVT (OR 54; 95% CI, 13–222) [76, 80]. Given the strong association, peripheral blood screening for JAK2 mutation is recommended in patients with idiopathic SVT [81].

Clinical presentation of SVT patients varies depending on the size and extent of thrombosis, vessels involved, chronicity of thrombosis and presence of bowel wall ischemia. Acute SVT presents with nausea, vomiting, diarrhea and sudden onset, colicky, mid-abdominal pain sometimes with signs of bowel infarction and peritonitis in up to two thirds of patients [82, 83]. In the subacute form, abdominal pain continues for days to weeks, however, without significant risk of bowel infarction. In the chronic setting of slow and progressive portal vein stenosis, most commonly from pancreatic cancer, patients do not complain of pain and present with nonspecific symptom of several months duration, and is sometimes even diagnosed incidentally. When the portal or splenic vein is severely stenosed or thrombosed, patients may have signs of portal hypertension including splenomegaly, ascites, hypersplenism and upper or lower GI bleeding from esophageal and mesenteric variceal hemorrhage, respectively [82]. Elevated mesenteric venous pressures can also cause bowel wall edema, which can result in malabsorption, weight loss and diarrhea. Distinguishing venous hypertensive bowel dysfunction and chronic mesenteric arterial ischemia is key in patients where tumors may be compressing both the SMA and the SMV.

Diagnosis of SVT is challenging since the clinical presentation overlaps with several other abdominal conditions; however, given a high mortality rate, a high degree of suspicion in patients with abdominal malignancy remains crucial to avoid delays in diagnosis. Doppler ultrasonography is excellent at depicting thrombus in the proximal portal, hepatic and mesenteric veins, however, it is highly operator dependent and may be obscured by shadowing artifacts from bowel gas. CT has been a widely established technique excellent at defining extent of bowel involvement, depicting bowel wall thickening, abnormal wall enhancement, filling defects in the vasculature and collateral circulation [84]. Late findings of pneumatosis and portal venous gas are sometimes seen radiographically, however, CT is excellent at ruling out other conditions that can cause abdominal symptoms (Fig. 11.23). CT can have false negatives if the thrombus is in a smaller, distal branch or related to suboptimal contrast timing opacifying the venous circulation. Mesenteric angiography is rarely performed as a diagnostic procedure and is reserved for those patients with a high suspicion of venous thrombosis with an intention to treat.

Treatment of SVT is not straightforward due to the challenging and complicated nature of affected patients and low level of evidence and lack of controlled trials. Several patients have underlying cirrhosis and the chronic form of SVT present with variceal bleeding, anticoagulation is not always indicated. However, if there are no major contraindications, anticoagulant therapy with LMWH or UFH along with Vitamin K antagonists is recommended for those presenting with acute symptomatic thrombosis [32, 76, 85]. More recently, direct thrombin inhibitors such as rivaroxaban has also been a cost effective alternative therapeutic option for those patients with preserved renal function. In general, treatment is recommended for at least 3 months, but in cases of un-resolving SVT for those patients in a persistent procoagulant state, the treatment is continued indefinitely. Acute SVT with evidence of ischemic bowel warrants immediate surgical management.

Given the risks associated with systemic thrombolysis, endovascular techniques for local thrombolysis is preferred for selective patients. Catheter directed thrombolysis, aspiration thrombectomy and stent placements have been described in several small case series' [86–94] for portal venous and mesenteric venous thrombosis (Fig. 11.24) with good long-term clinical success rates [95]. Pharmacological thrombolysis is performed with both urokinase and r-tPA with feared complications such as vessel perforation, worsening bowel ischemia, and gastrointestinal bleeding vary significantly, however, meticulous approach and technical improvements over the years have minimized major complications. Indirect methods such as intra-arterial infusion via the superior mesenteric artery (SMA) have also been performed, however, only in select patients with small venous thrombus burden, with longer infusion times and a larger dose of local thrombolytic [96, 97]. In patients with symptomatic portal vein stenosis, most commonly from tumor compression or after transplant, portal vein stenting is effective at reducing symptoms, thought have moderately high rates of stent thrombosis (43% at 16 months) [98].

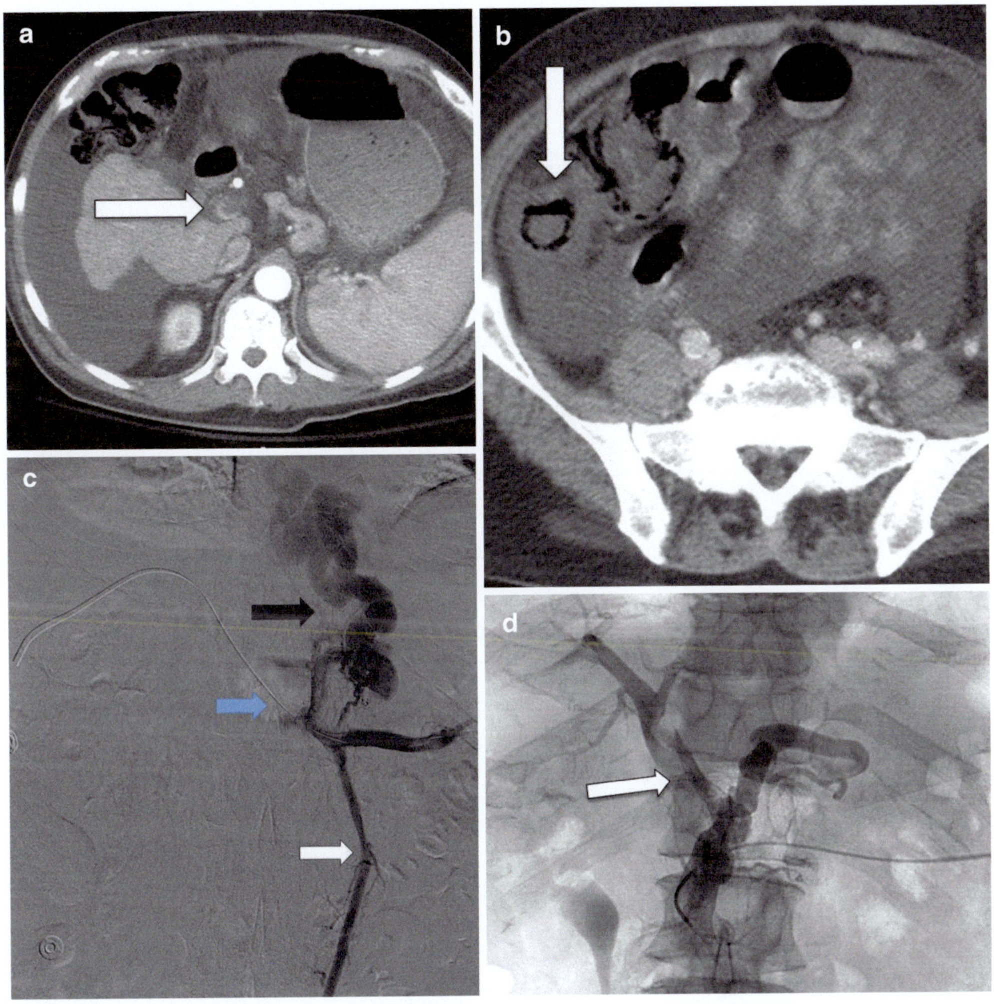

Fig. 11.23 (**a**) A Sixty-six year old male with cirrhosis, ascites presents with worsening abdominal pain. CT Abdomen with IV contrast shows occlusion of the extra-hepatic main portal vein. (**b**) CT Images of the lower abdomen in the same patient shows ileo-cecal pneumatosis, a sign of mesenteric ischemia. (**c**) Digital subtraction angiogram from transplenic venous access. Total occlusion of the portal vein (*blue arrow*) results in diminutive superior mesenteric vein (*white arrow*) and filling of esophageal and gastric varices (*black arrow*) via the coronary vein. Catheter directed thrombolysis was performed. (**d**) Venogram after transplenic catheter directed thrombolysis shows improved filling of the SMV with hepatopetal flow and filling of the portal vein. Filling defect in the portal vein persists (*arrow*), however, there is decreased filling of varices

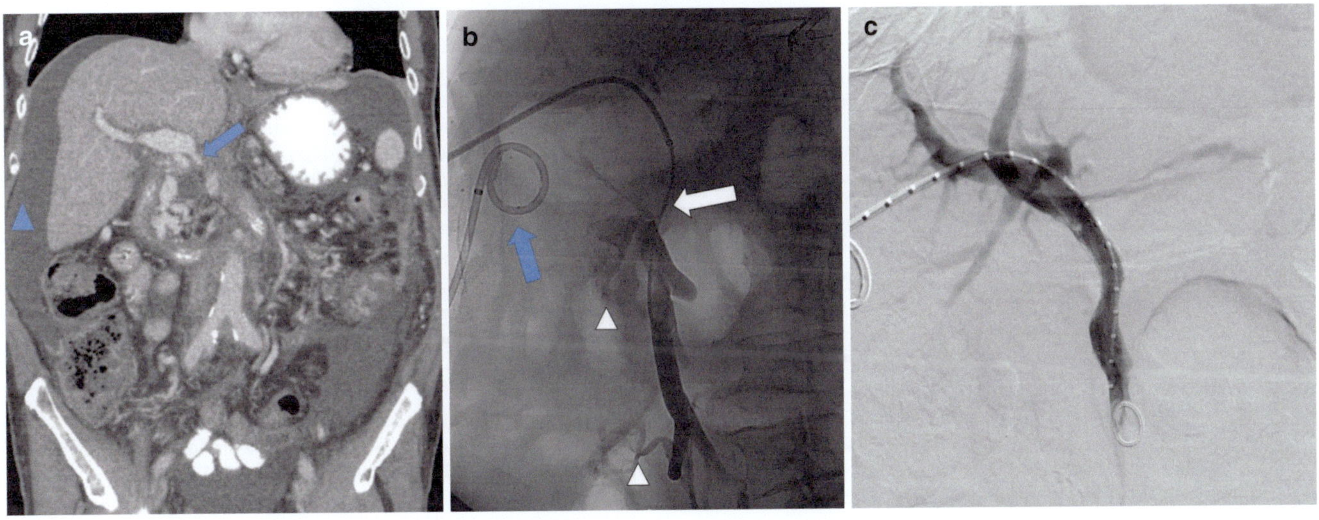

Fig. 11.24 (**a**) A 59 M with locally advanced pancreatic cancer causing occlusion of the main portal vein (*blue arrow*). Patient developed increasing ascites (*blue arrowhead*).(**b**) Transhepatic angiogram from the superior mesenteric vein showing no flow into the portal vein (*white arrow*). Elevated venous pressures result in varices and cavernous transformation of the portal vein (*white arrowheads*). An intraperitoneal drainage catheter (*blue*) was placed prior to transhepatic access. (**c**) Resotration of hepatopedal flow after placement of self-expanding metallic stent. Patients ascites volume decreased substantially

References

1. Trousseau A. Phlegmasia alba dolens. Lectures on clinical medicine, delivered at the Hotel-Dieu, Paris 1865;5:281–332.
2. Falanga A, Marchetti M, Russo L. The mechanisms of cancer-associated thrombosis. Thromb Res. 2015;135:S8–11.
3. Heit JA. The epidemiology of venous thromboembolism in the community. Arterioscler Thromb Vasc Biol. 2008;28(3):370–2.
4. Fuentes HE, Tafur AJ, Caprini JA. Cancer-associated thrombosis. Dis Mon. 2016;62(5):121–58.
5. Spencer FA, Emery C, Lessard D, Anderson F, Emani S, Aragam J, Goldberg RJ. The Worcester venous thromboembolism study. J Gen Intern Med. 2006;21(7):722–7.
6. Blom JW. Malignancies, prothrombotic mutations, and the risk of venous thrombosis. JAMA. 2005;293(6):715.
7. Walker AJ, Card TR, West J, Crooks C, Grainge MJ. Incidence of venous thromboembolism in patients with cancer – a cohort study using linked United Kingdom databases. Eur J Cancer. 2013;49(6):1404–13.
8. Fennerty A. Venous thromboembolic disease and cancer. Postgrad Med J. 2006;82:642–8.
9. Krutman M, Kuzniec S, Ramacciotti E, Varella AYM, Zlotnik M, Teivelis MP, Tachibana A, De Campos Guerra JC, Wolosker N. Rediscussing anticoagulation in distal deep venous thrombosis. Clin Appl Thromb Hemost. 2016;22:772–8.
10. Michelangelo S, Migliaccio L, Favaretto E, Palareti G, Cosmi B. Two years outcome of isolated distal deep vein thrombosis. Thromb Res. 2014;134(1):36–40.
11. Sartori M, Cosmi B, Legnani C, Favaretto E, Valdré L, Guazzaloca G, Rodorigo G, Cini M, Palareti G. The Wells rule and D-dimer for the diagnosis of isolated distal deep vein thrombosis. J Thromb Haemost. 2012;10(11):2264–9.
12. Galanaud J, Bosson J, Quéré I. Risk factors and early outcomes of patients with symptomatic distal vs. proximal deep-vein thrombosis. Curr Opin Pulm Med. 2011;17(5):387–91.
13. Vedantham S, Grassi CJ, Ferral H, et al. Reporting standards for endovascular treatment of lower extremity deep vein thrombosis. J Vasc Interv Radiol. 2005;17:417–34.
14. Meissner MN, Strandness DE. Pathophysiology and natural history of deep venous thrombosis. In: Rutherford RB, editor. Vascular surgery. 5th ed. Philadelphia: WB Saunders; 2000. p. 1920–37.
15. Delis KT, Bountouroglou B, Mansfield AO. Venous claudication in iliofemoral thrombosis: long-term effects on venous hemodynamics, clinical status, and quality of life. J Vasc Surg. 2004;239:1143.
16. Kahn SR. The post thrombotic syndrome. Thromb Res. 2011;127(Suppl 3):S89–92.
17. Kahn SR. How I treat postthrombotic syndrome. Blood. 2009;114:4624–31.
18. Heit JA. Predicting the risk of venous thromboembolism recurrence. Am J Hematol. 2012;87:S1.
19. Heit JA, Lahr BD, Petterson TM, Bailey KR, Ashrani AA, Melton LJ. Heparin and warfarin anticoagulation intensity as predictors of recurrence after deep vein thrombosis or pulmonary embolism: a population-based cohort study. Blood. 2011;118(18):4992–9.
20. Heit JA, O'Fallon WM, Petterson TM, Lohse CM, Silverstein MD, Mohr DN, Melton LJ. Relative impact of risk factors for deep vein thrombosis and pulmonary embolism. Arch Intern Med. 2002;162(11):1245.
21. Hull R, Hirsh J, Sackett DL, Taylor DW, Carter C, Turpie AG, Gent M. Clinical validity of a negative venogram in patients with clinically suspected venous thrombosis. Circulation. 1981;64(3):622–5. doi:10.1161/01.cir.64.3.622.
22. Arnoult A-C, Pernod G, Genty C, Galanaud J-P, Colonna M, Sevestre M-A, Bosson J-L. Low incidence of cancer after venous thromboembolism: an update from the French OPTIMEV Cohort. J Mal Vasc. 2016;41(3):169–75.
23. Chinsakchai K, Duis KT, Moll FL, Borst GJ. Trends in management of phlegmasia cerulea dolens. Vasc Endovascular Surg. 2010;45(1):5–14. doi:10.1177/1538574410388309.
24. Wells PS, Anderson DR, Rodger M, Stiell I, Dreyer JF, Barnes D, Forgie M, Kovacs G, Ward J, Kovacs MJ. Excluding pulmonary embolism at the bedside without diagnostic imaging: management of patients with suspected pulmonary embolism presenting to the emergency department by using a simple clinical model and d-dimer. Ann Intern Med. 2001;135(2):98–107. PMID: 11453709.
25. Wicki J, Perneger TV, Junod AF, Bounameaux H, Perrier A. Assessing clinical probability of pulmonary embolism in the emergency ward: a simple score. Arch Intern Med. 2001;161(1):92–7. doi:10.1001/archinte.161.1.92. PMID 11146703.
26. Schulman S, Kearon C, Kakkar AK, for the RE-COVER Study Group. Dabigatran versus warfarin in the treatment of acute venous thromboembolism. N Engl J Med. 2009;361(24):2342–52.
27. Schulman S, Kakkar AK, Goldhaber SZ, for the RE-COVER II Trial Investigators. Treatment of acute venous thromboembolism with dabigatran or warfarin and pooled analysis. Circulation. 2014;129(7):764–72.
28. Bauersachs R, Berkowitz SD, Brenner B, Buller HR, Decousus H, Gallus AS, Schellong S. Oral rivaroxaban for symptomatic venous thromboembolism. N Engl J Med. 2010;363(26):2499–510.
29. EINSTEIN-PE Investigators, Büller HR, Prins MH, Lensin AW, Decousus H, Jacobson BF, Minar E, Chlumsky J, Verhamme P, Wells P, Agnelli G, Cohen A, Berkowitz SD, Bounameaux H, Davidson BL, Misselwitz F, Gallus AS, Raskob GE, Schellong S, Segers A. Oral rivaroxaban for the treatment of symptomatic pulmonary embolism. N Engl J Med. 2012;366(14):1287–97.
30. Agnelli G, Buller HR, Cohen A, Curto M, Gallus AS, Johnson M, Masiukiewicz U, Pak R, Thompson J, Raskob GE, Weitz JI, AMPLIFY Investigators. Oral apixaban for the treatment of acute venous thromboembolism. N Engl J Med. 2013;369(9):799–808.
31. Hokusai-VTE Investigators, Büller HR, Décousus H, Grosso MA, Mercuri M, Middeldorp S, Prins MH, et al. Edoxaban versus warfarin for the treatment of symptomatic venous thromboembolism. N Engl J Med. 2013;369:1406–15.
32. Kearon C, Akl EA, Ornelas J, Blaivas A, Jimenez D, Bounameaux H, et al. Antithrombotic therapy for VTE disease: CHEST guideline and expert panel report. Chest. 2016;149(2):315–52.
33. Kearon C, Akl EA, Comerota AJ, Prandoni P, Bounameaux H, Goldhaber SZ, et al. Antithrombotic therapy for VTE disease. Chest. 2012;142(6):1698–704.
34. Braaten J, Goss R, Francis C, et al. Ultrasound reversibly disaggregates fibrin fibers. Thromb Haemost. 1997;78:1063–8.
35. Vedantham S, Thorpe PE, Cardella JF, et al. Quality improvement guidelines for the treatment of lower extremity deep vein thrombosis with use of endovascular thrombus removal. J Vasc Interv Radiol. 2006;17:435–48.
36. Patel N, Sacks D, Patel RI, et al. SIR reporting standards for the treatment of acute limb ischemia with use of transluminal removal of arterial thrombus. J Vasc Interv Radiol. 2003;14(Suppl):S453–65.
37. Vedantham S, Millward SF, Cardella JF, Hofmann LV, Razavi MK, Grassi CJ, et al. Society of Interventional Radiology Position Statement: treatment of acute iliofemoral deep vein thrombosis with use of adjunctive catheter-directed intrathrombus thrombolysis. J Vasc Interv Radiol. 2009;20(7 Suppl):S332–5.
38. Tapson VF. Acute pulmonary embolism. N Engl J Med. 2008;358(10):1037–52.
39. Attia J, Ray JG, Cook DJ, et al. Deep vein thrombosis and its prevention in critically ill adults. Arch Intern Med. 2001;161:1268e79.
40. Jaff MR, McMurtry MS, Archer SL, Cushman M, Goldenberg N, Goldhaber SZ, et al. Management of massive and submassive pulmonary embolism, iliofemoral deep vein thrombosis, and chronic thromboembolic pulmonary hypertension: a scientific statement from the American Heart Association. Circulation. 2011;123(16):1788–830.

41. Goldhaber SZ, Visani L, De Rosa M. Acute pulmonary embolism: clinical outcomes in the International Cooperative Pulmonary Embolism Registry (ICOPER). Lancet. 1999;353(9162):1386–9.
42. Agnelli G, Becattini C, Kirschstein T. Thrombolysis vs heparin in the treatment of pulmonary embolism: a clinical outcome-based meta-analysis. Arch Intern Med. 2002;162(22):2537–41.
43. Levine M, Hirsh J, Weitz J, et al. A randomized trial of a single bolus dosage regimen of recombinant tissue plasminogen activator in patients with acute pulmonary embolism. Chest. 1990;98(6):1473–9.
44. Dong B, Jirong Y, Wang Q, Wu T. Thrombolytic treatment for pulmonary embolism. Cochrane Database Syst Rev. 2006;(2):CD004437.
45. Wan S, Quinlan DJ, Agnelli G, Eikelboom JW. Thrombolysis compared with heparin for the initial treatment of pulmonary embolism: a meta-analysis of the randomized controlled trials. Circulation. 2004;110(6):744–9.
46. Meyer G, Vicaut E, Danays T, et al. Fibrinolysis for patients with intermediate-risk pulmonary embolism. NEJM. 2014;370:1402–11.
47. Goa G, Yang P, Liu M, et al. Thrombolysis for acute intermediate-risk pulmonary embolism: a meta-analysis. Thromb Res. 2015;136(5):932–7.
48. Sharifi M, Bay C, Skrocki L, et al. Moderate pulmonary embolism treated with thrombolysis (from the "MOPETT" Trial). Am J Cardiol. 2013;111:273–7.
49. Kuo W, Gould M, Louie J, et al. Catheter-directed therapy for the treatment of massive pulmonary embolism: systematic review and meta-analysis of modern techniques. J Vasc Interv Radiol. 2009;20(11):1431–40.
50. Piazza G, Hohlfelder B, Ouriel, et al. A prospective, single-arm, multicenter trial of ultrasound-facilitated, catheter-directed, low-dose fibrinolysis for acute massive and submassive pulmonary embolism: The SEATTLE II study. JACC Cardiovasc Interv. 2015 Aug 24;8(10):1382–92.
51. Kennedy R, Kenney H, Dunfee B, et al. Thrombus resolution and hemodynamic recovery using ultrasound-accelerated thrombolysis in acute pulmonary embolism. J Vasc Interv Radiol. 2013;24:841–8.
52. Bagla S, Smirniotopoulos J, van Breda A, et al. Ultrasound-accelerated catheter-directed thrombolysis for acute submassive pulmonary embolism. J Vasc Interv Radiol. 2015;26:1001–6.
53. Kuo W, Banerjee A, Kim P, et al. Pulmonary Embolism Response to Fragmentation, Embolectomy, and Catheter Thrombolysis (PERFECT): initial results from a Prospective Multicenter Registry. Chest. 2015 Sep;148(3):667–73.
54. Kuchar N, Boekstegers P, Muller O, et al. Randomized, controlled trial of ultrasound-assisted catheter directed thrombolysis for acute intermediate-risk pulmonary embolism (Ultima Trial). Circulation. 2014;129:479–86.
55. Molvar C. Inferior vena cava filtration in the management of venous thromboembolism: filtering the data. Semin Intervent Radiol. 2012;29(03):204–17.
56. Harvey JJ, Hopkins J, Mccafferty IJ, Jones RG. Inferior vena cava filters: what radiologists need to know. Clin Radiol. 2013;68(7):721–32.
57. PREPIC Study Group. Eight-year follow-up of patients with permanent vena cava filters in the prevention of pulmonary embolism: the PREPIC (Prevention du Risque d'Embolie Pulmonaire par Interruption Cave) randomized study. Circulation. 2005;112(3):416–22.
58. Mismetti P, Laporte S, Pellerin O, et al. Effect of a retrievable inferior vena cava filter plus anticoagulation vs anticoagulation alone on risk of recurrent pulmonary embolism: a randomized clinical trial. JAMA. 2015;313(16):1627–35.
59. Kim HS, Young MJ, Narayan AK, Hong K, Liddell RP, Streiff MB. A comparison of clinical outcomes with retrievable and permanent inferior vena cava filters. J Vasc Interv Radiol. 2008;19(3):393–9.
60. Greenfield LJ, Proctor MC. Suprarenal filter placement. J Vasc Surg. 1998;28:432–8, discussion 438
61. Kalva S, Chlapoutaki C, Wicky S, Greenfield AJ, Waltman AC, Athanasoulis CA. Suprarenal inferior vena cava filters: a 20-year single-center experience. J Vasc Interv Radiol. 2008;19(7):1041–7.
62. Owens CA, Bui JT, Knuttinen MG, et al. Pulmonary embolism from upper extremity deep vein thrombosis and the role of superior vena cava filters: a review of the literature. J Vasc Interv Radiol. 2010;21:779e87.
63. Mansour A, Ismael Y, Abdel-Razeq H. Inferior vena cava filters in patients with advanced-stage cancer. Hematol Oncol Stem Cell Ther. 2014;7(4):136–41.
64. Jarrett BP, Dougherty MJ, Calligaro KD. Inferior vena cava filters in malignant disease. J Vasc Surg. 2002;36(4):704–7.
65. Wallace MJ, Jean JL, Gupta S, Eapen GA, Johnson MM, Ahrar K, et al. Use of inferior vena caval filters and survival in patients with malignancy. Cancer. 2004;101(8):1902–7.
66. Hunter W, Johnston W. The history of an aneurysm of the aorta, with some remarks on aneurysms in general. London: William Johnston; 1757.
67. Wilson LD, Detterbeck FC, Yahalom J. Clinical practice. Superior vena cava syndrome with malignant causes. N Engl J Med. 2007;356:1862–9.
68. Rice TW, Rodriguez RM, Light RW. The superior vena cava syndrome: clinical characteristics and evolving etiology. Medicine (Baltimore). 2006;85:37–42.
69. Kishi K, Sonomura T, Mitsuzane K, Nishida N, Yang RJ, Sato M, et al. Self-expandable metallic stent therapy for superior vena cava syndrome: clinical observations. Radiology. 1993;189(2):531–5.
70. Yu JB, Wilson LD, Detterbeck FC. Superior vena cava syndrome: a proposed classification system and algorithm for management. J Thorac Oncol. 2008;3(811–814):8.
71. Schafer S. Oncologic complications. In: Otto S, editor. Oncology nursing. 3rd ed. St. Louis: Mosby Yearbook; 1997. p. 406–74.
72. Davenport D, Ferree C, Blake D, Raben M. Radiation therapy in the treatment of superior vena caval obstruction. Cancer. 1978;42:2600–3. doi:10.1002/1097-0142(197812)42:6<2600.
73. Straka C, Ying J, Kong F, Willey CD, Kaminski J, Kim DW. Review of evolving etiologies, implications and treatment strategies for the superior vena cava syndrome. SpringerPlus. 2016;5(1) doi:10.1186/s40064-016-1900-7.
74. Gwon DI, Ko G-Y, Kim JH, Shin JH, Yoon H-K, Sung K-B. Malignant superior vena cava syndrome: a comparative cohort study of treatment with covered stents versus uncovered stents. Radiology. 2013;266(3):979–87.
75. Rachapalli V, Boucher LM. Superior vena cava syndrome: role of the interventionalist. Can Assoc Radiol J. 2014;65:168–76. doi:10.1016/j. carj.2012.09.003.
76. Riva N, Donadini MP, Dentali F, Squizzato A, Ageno W. Clinical approach to splanchnic vein thrombosis: Risk factors and treatment. Thromb Res. 2012;130(Suppl. 1):S1–3.
77. Thatipelli MR, McBane RD, Hodge DO, Wysokinski WE. Survival and recurrence in patients with splanchnic vein thromboses. Clin Gastroenterol Hepatol. 2010;8:200–5.
78. Kralovics R, Passamonti F, Buser AS, Teo SS, Tiedt R, Passweg JR, et al. A gain-of-function mutation of JAK2 in myeloproliferative disorders. N Engl J Med. 2005;352(17):1779–90.
79. Colaizzo D, Amitrano L, Tiscia GL, Scenna G, Grandone E, Guardascione MA, et al. The JAK2 V617F mutation frequently occurs in patients with portal and mesenteric venous thrombosis. J Thromb Haemost. 2007;5(1):55–61.
80. Dentali F, Squizzato A, Brivio L, Appio L, Campiotti L, Crowther M, et al. JAK2V617F mutation for the early diagnosis of Ph- myeloproliferative neoplasms in patients with venous thromboembolism: a meta-analysis. Blood. 2009;113:5617–23.

81. Xavier SG, Gadelha T, Rezende SM, Zalcberg IR, Spector N. JAK2V617F mutation in patients with thrombosis: to screen or not to screen? Int J Lab Hematol. 2011;33:117–24.
82. Kumar S, Sarr MG, Kamath PS. Mesenteric venous thrombosis. N Engl J Med. 2001;345:1683–8.
83. Boley SJ, Kaleya RN, Brandt LJ. Mesenteric venous thrombosis. Surg Clin North Am. 1992;72:183–201.
84. Duran R, Denys AL, Letovanec I, Meuli RA, Schmidt S. Multidetector CT features of mesenteric vein thrombosis. Radiographics. 2012;32(5):1503–22. doi:10.1148/rg.325115100.
85. de Franchis R, on behalf of the Baveno V Faculty. Revising consensus in portal hypertension: report of the Baveno V consensus workshop on methodology of diagnosis and therapy in portal hypertension. J Hepatol. 2010;53:762–8.
86. Poplausky M, Kaufman J, Geller S, et al. Mesenteric venous thrombosis treated with urokinase via the superior mesenteric artery. Gastroenterology. 1996;110:1633–5.
87. Hoffer E, Krohmer S, Gemery J, et al. Endovascular recanalization of symptomatic portomesenteric venous obstruction after pancreaticoduodenectomy and radiation. J Vasc Interv Radiol. 2009;20(12):1633–7.
88. Haskal Z. Power – pulse thrombolysis, thrombectomy, and TIPS formation for the accelerated treatment of portosplenomesenteric thrombosis in Budd Chiari syndrome. J Vasc Interv Radiol. 2007;18(11):1458–60.
89. Kim H, Patra A, Khan J, et al. Transhepatic catheter directed thrombectomy and thrombolysis of acute superior mesenteric venous thrombosis. J Vasc Interv Radiol. 2005;16(12):1685–91.
90. Luo J, Yan Z, Wang J, et al. Endovascular treatment for non-acute symptomatic portal venous thrombosis through intrahepatic portosystemic shunt approach. J Vasc Interv Radiol. 2011;22(1):61–9.
91. Jia Z, Jiang G, Tian F, et al. Early endovascular treatment of superior mesenteric occlusion secondary to thromboemboli. Eur J Vasc Endovasc Surg. 2014;47(2):196–203.
92. Hollingshead M, Burke C, Mauro M, et al. Transcatheter thrombolytic therapy for acute mesenteric and portal vein thrombosis. J Vasc Interv Radiol. 2005;16(5):651–61.
93. Liu FY, Wang MQ, Fan QS, et al. Interventional treatment for symptomatic acute-subacute portal and superior mesenteric vein thrombosis. World J Gastroenterol. 2009;15(40):5028–34.
94. Yamakado K, Nakatsuka A, Tanaka N, et al. Portal venous stent placement in patients with pancreatic and biliary neoplasms invading portal veins and causing portal hypertension: initial experience. Radiology. 2001;220:150–6.
95. Keussen I. Interventional treatment of mesenteric venous occlusion. Pol J Radiol. 2014;79:233–8. doi:10.12659/pjr.890990.
96. Wang MQ, Guo LP, Lin HY, et al. Transradial approach for transcatheter selective superior mesenteric artery urokinase infusion therapy in patients with acute extensive portal and superior mesenteric vein thrombosis. Cardiovasc Intervent Radiol. 2010;33:80–9.
97. Safieddine N, Mamazza J, Common A, et al. Splenic and superior mesenteric artery thrombolytic infusion therapy for acute portal and mesenteric vein thrombosis. Can J Surg. 2007;50:68–9.
98. Cao G, Ko GY, Sung KB, et al. Treatment of postoperative main portal vein and superior mesenteric vein thrombosis with balloon angioplasty and/or stent placement. Acta Radiol. 2013;54:526–32.

12 Cardiac Masses

Bader S. Alshammari and Dipan J. Shah

Abstract

Cardiac magnetic resonance (CMR) imaging plays a pivotal role in the investigation and diagnosis of cardiac masses. In this chapter, we will present some illustrative cases.

Keywords

Cardiac magnetic resonance (CMR) imaging • Tumor • Thrombus • Mass

Introduction

Primary cardiac tumors are uncommon (0.02–3%) [1, 2]. Cardiac masses and pseudomasses represent a diagnostic challenge to multiple imaging modalities. Echocardiography, cardiac magnetic resonance (CMR), and computed tomography (CT) are very important for detection of cardiac masses. Most primary cardiac tumors are benign [1]. Atrial myxoma is a benign tumor and by far the most common primary cardiac tumor while the majority of primary malignant cardiac tumors are angiosarcomas in adults or rhabdomyosarcomas in children. It is important to remember that cardiac metastases are 10–40 times more frequent than primary cardiac tumors, melanoma being the most common tumor preferentially metastasize to the heart [2].

Most cardiac masses are initially detected by echocardiography, which is a first line modality for imaging of the heart for a variety of conditions. However, echocardiography has several limitations: poor image quality in those with difficult acoustic windows, limited field of view, and limited tissue characterization [1, 2]. Cardiac MR (CMR) has become the modality of choice in this setting because of its excellent spatial resolution, ability to obtain multiple imaging planes, precise localization, and excellent tissue characterization which allows a more comprehensive characterization of the mass and aids in generation of a differential diagnosis.

B.S. Alshammari, M.D. (✉) • D.J. Shah, M.D.
Houston Methodist DeBakey Heart and Vascular Center, Houston, TX, USA
e-mail: badralshmry@gmail.com

Role of CMR in the Evaluation of Cardiac Masses

The excellent soft tissue definitions that CMR provides allow clear delineation of the myocardium, pericardium and vascular structures, which facilitates the identification of abnormal mass. In addition, tissue characterization by CMR can assist in generating a differential diagnosis, and can distinguish different types of cardiac tumors. Tissue characterization is done by imaging the mass using a variety of different MR sequences (e.g. T1 weighted, T2 weighted, first pass perfusion or delayed contrast enhancement), which can assist in generating a differential diagnosis of cardiac masses (Table 12.1).

Typical magnetic resonance protocol used in assessment of cardiac masses consists of:

1. Multiplanar locator in order to know the position of the heart in the thorax.
2. Functional sequences, cine-MRI, of “bright blood” based on gradient echo, (fast imaging with steady-state precession, SSFP). They are sequences with mixed T2 and T1 weighting (T2/T1), with great differentiation in the signal intensity of the blood and the myocardium, which facilitates the detection of intracavitary lesion.

S.W. Yusuf, J. Banchs (eds.), *Cancer and Cardiovascular Disease*, https://doi.org/10.1007/978-3-319-62088-6_12

Table 12.1 CMR characteristics of cardiac masses

Cardiac mass	T 1 Weighted	T2 Weighted	Post contrast
Myxoma	Isointense, heterogeneous	Hyperintense, heterogeneous	Heterogeneous enhancement
Papillary fibroelastoma	Isointense	Slightly hyperintense	Hyperintense
Rhabdomyoma	Iso- or hyperintense	Slightly hyperintense	Hypointense or isointense
Fibroma	Iso- or hyperintense	Hypointense	Hyperintense
Hemagioma	Isointense	Hyperintense or heterogeneous	Hyperintense or heterogeneous
Paraganglioma	Iso- or hypointense	Hyperintense	Hyperintense
Intravenous leiomyomatosis	Isointense	Isointense	Heterogeneous
Bronchogenic cyst	Hypointense	Hyperintense	None
Angiosarcoma	Isointense, with hyperintense areas	Iso- or hyperintense	Hyperintense
Undifferentiated sarcoma	Isointense	Isointense	Nonspecific
Rhabdomyosarcoma	Isointense	Isointense, heterogeneous	Central nonenhancing areas
Osteosarcoma	Hyperintense	Hyperintense	Nonspecific
Malignant fibrous histiocytoma	Isonintense	Hyperintense, heterogeneous	Nonspecific
Leiomyosarcoma	Isointense	Hyperintense	Nonspecific
Fibrosarcoma	Isointense, heterogeneous	Hyperintense	Central nonenhancing areas
Lymphoma	Hypo- or isointense	Hyperintense	Variable

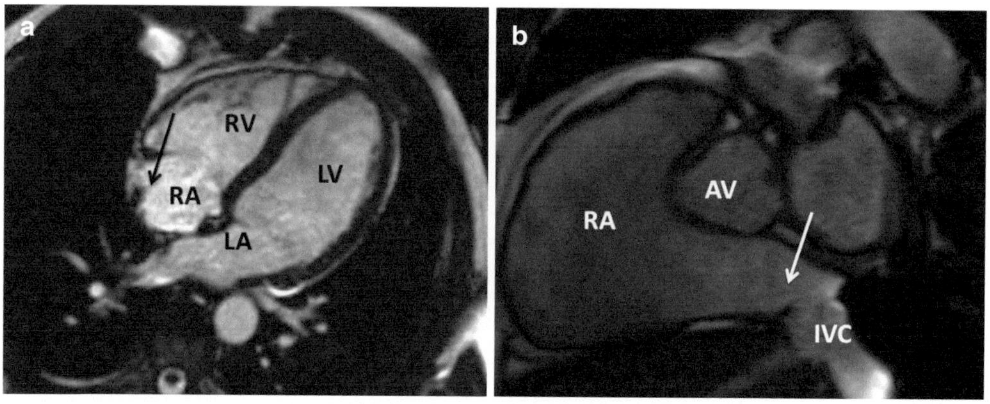

Fig. 12.1 (**a**) Cine steady-state free procession in the four-chambers view showing a prominent crista terminalis in the RA (*black arrow*)—a normal structure in the right atrium that can appear as a cardiac mass on echocardiography. (**b**) Cine steady-state free procession of Eustachian valve showing a thin, mobile membrane (*white arrow*) extending from the inferior vena cava into the right atrium. *RV* right ventricle, *RA* right atrium, *LV* left ventricle, *LA* left atrium, *AV* aortic valve, *IVC* inferior vena cava

3. Morphological and tissue characterization sequences based on spin echo. T1 and T2 weighted sequences will be obtained with or without fat suppression sequences.
4. First-pass perfusion during rapid IV administration of gadolinium to assess for mass vascularity.
5. Late gadolinium enhancement (LGE) sequences (T1-weighted sequences). They can be fast gradient echo or phase-sensitive inversion-recovery (PSIR) sequences. The inversion time for this sequence ranges from 150 to 300 ms. However, 500–600 ms inversion time is very useful to identify thrombi.

Cardiac Pseudomasses

There are a number of normal structures that are not true masses but can mimic a cardiac or paracardiac masses. The most common of these is a right atrial pseudotumor produced by a prominent crista terminalis, which can appear as a right atrial mass on echocardiography (Fig. 12.1a).

A prominent Chiari malformation or Eustachian valve can also be mistaken as a right atrial mass; these can easily visualized by CMR (Fig. 12.1b).

Extracardiac structures that can simulate cardiac pathology include a large hiatal hernia that can compress the atria. CMR is superior to echocardiography in identifying hiatal hernia as a true extra-cardiac mass (Fig. 12.2).

Intracavitary Thrombi

The diagnosis of intracavitary thrombus may be suspected from echocardiographic findings (such as LV apical location or association with wall motion abnormality). However, it can occur within any cardiac chamber. By far intracavitary thrombus is the most common intra-cardiac mass [3, 4]. Left atrial appendage thrombus is most commonly associated with atrial fibrillation [2].

Intraventricular thrombus usually occurs in the setting of cardiomyopathy, because decrease contractility predisposes to sluggish blood flow and can be a substrate for thrombus formation as shown in Fig. 12.3.

CMR enables thrombus to be detected based on intrinsic tissue characteristics related to avascular tissue composition. CMR is more sensitive and specific than echocardiography for detecting ventricular or atrial thrombi [3]. The sensitivity is significantly improved by administration of intravenous contrast material. Post-contrast delayed enhancement inversion recovery images with a long inversion time are exquisitely sensitive for detection of even small thrombi [5].

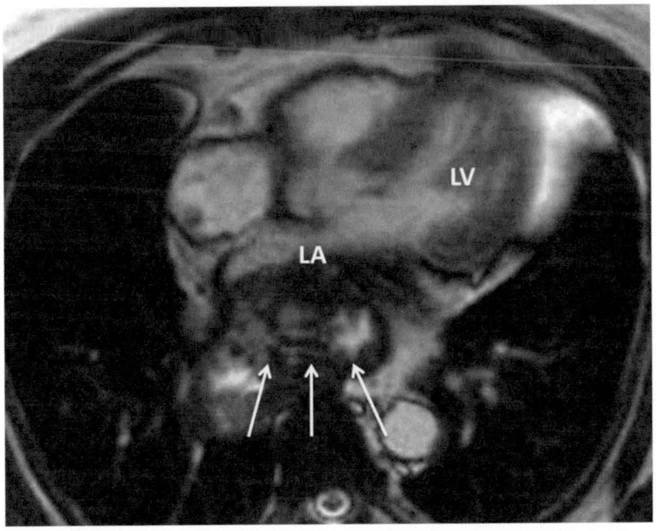

Fig. 12.2 Showing an axial Cine steady-state free procession in the chest with a large hiatal hernia (*white arrows*), which is compressing upon left atrium. *LA* left atrium, *LV* left ventricle

The long inversion time allows recovery of signal by virtually all tissue except thrombus, which remains low in signal intensity and therefore dark on imaging as demonstrated in Fig. 12.3.

Benign Primary Cardiac Tumors

Benign cardiac tumors are usually classified pathologically according to histologic features. They can have an intracavitary location and be attached to endocardium or myocardium. They can also be intra-myocardial. Myxoma, papillary fibroelastoma, and lipoma are the most frequent ones.

Myxoma

Cardiac myxoma is the most frequent primary cardiac tumor (25–50%) [1]. The vast majority are sporadic and occur in adults between 40 and 70 years of age. They are usually asymptomatic or they can be associated with heart failure, systemic embolism, syncope or sudden death [6]. Nearly 7% of cardiac myxomas can exist as part of the carney complex which is an autosomal dominant syndrome characterized by myxoma, hyperpigmentation and extra-cardiac tumors [7].

They are most commonly located in the left atrium (75%), they are usually attached by a pedicle to the interatrial septum, close to fossa ovalis and they can prolapse through the atrial-ventricular valves. Ventricular origin for myxoma is very rare (<2%) but can occur, as is right atrial origin [3].

Cardiac myxomas are heterogeneous masses of variable sizes (1–15 cm), due to the presence necrosis, calcification, bleeding, cystic formations or fibrosis [8].

CMR features of myxoma are shown in Fig. 12.4.

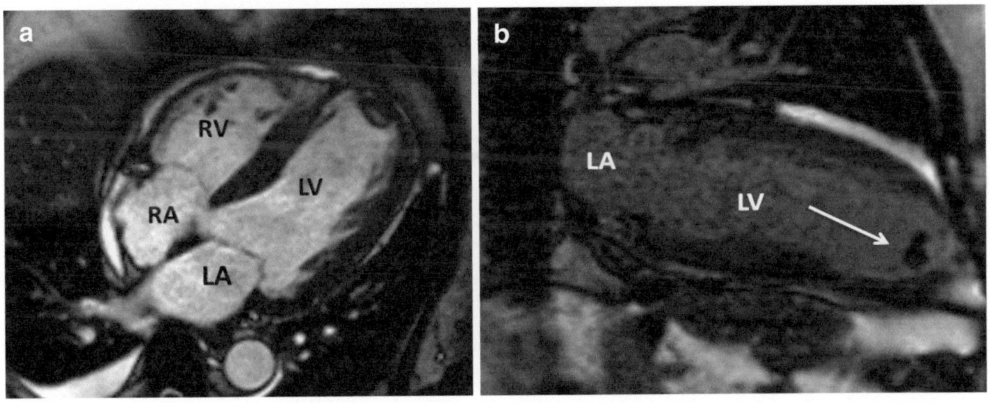

Fig. 12.3 A fifty-eight year-old male who presented with acute myocardial infarction and underwent angioplasty of LAD who underwent cardiac MRI. (**a**) Cine steady-state free procession showing a large apical thrombus. (**b**) Showing a thrombus (*arrow*) after gadolinium injection of the same patient performed 15 min after administration of gadolinium, using long inversion time (TI). *LAD* left anterior descending artery, *RV* right ventricle, *RA* right atrium, *LV* left ventricle, *LA* left atrium

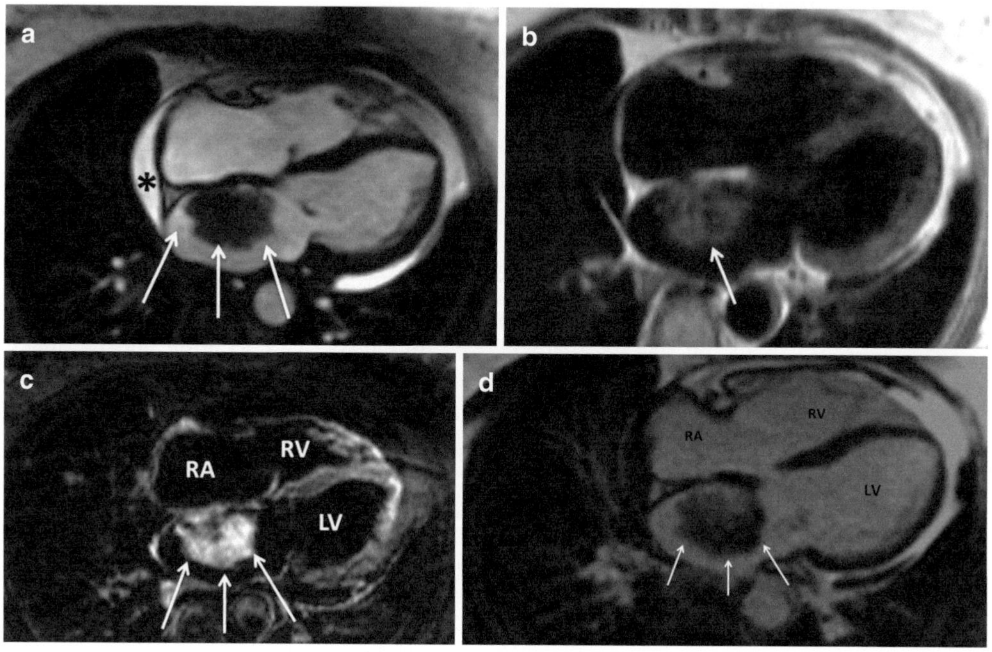

Fig. 12.4 Myxoma in a 68-year-old asymptomatic male who underwent cardiac MRI. Cine steady-state free procession images in the four-chamber view, (**a**) demonstrates a well-outlined and intracavitary mass (*white arrows*) in the left atrium. Note a small pericardial effusion (*asterisk*). (**b**) In T1-weighted fast spin echo the mass can be identified in the left atrium well-outlined and of intermediate signal. LA myxoma appears hyperintense to myocardium on T2-weighted sequence (**c**); and heterogeneous enhancement after gadolinium injection (**d**). *RV* right ventricle, *RA* right atrium, *LV* left ventricle, *LA* left atrium

Papillary Fibroelastoma

Papillary fibroelastomas are benign avascular papillomas of the endocardium. They account for 10% of primary cardiac tumors [9, 10].

They are small (<1 cm), well-defined lesions, usually asymptomatic and usually detected incidentally by echocardiography that is performed for another indication. Most of them are usually located on the endocardial surface of the aortic (29%) or mitral (25%) valves [7].

CMR features of papillary fibroelastomas are shown in Fig. 12.5.

Lipoma

Cardiac lipomas are benign neoplasms composed of encapsulated mature adipose tissue, similar to extracardiac lipomas [3]. They can be detected at any age. Multiple cases have been described associated with tuberous sclerosis [11].

The most common location is the right atrium and the left ventricle. Other locations are cardiac valves, intramyocardial or pericardial [12].

Most lipomas do not cause any symptoms, but occasionally can lead to dyspnea if there is obstruction of blood flow, and/or arrhythmias if there is involvement of the cardiac conduction system [13, 14]. Given their fatty nature, cardiac lipomas are high in signal intensity on T1-weighted sequences with low signal intensity on fat saturation pulses sequences (e.g. T1 or T2-weighted spin echo).

CMR features of cardiac lipomas are shown in Fig. 12.6.

Lipomatous Hypertrophy of the Inter-Atrial Septum

Lipomatous hypertrophy of inter-atrial septum is not a true neoplasm. It is due to hyperplasia of otherwise normal fatty cells within the inter-atrial septum. The diagnosis is based on the finding of fatty deposits in the inter-atrial septum, resulting in a diameter exceeding 2 cm in the transverse dimensions. The exact etiology is unknown but it appears to be associated with obesity and advanced age. The exact incidence of this disorder is difficult to discern but incidences of lipomatous hypertrophy of the inter-atrial septum were 1% in autopsy series [19].

Lipomatous hypertrophy of the inter-atrial septum is associated with atrial arrhythmia [20].

CMR features of cardiac lipomatous hypertrophy of inter-atrial septum are shown in Fig. 12.7.

Fibroma

Cardiac fibromas are congenital neoplasms that typically affect children. However, 15% of cardiac fibromas occur in adults [15].

Approximately one-third of patients present with arrhythmias, one-third with heart failure or cyanosis, and one-third are detected incidentally [15].

They are well-circumscribed tumors located within ventricular myocardium as shown in Fig. 12.8.

The key findings are that they demonstrate reduced signal on T 2-weighted imaging (due to their limited water content) and demonstrate very high signal intensity on LGE imaging (due to their high collagen content) [16].

CMR features of cardiac fibromas are shown in Fig. 12.8.

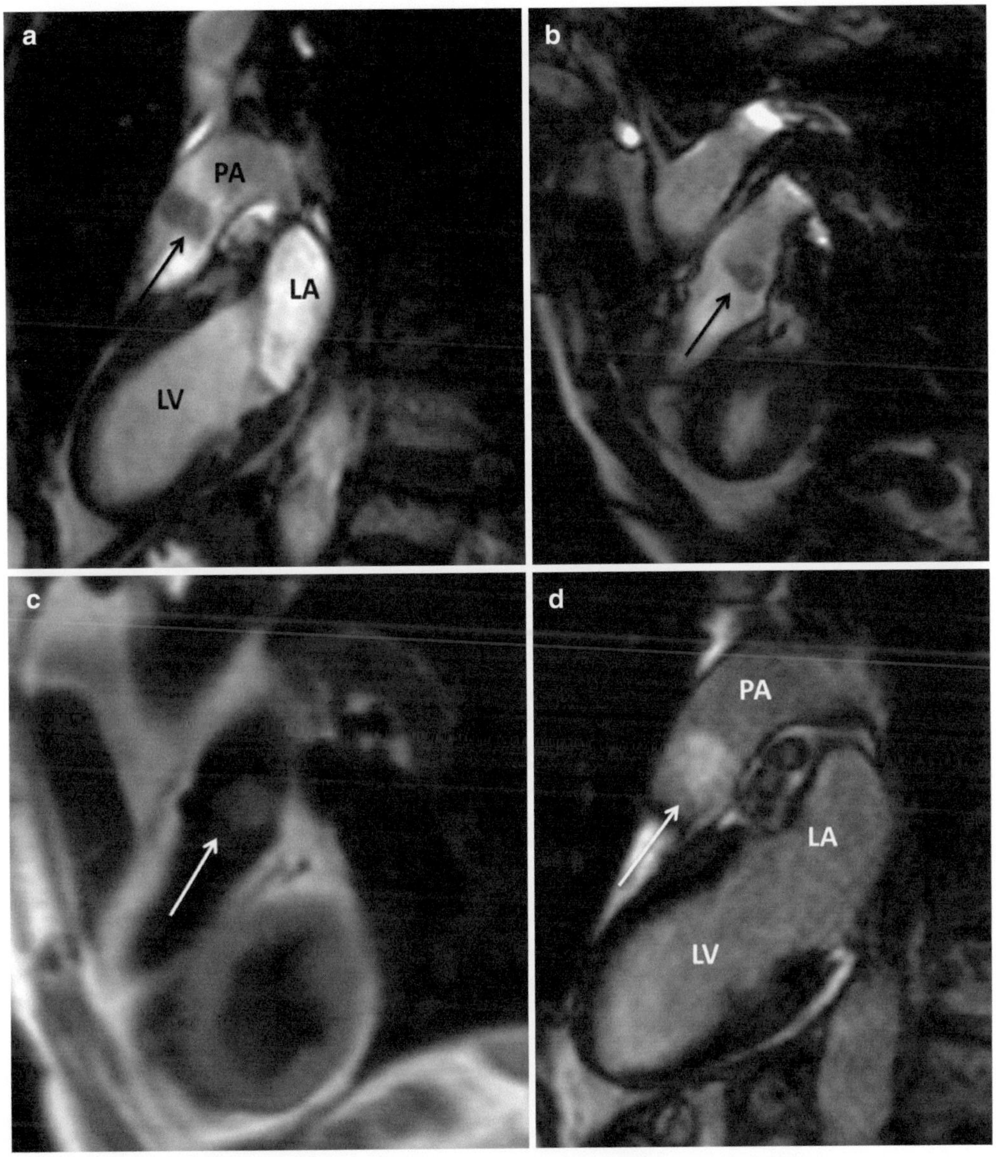

Fig. 12.5 Papillary fibroelastoma of the pulmonic valve (*arrow*) demonstrated on cine steady-state free procession (**a**, **b**). Papillary fibroelastoma of the pulmonic valve demonstrating isointense signal on T1-weighted fast spin echo (**c**). After gadolinium injection imaging demonstrates intense contrast uptake by the mass (**d**). *PA* pulmonary artery, *LA* left atrium, *LV* left ventricle

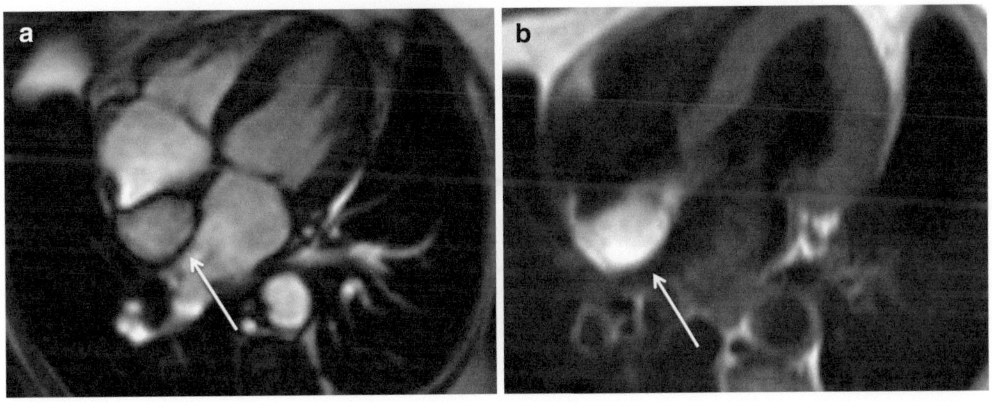

Fig. 12.6 Lipoma in a 53 year-old woman with incidental finding of a mass on echocardiography who underwent cardiac MRI. (**a**) Cine steady-state free procession demonstrating a well-defined uniformly high signal lesion within the inter-atrial septum (*arrow*). (**b**) Four-Chamber T1-weighted fast spin echo image again showing the lesion as having uniformly high signal in keeping with a fat composition due to lipoma

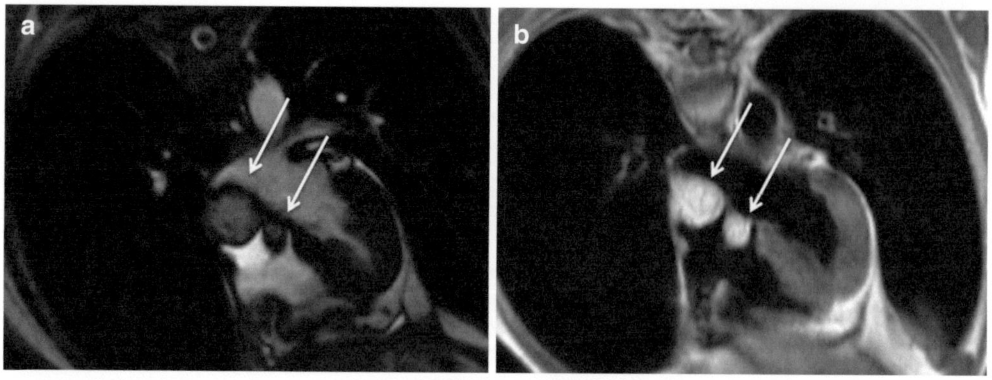

Fig. 12.7 Cine steady-state free procession demonstrates lipomatous hypertrophy of the inter-atrial septum (**a**, *arrow*), and hyperintense on T1-weighted fast spin echo due to high fat content of the inter-atrial septum(**b**)

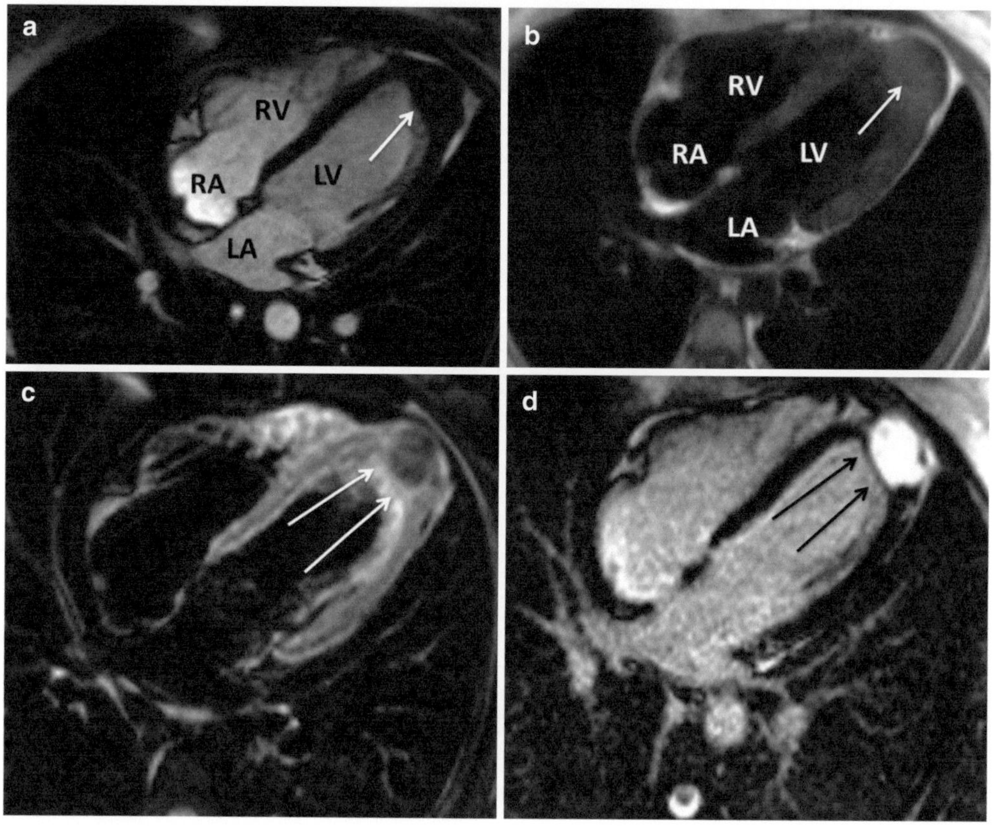

Fig. 12.8 Fibroma in asymptomatic 22 year-old female. Cine steady-state free procession in the four-chambers (**a**) and T-2 weighted imaging (**b**) demonstrating a homogenous myocardial mass in LV apex which appears isointense on T2-weighted imaging. Cardiac fibroma appears hypointense on T2-weighted images (**c**). The most characteristic feature of cardiac fibroma is diffuse homogeneous enhancement after gadolinium injection (**d**). *RV* right ventricle, *RA* right atrium, *LV* left ventricle, *LA* left atrium

Rhabdomyoma

Rhabdomyomas are the most frequent cardiac tumor in children. They are intramural tumors and can occur in isolation or associated with tuberous sclerosis [17]. They are usually asymptomatic but can cause obstruction of the ventricular outflow tract or arrhythmias [18].

CMR features of rhabdomyomas are described in Table 12.1 and in Fig. 12.9 [26].

Paraganglioma

Cardiac paragangliomas are exceptionally rare neuroendocrine neoplasms. Most of these lesions present with symptoms of catecholamine excess (hypertension, tachyarrythmias, and heart failure). They usually occur between 10 and 60 years of age. Their usual location in the atria and at the root of the great vessels. They can be isolated or associated with paragangliomas in other locations (20%) [7].

CMR features of cardiac paragangliomas are shown in Fig. 12.10.

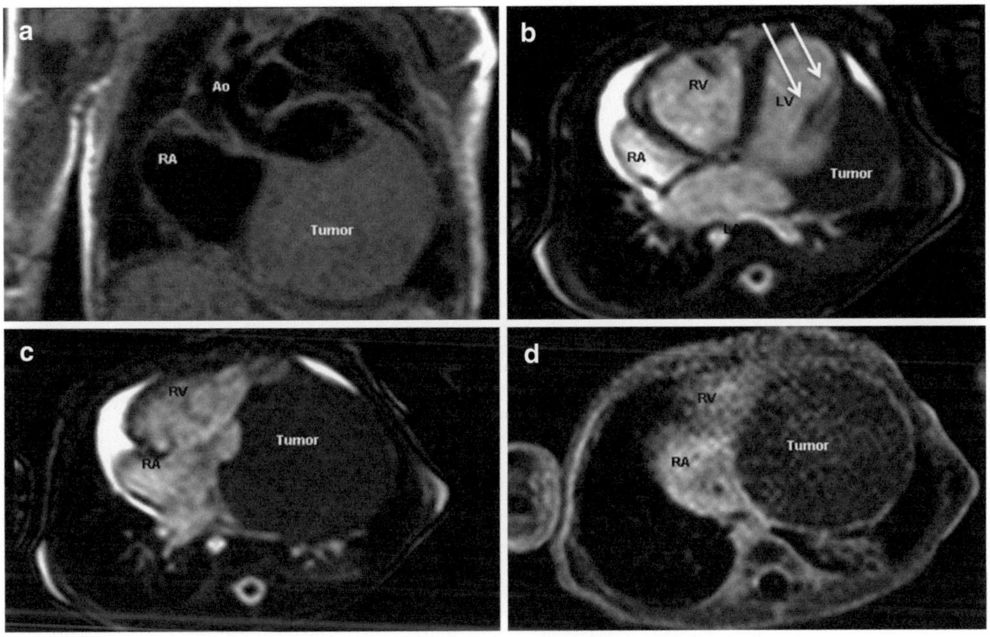

Fig. 12.9 Intramural left ventricular rhabdomyoma in a new born. (**a**) T1-weighted fast spin echo showing a large homogeneous isointense mass involving the LV wall. (**b**) Cine steady-state free procession in axial plane, showing the cardiac mass involving the interventricular septum. (**c**) Cine steady state free procession in four-chamber view, showing no intracardiac obstruction. (**d**) After gadolinium injection, no mass hyperenhancement is visible. *Ao* indicates aorta, *RA* right atrium, *RV* right ventricle, *LA* left atrium, *LV* left ventricle. Source: Reproduced with permission from [26] © 2011 Wolters Kluwer Health

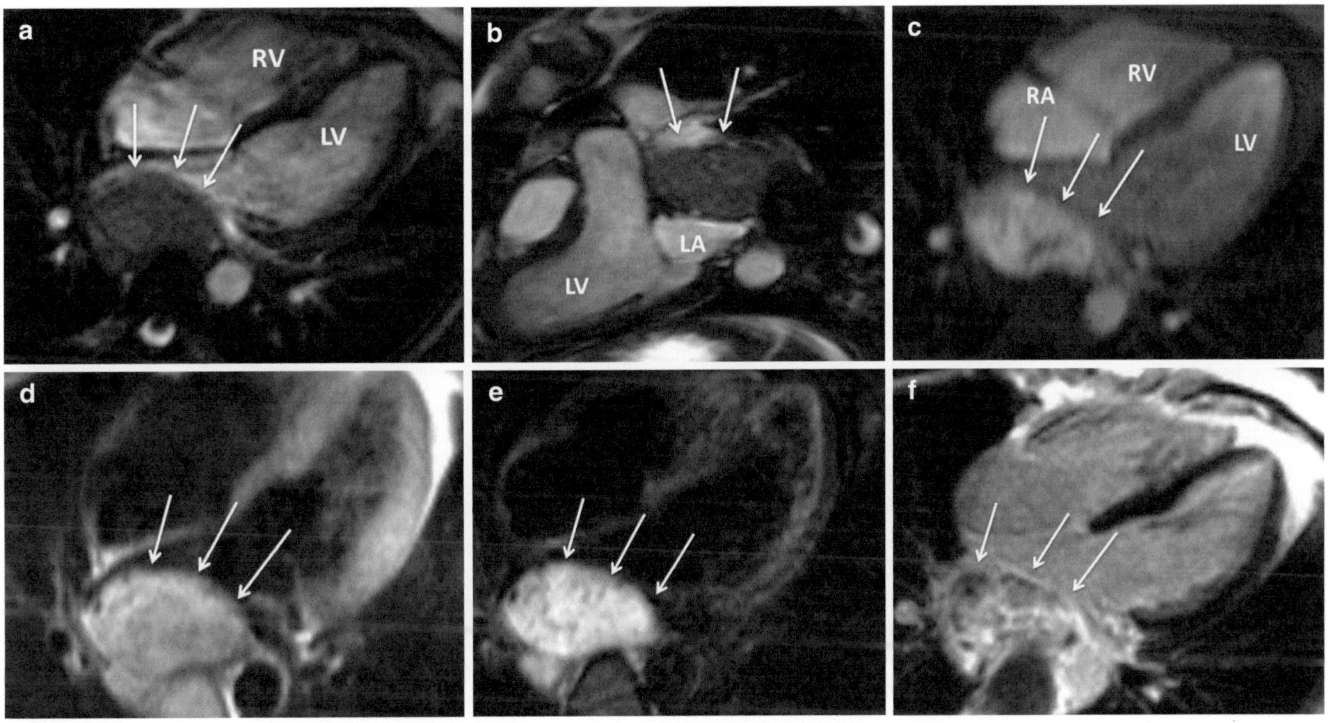

Fig. 12.10 Paraganglinoma in a 42 year-old male with dyspnea who underwent cardiac MRI. Cine steady-state free procession demonstrating a large left atrial mass and extending along the inter-atrial septum (**a**, **b**). Paraganglinoma on perfusion imaging (**c**) demonstrating first pass perfusion comparable to myocardium after gadolinium injection. The mass is isointense to myocardium on T1-weighted fast spin echo in axial plane (**d**), hyperintense to myocardium on T2-weighted imaging in axial plane (**e**), and demonstrates heterogeneous uptake after gadolinium injection in axial plane (**f**). *RA* right atrium, *RV* right ventricle, *LV* left ventricle, *RV* right ventricle, *LA* left atrium, *LV* left ventricle, *SVC* superior vena cava

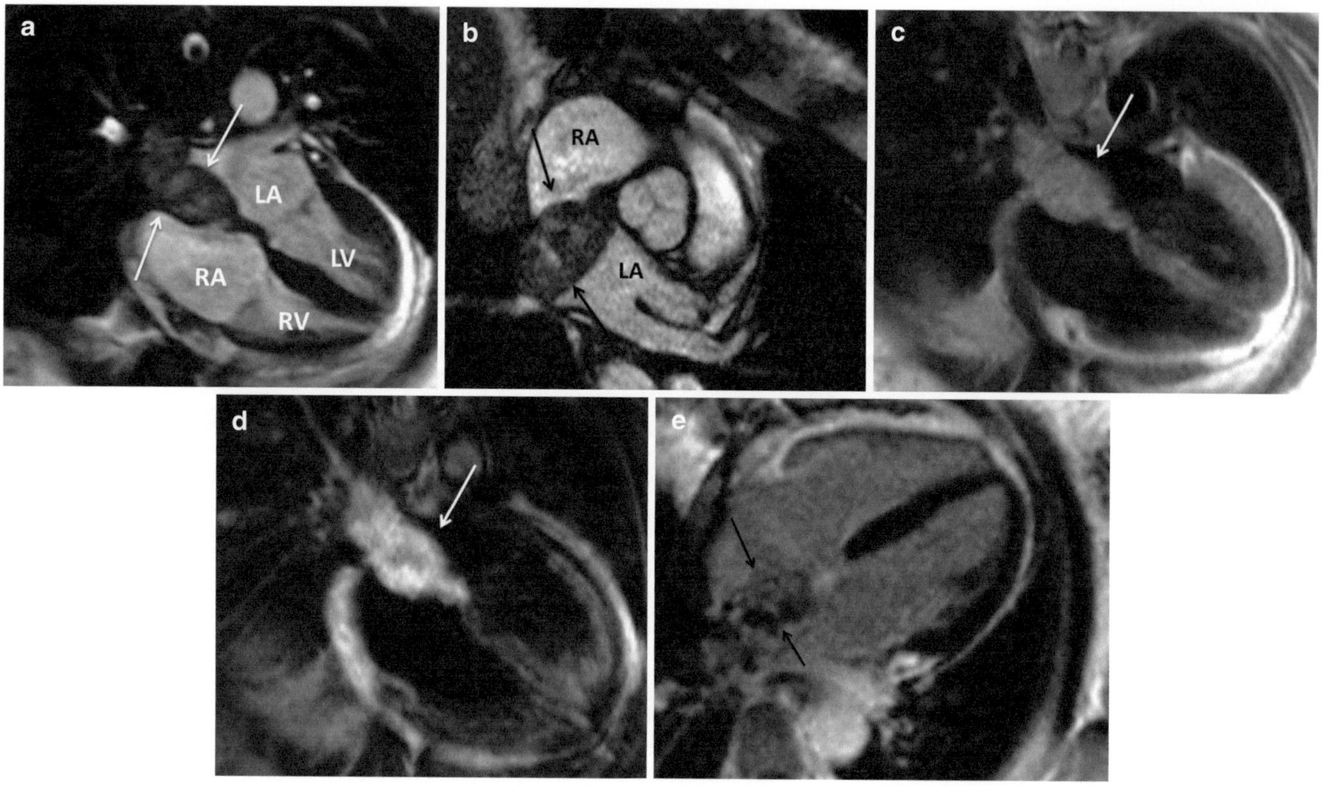

Fig. 12.11 Primary angiosarcoma in a 58 year-old male with dyspnea, peripheral edema and weight loss. (**a**) Cine steady-state free procession in axial plane shows a heterogeneous mass with invasion into the inter-atrial septum with partial obstruction of the SVC (**b**). Angiosarcoma appears isointense on T1-weighted fast spin echo image (**c**), and hyper-intense on T-2 weighted imaging (**d**). Primary angiosarcoma demonstrates heterogeneous uptake (**e**) after gadolinium injection (*arrows*). *RV* right ventricle, *RA* right atrium, *LV* left ventricle, *LA* left atrium

Malignant Primary Cardiac Tumors

Malignant tumors comprise approximately 25% of primary cardiac neoplasms [3]. They are classified by tissue type as mesenchymal (sarcoma), which represents the majority, or lymphoid with lymphoma making up most of the reminder. Imaging characteristics of malignant tumors are quite similar, with most lesions demonstrating invasion of surrounding structures and myocardium, poor border definition, and frequent coexisting pericardial effusion. Various cardiac sarcomas have many features in common with similar CMR features [3].

Angiosarcoma

Angiosarcoma is the most common form of cardiac sarcoma, accounting for approximately 40% of cases. Angiosarcoma has a predilection for the right atrium with more than 90% originating at this location [21].

Other forms of sarcomas (undifferentiated sarcomas, malignant fibrous histiocytoma, osteosarcoma, leiomyosarcoma, or rhabdomyosarcoma) are bulky and infiltrating masses with a predilection to arise in the left atrium [22].

CMR features of angiosarcoma are shown in Fig. 12.11.

Lymphoma

Cardiac lymphomas are almost always aggressive B-cell lymphomas. These neoplasms have increased prevalence in immunocompromised patients, but also can occur in immunocompetent patients. The average age of presentation is approximately 58 years. Males appear to have a slight predominance [3]. Clinical features are typically of dyspnea, arrhythmia, superior vena cava obstruction or cardiac tamponade due to frequent involvement in the pericardium resulting in pericardial effusion. They are commonly involving right atrium, followed by right ventricle [7].

CMR features of cardiac lymphomas are shown in Fig. 12.12.

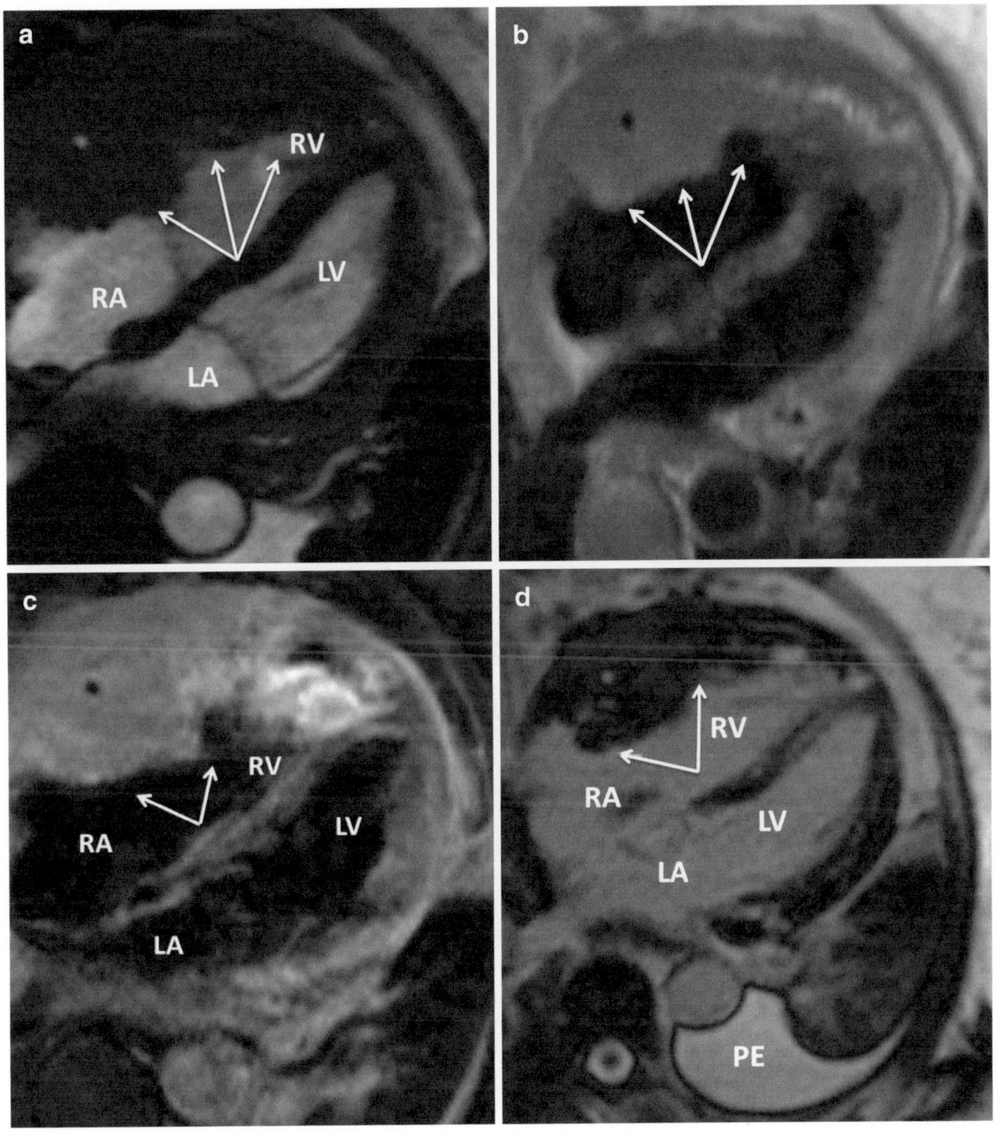

Fig. 12.12 Seventy-year-old male with cardiac B-cell lymphoma. Cine steady-state free procession in axial plane demonstrates a large tumor (*arrows*) originating in the right sided chambers not only involve cardiac chamber cavities but also within the myocardium (**a**). Cardiac lymphoma appears isointense T1-weighted fast spin echo imaging (**b**). Cardiac lymphoma demonstrates heterogeneous hyperintense on T-2 imaging (**c**) and heterogeneous uptake on post-contrast imaging (**d**). *RV* right ventricle, *RA* right atrium, *LV* left ventricle, *LA* left atrium, *PE* pleural effusion

Secondary Cardiac Tumors

Secondary cardiac tumors are 20 times more common than primary cardiac tumors [27]. Metastatic disease may result from contiguous extension, lymphangitic spread, transvenous route, or hematogenous spread [23]. Tumors metastasizing to the heart often involve the pericardium also. Metastatic malignant melanoma has the highest rate of cardiac metastasis [24]. Metastases to the heart and pericardium are discovered at autopsy in 10–12% of all patients with malignancies [25].

Direct extension to involve the heart or the pericardium is often observed in lung carcinoma and breast. Hematogenous spread is usual for melanoma, leukemia, or sarcomas. CMR features of cardiac metastasis are shown in Fig. 12.13.

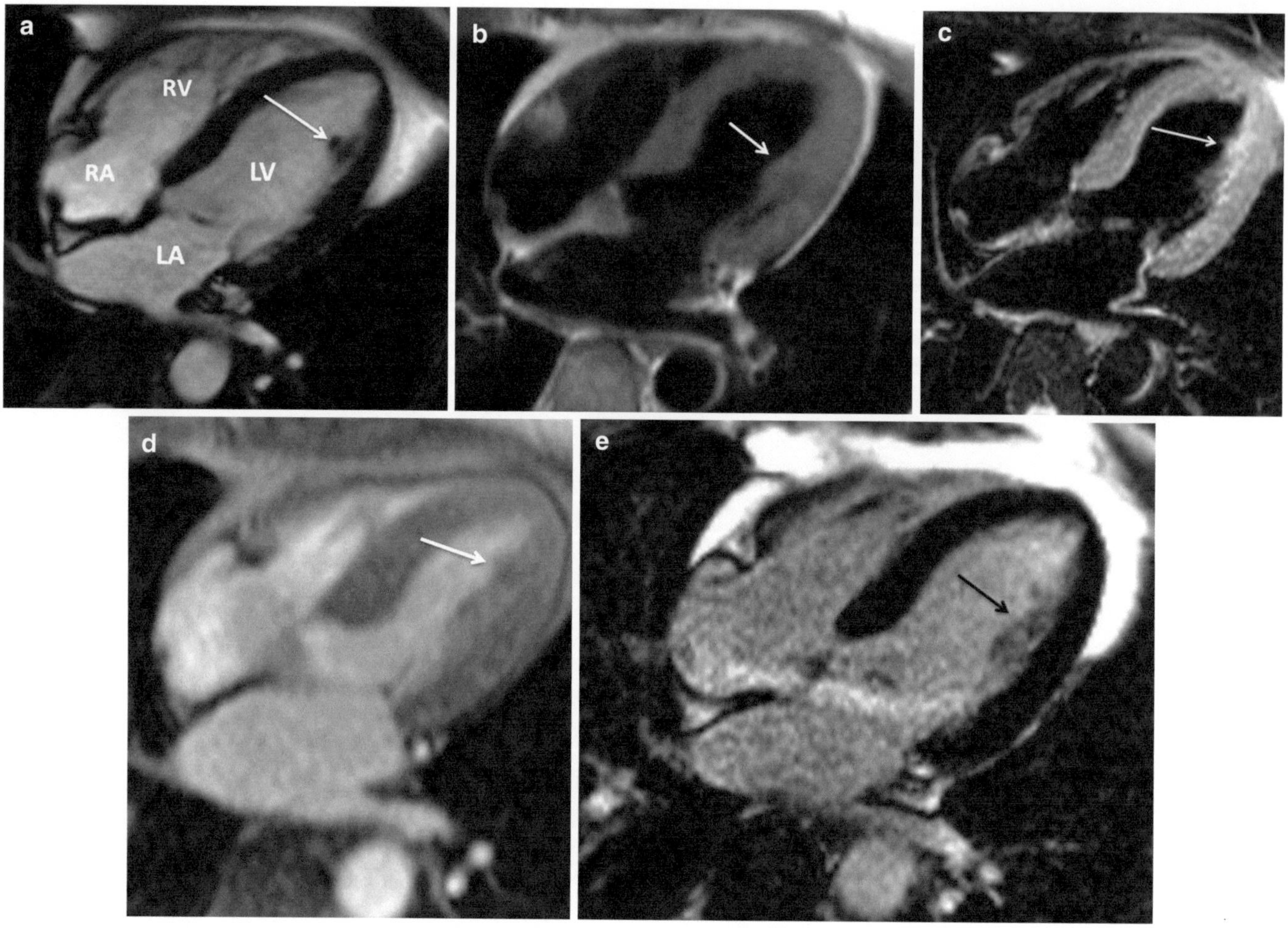

Fig. 12.13 Metastasis from skin melanoma in a 74 year-old female with palpitations demonstrating a well circumscribed intracavitary mass in LV on cine steady-state free procession in axial plane (*arrow*, **a**). The mass is isointense to myocardium on T1-weighted fast spin echo imaging (**b**). Also demonstrates a slight hyperintense lesion on T-2 weighted imaging (*arrow*, **c**) and hypoperfusion in comparison to myocardium on first pass imaging (*arrow*, **d**). Cardiac metastasis showing mild enhancement after gadolinium injection (*arrow*, **e**). *RV* right ventricle, *RA* right atrium, *LV* left ventricle, *LA* left atrium

References

1. Motwani M, Kidambi A, Herzog BA, Uddin A, Greenwood JP, Plein S. MR imaging of cardiac tumors and masses: a review of methods and clinical applications. Radiology. 2013;268:26–43.
2. Sparrow PJ, Kurian JB, Jones TR, Sivananthan MU. MR imaging of cardiac tumors. Radiographics. 2005;25:1255–76.
3. Grizzard JD, Ang GB. Magnetic resonance imaging of pericardial disease and cardiac masses. Magn Reson Imaging Clin N Am. 2007;15(4):579–607, vi.
4. Schvartzman PR, White RD. Imaging of cardiac and paracardiac masses. J Thorac Imaging. 2000;15(4):265–73.
5. Weinsaft JW, Kim HW, Shah DJ, Klem I, Crowley AL, Brosnan R, James OG, Patel MR, Heitner J, Parker M, Velazquez EJ, Steenbergen C, Judd RM, Kim RJ. Detection of left ventricular thrombus by delayed-enhancement cardiovascular magnetic resonance prevalence and markers in patients with systolic dysfunction. J Am Coll Cardiol. 2008;52(2):148–57.
6. Butany J, Nair V, Naseemuddin A, Nair GM, Catton C, Yau T. Cardiac tumours: diagnosis and management. Lancet Oncol. 2005;6:219–28.
7. Araoz PA, Mulvagh SL, Tazelaar HD, Julsrud PR, Breen JF. CT and MR imaging of benign primary cardiac neoplasms with echocardiographic correlation. Radiographics. 2000;20:1303–19.
8. Masui T, Takahashi M, Miura K, Naito M, Tawarahara K. Cardiac myxoma: identification of intratumoral hemorrhage and calcification on MR images. AJR Am J Roentgenol. 1995;164:850–2.
9. Randhawa K, Ganeshan A, Hoey ET. Magnetic resonance imaging of cardiac tumors: part 2, malignant tumors and tumor-like conditions. Curr Probl Diagn Radiol. 2011;40:169–79.
10. Burke A, Virmani R. Classification and incidence of cardiac tumors. In: Burke A, Virmani R, editors. Tumors of the heart and great vessels: atlas of tumor pathology, vol. 16. 3rd ed. Washington, DC: Armed Forces Institute of Pathology; 1996. p. 1–11.
11. Ghadimi Mahani M, Lu JC, Rigsby CK, Krishnamurthy R, Dorfman AL, Agarwal PP. MRI of pediatric cardiac masses. AJR Am J Roentgenol. 2014;202:971–81.
12. Rodríguez E, Soler R, Gayol A, Freire R. Massive mediastinal and cardiac fatty infiltration in a young patient. J Thorac Imaging. 1995;10:225–6.
13. Zingas AP, Carrera JD, Murray CA III, Kling GA. Lipoma of the myocardium. J Comput Assist Tomogr. 1983;7(6):1098–100.

14. Conces DJ Jr, Vix VA, Tarver RD. Diagnosis of a myocardial lipoma by using CT. AJR Am J Roentgenol. 1989;153(4):725–6.
15. Burke AP, Rosado-de-Christenson M, Templeton PA, Virmani R. Cardiac fibroma: clinicopathologic correlates and surgical treatment. J Thorac Cardiovasc Surg. 1994;108:862–70.
16. Yan AT, Coffey DM, Li Y, Chan WS, Shayne AJ, Luu TM, Skorstad RB, Khin MM, Brown KA, Lipton MJ, Kwong RY. Images in cardiovascular medicine. Myocardial fibroma in gorlin syndrome by cardiac magnetic resonance imaging. Circulation. 2006;114(10):e376–9.
17. Nir A, Tajik AJ, Freeman WK, Seward JB, Offord KP, Edwards WD, et al. Tuberous sclerosis and cardiac rhabdomyoma. Am J Cardiol. 1995;76:419–21.
18. Tao TY, Yahyavi-Firouz-Abadi N, Singh GK, Bhalla S. Pediatric cardiac tumors: clinical and imaging features. Radiographics. 2014;34:1031–46.
19. Reyes CV, Jablokow VR. Lipomatous hypertrophy of the cardiac interatrial septum: a report of 38 cases and review of the literature. Am J Clin Pathol. 1979;72(5):785–8.
20. Hutter AM, Page DL. Atrial arrhythmias and lipomatous hypertrophy of the cardiac interatrial septum. Am Heart J. 1971;82(1):16–21.
21. Best AK, Dobson RL, Ahmad AR. Best cases from the AFIP: cardiac angiosarcoma. Radiographics. 2003;23(Spec no):S141–5.
22. Araoz PA, Eklund HE, Welch TJ, Breen JF. CT and MR imaging of primary cardiac malignancies. Radiographics. 1999;19(6):1421–34.
23. Chiles C, Woodard PK, Gutierrez FR, et al. Metastatic involvement of the heart and pericardium: CT and MR imaging. Radiographics. 2001;21(2):439–49.
24. Glancy DL, Roberts WC. The heart in malignant melanoma. A study of 70 autopsy cases. Am J Cardiol. 1968;21(4):555–71.
25. Abraham KP, Reddy V, Gattuso P. Neoplasms metastatic to the heart: review of 3314 consecutive autopsies. Am J Cardiovasc Pathol. 1990;3:195–8.
26. Padalino MA, Vida VL, Bhattarai A, Reffo E, Milanesi O, Thiene G, Stellin G. Cristina Basso. Circulation. 2011;124:2275–7.
27. Lam KY, Dickens P, Chan AC. Tumors of the heart. A 20-year experience with a review of 12,485 consecutive autopsies. Arch Pathol Lab Med. 1993;117:1027–31.

Surgical Treatment for Cardiac Sarcomas

13

Ross M. Reul and Michael J. Reardon

Abstract

In this chapter we have presented some cases of cardiac sarcomas and outlined the general approach and surgical treatment of this condition.

Keywords

Cardiac tumor • Sarcoma • Cardiac auto transplantation

Introduction

Cardiac tumors are a rare entity, comprised of tumors with a diverse histology and natural history. They are divided into primary and secondary tumors. Primary cardiac tumors are rare, with an autopsy incidence of 0.002–0.3% [1–3]. Primary cardiac tumors include benign or malignant neoplasms that may arise from any cardiac tissue. Secondary or metastatic cardiac tumors are about 30 times more common than the primary neoplasm with an autopsy incidence of 1.7–14% [4].

Another two possible categories one could think of is infra-diaphragmatic tumors that invade by direct extension and secondly tumors that extend from the mediastinal space invading directly usually involving pericardial layers. Infra-diaphragmatic tumors can occur with almost any cell type, but the large majority of these have been attributed to renal cell carcinoma (RCC) where as much as 10% of patients with have tumor extension into the inferior vena cava [5] and in patients with RCC, involvement of the right atrium (RA) is encountered in up to 5% of cases, pulmonary artery tumor emboli is even more rarely observed [6, 7]. Other sources for this route of invasion include uterine malignancies [8], and hepatocellular carcinoma [9].

In this chapter we will illustrate cardiac tumors focusing on primary, right and left, cardiac sarcomas.

R.M. Reul, M.D. • M.J. Reardon, M.D. (✉)
Department of Cardiovascular Surgery, Houston Methodist DeBakey Heart and Vascular Center, Houston, TX, USA
e-mail: mreardon@houstonmethodist.org

Right Heart Sarcomas

Right heart tumors tend to be large, bulky, and infiltrative at the time of presentation. They usually do not cause symptomatic obstruction to intra-cardiac blood flow until they are advanced. We prefer to obtain tissue for histologic diagnosis prior to definitive resection of right heart tumors when the patient's condition permits. When sarcoma is confirmed patients are treated with neoadjuvant chemotherapy with Adriamycin and Ifosfamide. This allows us to evaluate the patient's response to treatment and, if responsive, to shrink the tumor to increase the likelihood of performing R0 resection. We have found that right heart sarcomas that do not have an appreciable chemotherapy response are unlikely to have a reasonable survival after surgery. Our series of right heart sarcomas is currently the largest reported and we have shown that R0 resection (patients with negative surgical margins) doubles survival and that neoadjuvant therapy significantly increases R0 resection rates [10].

Case 1

The patient is a 46 year old male who presented with chest pain and dyspnea. Investigations revealed a large right heart tumor, pericardial effusion, and several small pulmonary nodules. He had drainage of the pericardial effusion and histology was positive for angiosarcoma. He underwent six rounds of Chemotherapy with Adriamycin and Ifosfamide which led to complete resolution of the pulmonary masses and significant reduction of the size of the right heart tumor.

S.W. Yusuf, J. Banchs (eds.), *Cancer and Cardiovascular Disease*, https://doi.org/10.1007/978-3-319-62088-6_13

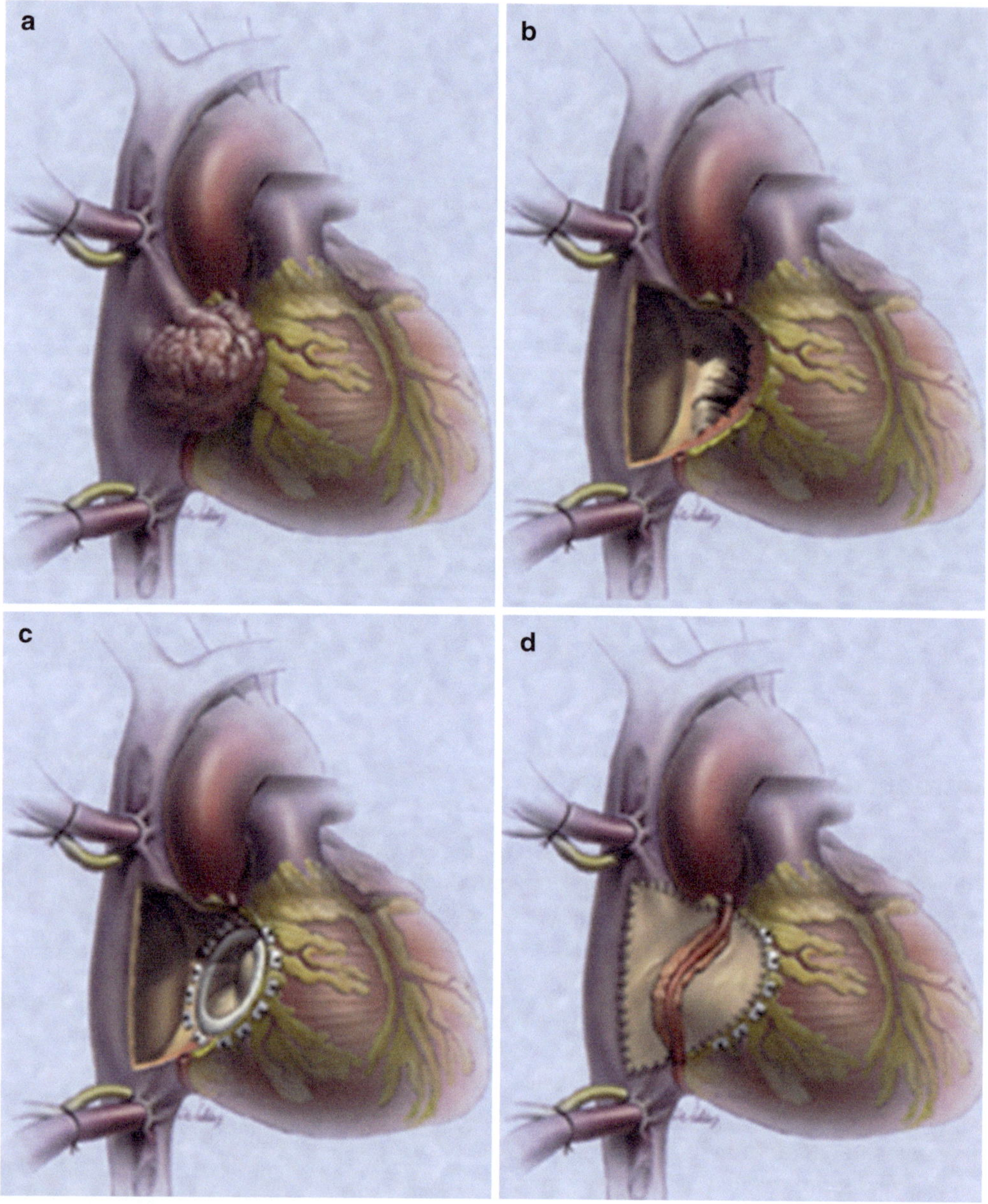

Fig. 13.1 (**a**) Right heart tumor. (**b**) Tumor resected. (**c**) Tricuspid valve replaced. (**d**) Completed reconstruction

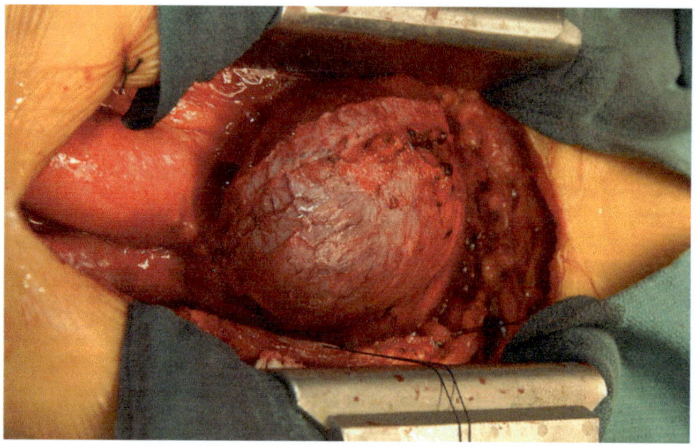

Fig. 13.2 Operative photograph of the right heart tumor

Following the six rounds of chemotherapy the response of the tumor slowed and surgical resection was recommended.

The residual tumor was a very large mass located in the right atrial/right ventricular groove (Figs. 13.1a and 13.2). An extensive resection was required for complete removal including excision of most of the right atrium, the tricuspid valve, the right coronary artery, and a portion of the right ventricle (Fig. 13.1b). The tricuspid valve was replaced with a bioprosthetic valve (Figs. 13.1c and 13.3). The final reconstruction was done using bovine pericardium for the right atrium and the segment of resected coronary artery was replaced with an interposed mammary artery graft (Figs. 13.1d and 13.4). The patient recovered well and survived for 47 months before he expired from metastatic disease.

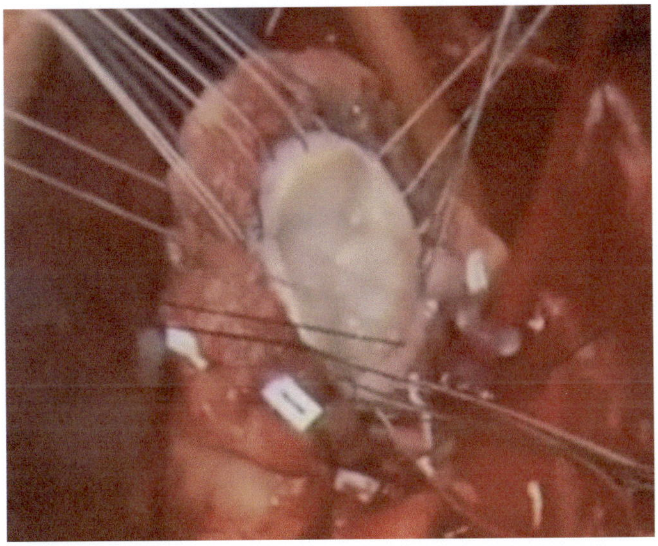

Fig. 13.3 Operative photograph of tricuspid valve replacement

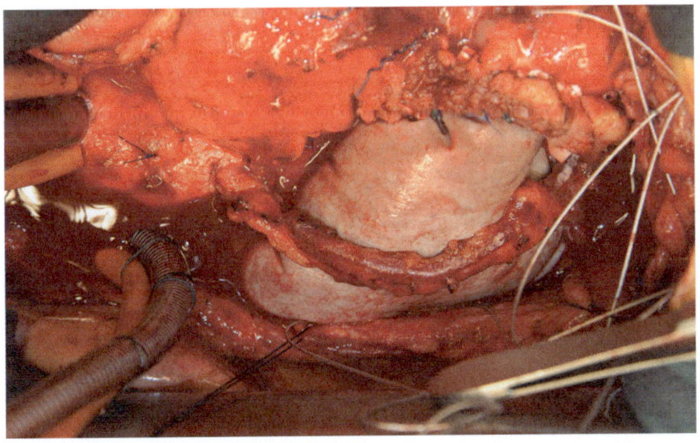

Fig. 13.4 Operative photograph showing final reconstruction

Pulmonary Artery Sarcomas

Our cardiac tumor group has a long-standing interest in pulmonary artery (PA) sarcomas [11–13]. PA sarcomas are usually asymptomatic until they reach a large size and cause symptoms due to obstruction of pulmonary blood flow (Fig. 13.5). This usually leads to the need for urgent surgical resection. PA sarcomas often begin at the level of the pulmonary valve (Fig. 13.6) and extend distally, expanding within the lumen without penetrating the wall of the PA (Fig. 13.7).

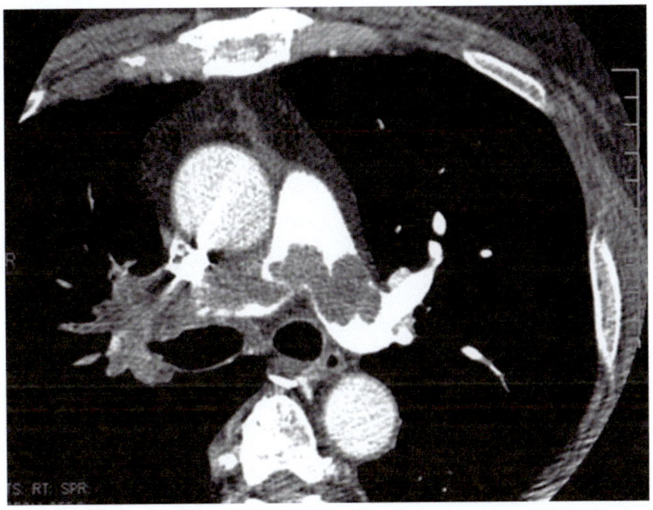

Fig. 13.5 CT scan showing pulmonary artery sarcoma

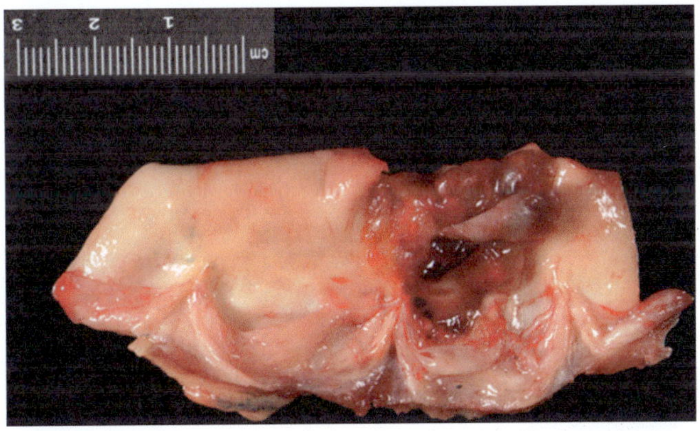

Fig. 13.6 Operative specimen showing sarcoma attached to the pulmonary root near the pulmonary valve

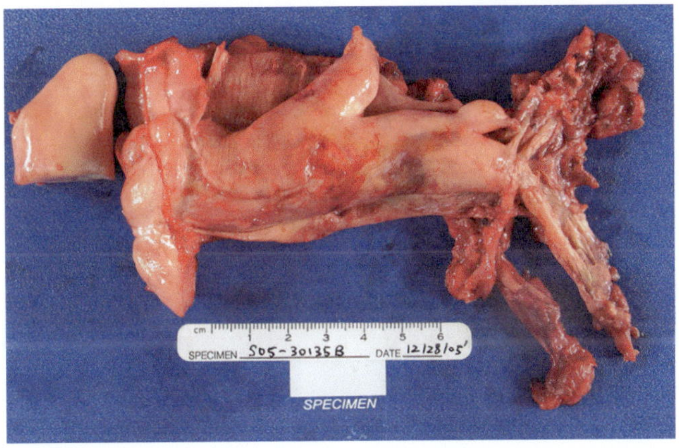

Fig. 13.7 Operative specimen showing sarcoma filling the pulmonary artery without transgressing the artery wall

Case 2

A 38 year old patient presented with severe dyspnea that had progressed rapidly during the month prior to presentation. The CT at presentation showed a large mass within the main PA protruding into the left PA and filling the right PA (Fig. 13.5). Cardiac MRI showed the large mass within the PA and contrast enhancement suggesting perfusion of the mass helped to define the mass as tumor and not thrombus. The patient was evaluated by the Houston Methodist DeBakey Heart & Vascular Center/M. D. Anderson Cancer Center multidisciplinary heart team and surgical resection was recommended. Complete resection of the tumor would have to include the pulmonary root, main PA, and the entire right PA (Fig. 13.8). At surgery the entire pulmonary root was resected into the right ventricular outflow tract and the pulmonary root, main PA, entire right PA, and the right lung were resected successfully *en bloc* (Fig. 13.9). Reconstruction was performed with an allograft root sewn into the right ventricular outflow tract (Fig. 13.10) with a Dacron tube graft to the left main PA. The patient recovered well from surgery and remains alive 3 years later.

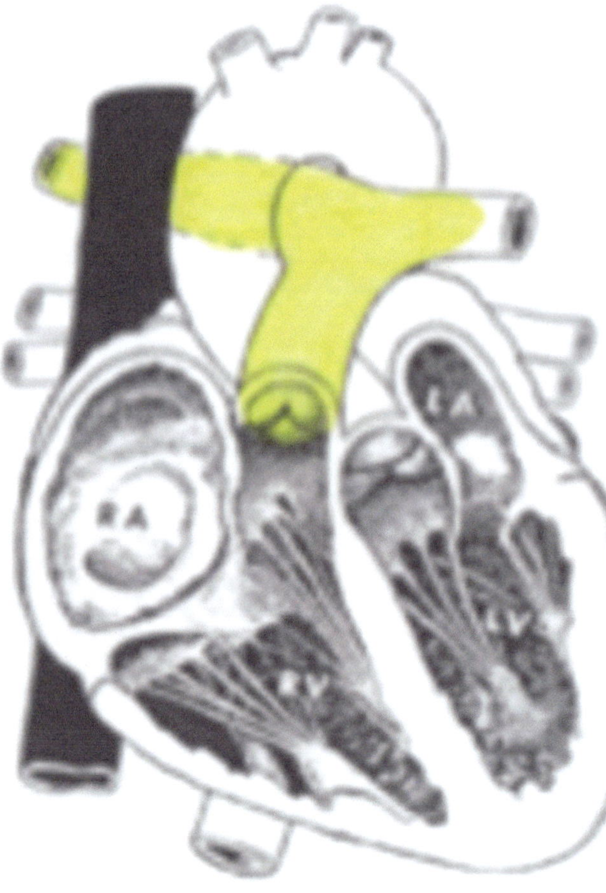

Fig. 13.8 Extent of the required section

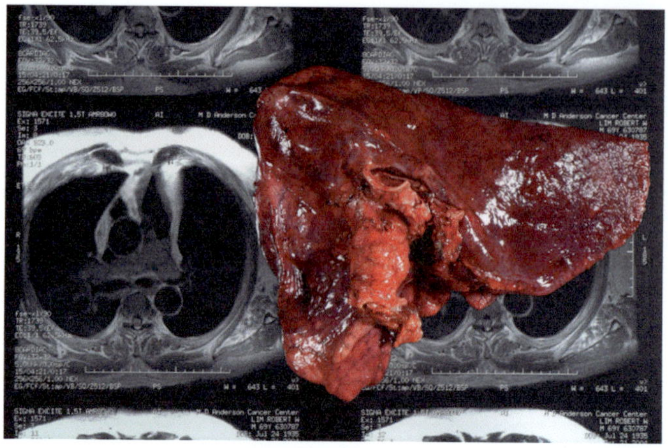

Fig. 13.9 Operative specimen against the preoperative CT scan

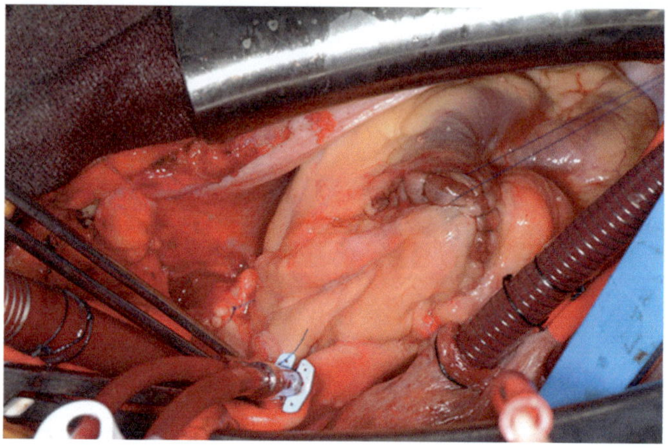

Fig. 13.10 Operative photograph showing the allograft root replacement

Left Heart Sarcomas

Case 3

A 52 year old female presented with severe shortness of breath and was started on treatment for asthma. After 2 weeks her symptoms were worsening so she went to her local ER where an echocardiogram was ordered which revealed a large left atrial mass. Cardiac surgery was consulted and this was thought to be a large left atrial myxoma and immediate surgery was performed. During the operation a broad-based left atrial mass was found and as much of the tumor as possible was resected and the atrium reconstructed with pericardium. Pathology from this operation revealed undifferentiated sarcoma with positive margins. She was followed without further treatment and had recurrence of the tumor seen on echocardiogram 6 months later (Fig. 13.11). She was then referred to the Houston Methodist DeBakey Heart & Vascular Center/M. D. Anderson Cancer Center multidisciplinary heart team. Because of the large size and location of her tumor surgical resection with cardiac auto-transplant was recommended.

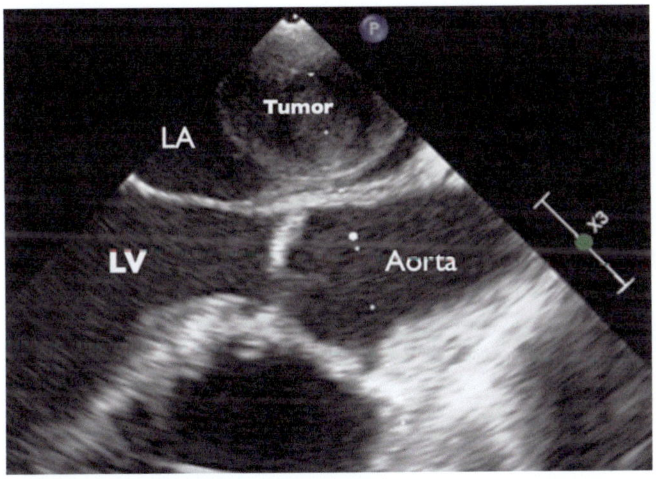

Fig. 13.11 Echocardiogram of recurrent left atrial sarcoma

Cardiac auto-transplant was developed by our cardiac tumor team with our first case performed in 1998 [14] and we currently have the largest global series [15]. Although we prefer to begin appropriate chemotherapy before surgical resection whenever possible, large left sided sarcomas do not always allow for this. We begin with a median sternotomy and direct cannulation of the superior vena cava and inferior vena cava leaving enough room to divide these and allow subsequent reconnection (Fig. 13.12). The superior vena cava, aorta and pulmonary artery are divided and the left atrium opened first to see if this will allow adequate visualization for complete resection (Fig. 13.13). In this case the tumor could be seen but ade-

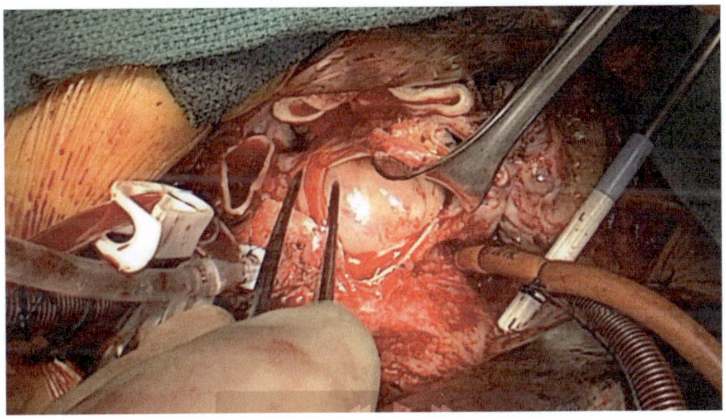

Fig. 13.13 Operative photograph of left atrial tumor exposure

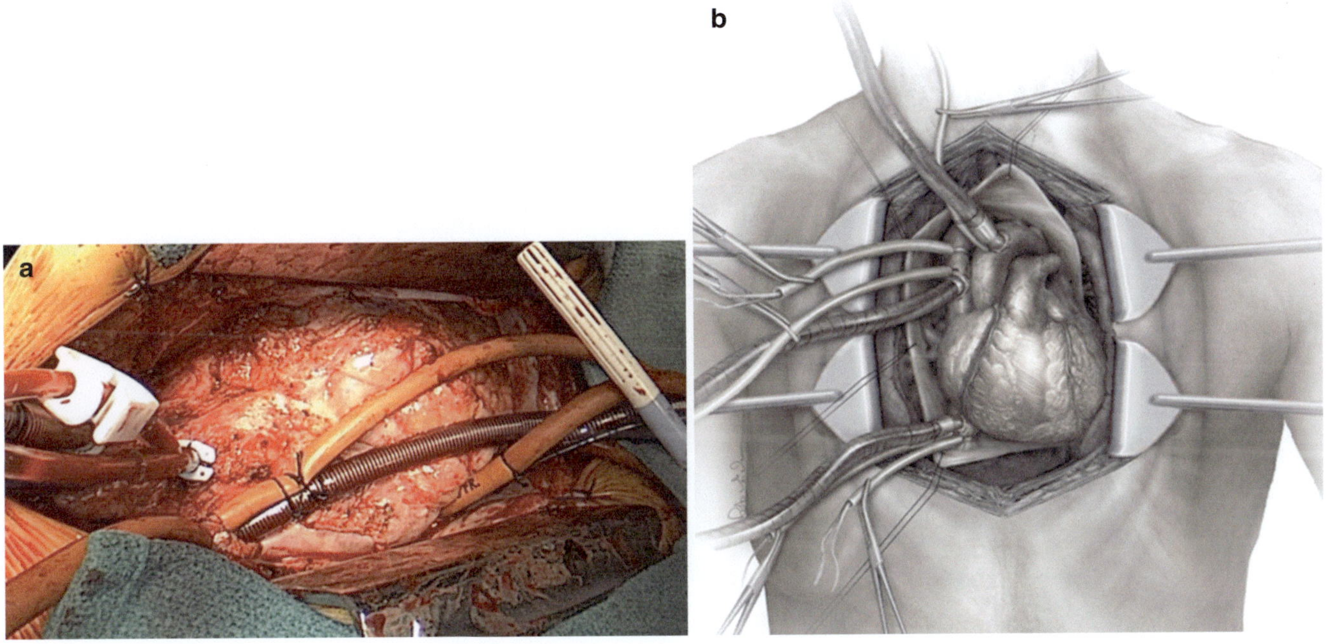

Fig. 13.12 (**a**) Operative photograph of cannulation. (**b**) Drawing of cannulation technique

quate exposure for radical resection was not achieved so the inferior vena cava/ right atrial junction was divided also and the heart removed (Fig. 13.14). This allowed complete exposure of the posterior left atrium and complete tumor removal (Fig. 13.15). The posterior atrium was then reconstructed with bovine pericardium. The pulmonary veins can be connected in a variety of ways. In this case they were connected as a cuff (Fig. 13.16). The entire anterior left atrium can also be removed but in this case only a portion was needed and this was reconstructed with bovine pericardium (Fig. 13.17). The heart was then sewn back into place much like a standard transplant (Fig. 13.18). Once all anastomoses were complete (Fig. 13.19) the patient was weaned from cardiopulmonary bypass without problem. She was transferred to the floor on postoperative day 1 and discharged on day 10. She is currently on a regimen of Adriamycin and Ifosfamide and has no evident disease.

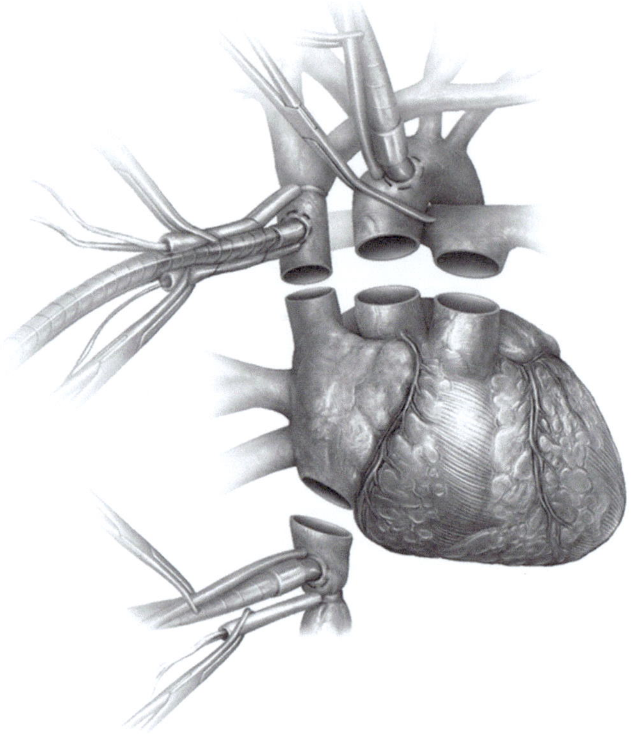

Fig. 13.14 Drawing of technique for removal of the heart

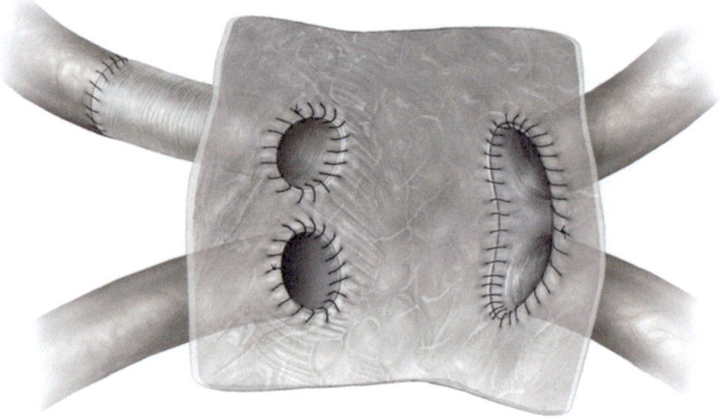

Fig. 13.16 Posterior left atrial reconstruction techniques

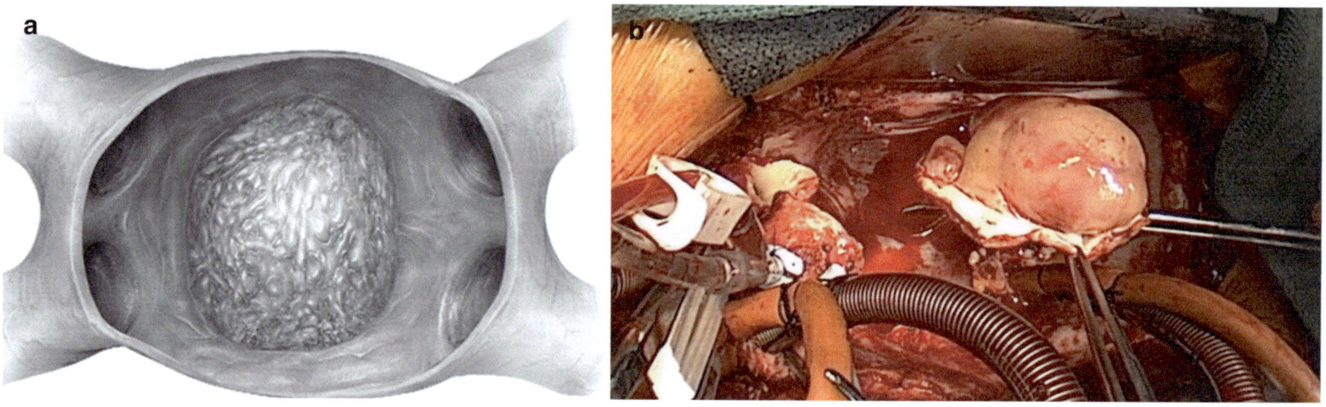

Fig. 13.15 (**a**) Drawing of tumor exposure after cardiac removal. (**b**) Operative picture of tumor

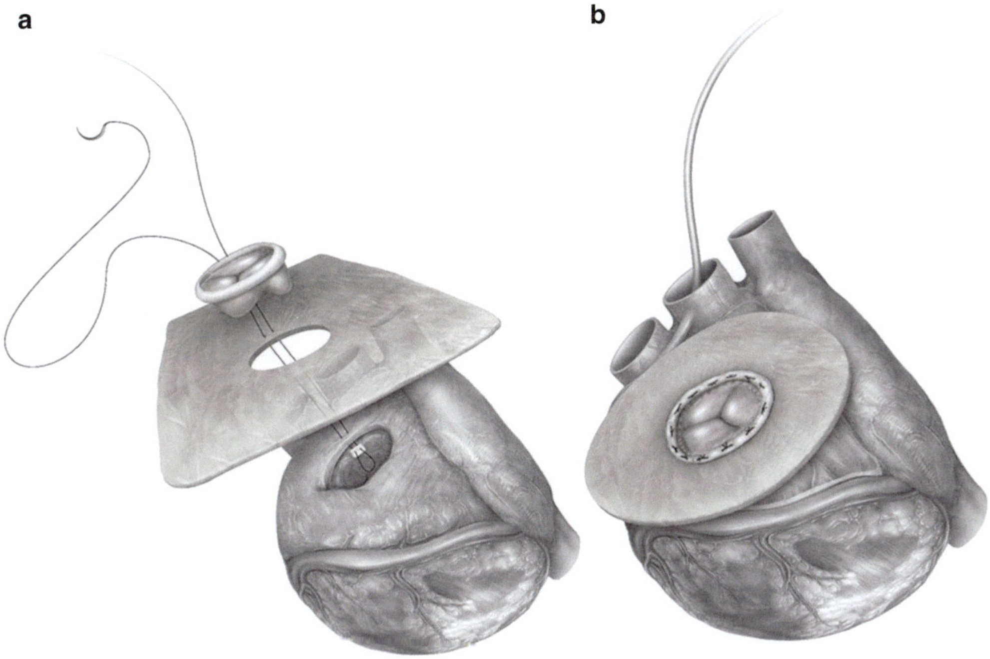

Fig. 13.17 (**a**, **b**) Technique for removal of the anterior left atrium when needed

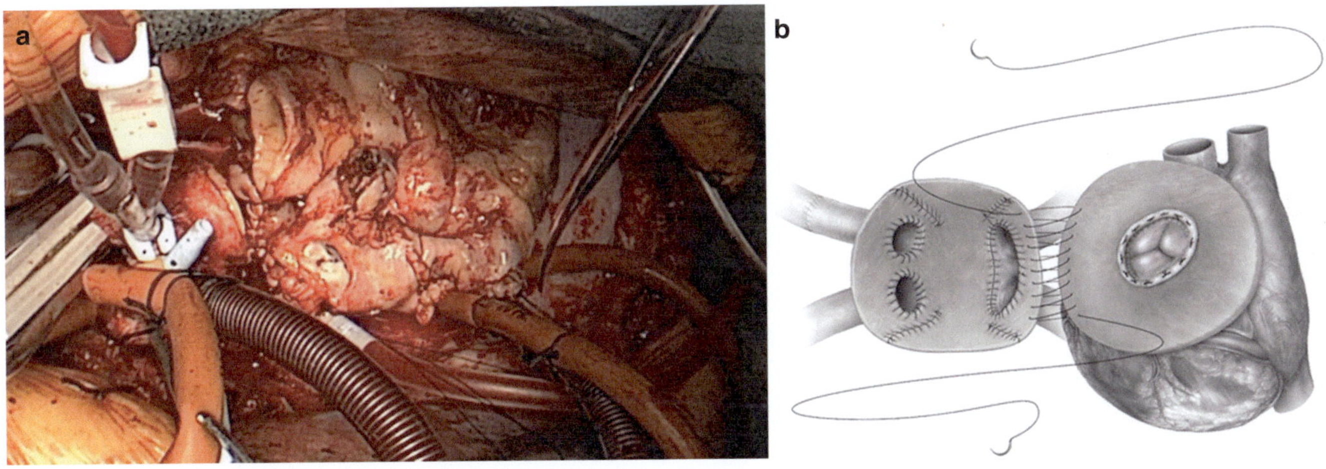

Fig. 13.18 (**a**) Operative photo of cardiac implantation. (**b**) Drawing of cardiac implantation

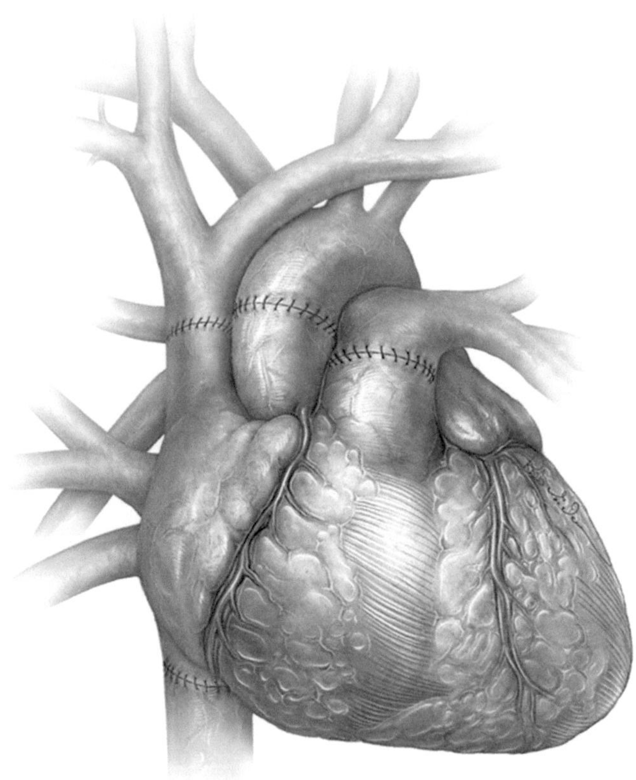

Fig. 13.19 Heart reconnected

References

1. Virmani R, Burke A, Farb A. Atlas of cardiovascular pathology. Philadelphia: Saunders; 1996.
2. Al-Mamgani A, Baartman L, Baaijens M, et al. Cardiac metastases. Int J Clin Oncol. 2008;13:369–72.
3. Eisenhauer EA, et al. New response evaluation criteria in solid tumors: revised RECIST guideline. Eur J Cancer. 2009;45: 228–47.
4. Marshall VF, Middleton RG, Holswade GR, et al. Surgery for renal cell carcinoma in the vena cava. J Urol. 1970;103:414–20.
5. Hanfling SM. Metastatic cancer to the heart: Review of the literature and report of 127 cases. Circulation. 1960;2:474.
6. Columbus MR. De Re Anatomica, Liber XV, Venice, N Bevilacque; 1559. p. 269.
7. Xu ZF, Yong F, Chen YY, et al. Uterine intravenous leiomyomatosis with cardiac extension: Imaging characteristics and literature review. World J Clin Oncol. 2013;4(1):25–8. doi:10.5306/wjco.v4.i1.25.
8. Jun CH, Sim da W, Kim SH, et al. Risk factors for patients with stage IVB hepatocellular carcinoma and extension into the heart: prognostic and therapeutic implications. Yonsei Med J. 2014;55(2):379–86. doi:10.3349/ymj.2014.55.2.379.
9. Steinberg C, Boudreau S, Leveille F, et al. Advanced hepatocellular carcinoma with subtotal occlusion of the inferior vena cava and a right atrial mass. Case Rep Vasc Med. 2013;2013:489373. doi:10.1155/2013/489373. Epub 11 Apr 2013.
10. Abu Saleh WK, Ramlawi B, Shapira OM, Al Jabbari O, Ravi V, Benjamin R, Durand JB, Leja MJ, Blackmon SH, Bruckner BA, Reardon MJ. Improved outcomes with the evolution of a neoadjuvant chemotherapy approach to right heart sarcoma. Ann Thorac Surg. 2017;104:90–96.
11. Blackmon SH, Rice DC, Correa AM, et al. Management of primary pulmonary artery sarcomas. Ann Thorac Surg. 2009;87: 977–84.
12. Blackmon SH, Reardon MJ. Pulmonary artery sarcoma. Methodist Debakey Cardiovasc J. 2010;6:38–43.
13. Blackmon SH, Reardon MJ. Primary pulmonary artery sarcoma extending retrograde into the superior vena cava. Tex Heart Inst J. 2011;38:320. author reply 320–1
14. Reardon MJ, DeFelice CA, Sheinbaum R, Baldwin JC. Cardiac autotransplant for surgical treatment of a malignant neoplasm. Ann Thorac Surg. 1999;67:1793–5.
15. Ramlawi B, Leja MJ, Abu Saleh WK, et al. Surgical Treatment of Primary Cardiac Sarcomas: Review of a Single-Institution Experience. Ann Thorac Surg. 2015;101:698–702.

Cardiac Arrhythmia and Device Management in Patients with Cancer

14

Kaveh Karimzad

Abstract
In this chapter we have briefly discussed the management of torsade de pointe and cardiac devices, in patients with cancer.

Keywords
Torsade de pointes • Cardiac devices

Introduction

Prolong QTc interval and related arrhythmia is not uncommon in patient afflicted with malignancy. Various chemotherapy agents prolong the QTc interval and these patients are frequently on multiple antibiotics and antifungal agents, some of which are also QTc prolonging agents.

Another group of patients who are particularly susceptible to complications of cancer therapy, are patients with intracardiac devices, who are to undergo radiation therapy or cardiac magnetic resonance imaging (MRI) investigation.

In this chapter we briefly discuss this two common clinical scenario.

Management of Cardiac Devices During Radiation Therapy

Introduction

With an aging population, increasing number of cancer survivors and increased use of pacemaker and Implantable cardioverter defibrillator (ICD), it is not surprising that the number of patients with these devices who present for radiation therapy is increasing.

Radiation therapy has several potential damaging effects on cardiac devices. Modern devices have mental oxide semi-conductors. These semi-conductors have enabled us to have devices with smaller size, but the same semi-conductors have made these devices more susceptible to damage by radiation. Damage usually occurs in silicon and silicon oxide insulators of cardiac devices [1].

K. Karimzad, M.D.
Department of Cardiology, University of Texas MD Anderson Cancer Center, Houston, TX 777030, USA
e-mail: kkarimzad@mdanderson.org

Device Reset

Therapeutic radiation can commonly cause device reset. Reset is a safety backup mode of pacing in case of catastrophic failure of the device. The pacing parameter during reset mode is unique to each manufacturer. These pacing parameters are not necessarily optimal, but they are neither unsafe. A programmer is required to restore the programming to the original setting [2].

Radiation and Defibrillators

Radiation therapy can affect detection and charge time of defibrillators. It can also cause damage to ICD memory. It is very important to estimate the absorb radiation dose to the device before initiation of radiation. Each manufacturer has recommended tolerance dose for their ICD devices.

Defibrillator Deactivation

A controversial issue regarding management of cardiac devices during radiation therapy is the deactivation of tachytherapy with magnet during radiation. Defibrillator shock due to electromagnetic interference (EMI) during radiation is extremely rare. It has only been reported in in-vitro studies.

S.W. Yusuf, J. Banchs (eds.), *Cancer and Cardiovascular Disease*, https://doi.org/10.1007/978-3-319-62088-6_14

There are different practices in high-volume centers regarding deactivation of tachy-therapy with magnet [3]. Here at MD Anderson, we do not recommend it, as there is no evidence that radiation causes inappropriate defibrillator shock due to over sensing.

Scatter Radiation
Scatter radiation can also cause reset due to neutron exposure. Scatter neutrons increase with increased in photon beam energy. Conventional shielding options usually does not protect against scattered ration [4]. Hurkmans et al. demonstrated that effect of radiation dose on defibrillators is unpredictable. In this in-vitro study, investigators exposed 11 defibrillators directly to radiotherapy. Although most of these defibrillators didn't fail below 80 Gy of radiation, some of them failed at very low dose of 0.5–1.5 Gy [5].

Pulse Check Method
Pulse check method is a method that we use here at MD Anderson to minimize frequent visits to device clinic during radiation therapy. We program lower rate slightly faster than the reset mode and we ask the radiation therapy team to check the heart rate after each radiation fraction. If the detected heart rate is less than the program lower rate, we immediately check device for any damage or reset. This method is very useful in a pacemaker dependent patient, but it is not very helpful if the intrinsic rate is faster than programed lower rate.

Device Repositioning
There are certain situations that we consider repositioning of the device. If the pacemaker or defibrillator generator is located directly in the therapy beam, or if we have a patient with estimated absorbed dose to the device more than 5 Gy. Pacemaker dependency and a device interfering with the effective radiation to the tumor are other scenarios in which we consider repositioning. Before making the decision to the reposition a device, we always consider potential complication of device re-implantation. Here at MD Anderson, We use lead extenders and subcutaneous tunneling technique across the chest to reposition the device to contralateral pectoral site, as shown in Fig. 14.1.

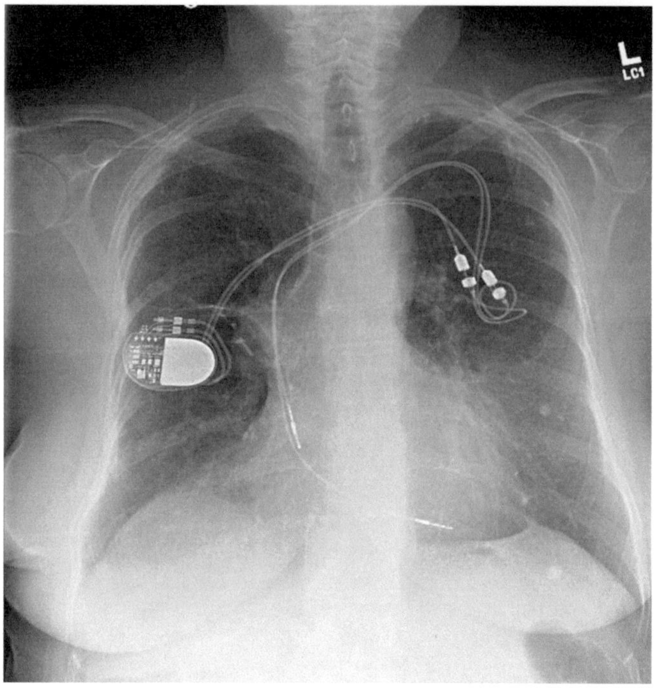

Fig. 14.1 A chest-x-ray showing the device on the contralateral pectoral site

MD Anderson Practice

We use a management algorithm for patients with cardiac devices undergoing radiation therapy at MD Anderson. All of these patients visit cardiac device clinic for device check before radiation therapy. After discussing with radiation oncology team, first we determine if the device is in the direct radiation field or not. If we conclude that the device is in the direct radiation field, we consider device relocation. Factors favoring relocation of the device are pacemaker dependency and device interfering with the effective radiation dose to the tumor. If we determine that the device is not in the direct radiation field, we use pulse check method. We program the pacing rate at 75 beats per minute which is a slightly faster than the reset mode for all device manufacturers. Subsequently, patient will proceed with the radiation and we ask radiation therapy team to the check the heart rate after each radiation fraction. If the heart rate is less than 75 beats per minute, we immediately check the device for damage or reset. But if the heart rate is more than 75 beats per minute after each radiation fraction, we proceed with the next step. When pulse check method is not possible, we have to do more frequent device checks: device check after each session for pacemaker dependent or ICD and weekly check for non-pacemaker dependent patient. Pulse check method is extremely helpful in decreasing the frequency of device checks during radiation, as shown in Fig. 14.2.

Knowledge Gap

There are several knowledge gaps in regard to management of cardiac devices during radiation therapy. There is no randomized clinical trial which addresses this issue. The current recommendations are based on experience in high-volume centers and there is no complete agreement between different centers, especially on issues like deactivation of defibrillator during radiation therapy and device manufacturers have diverging opinions about this.

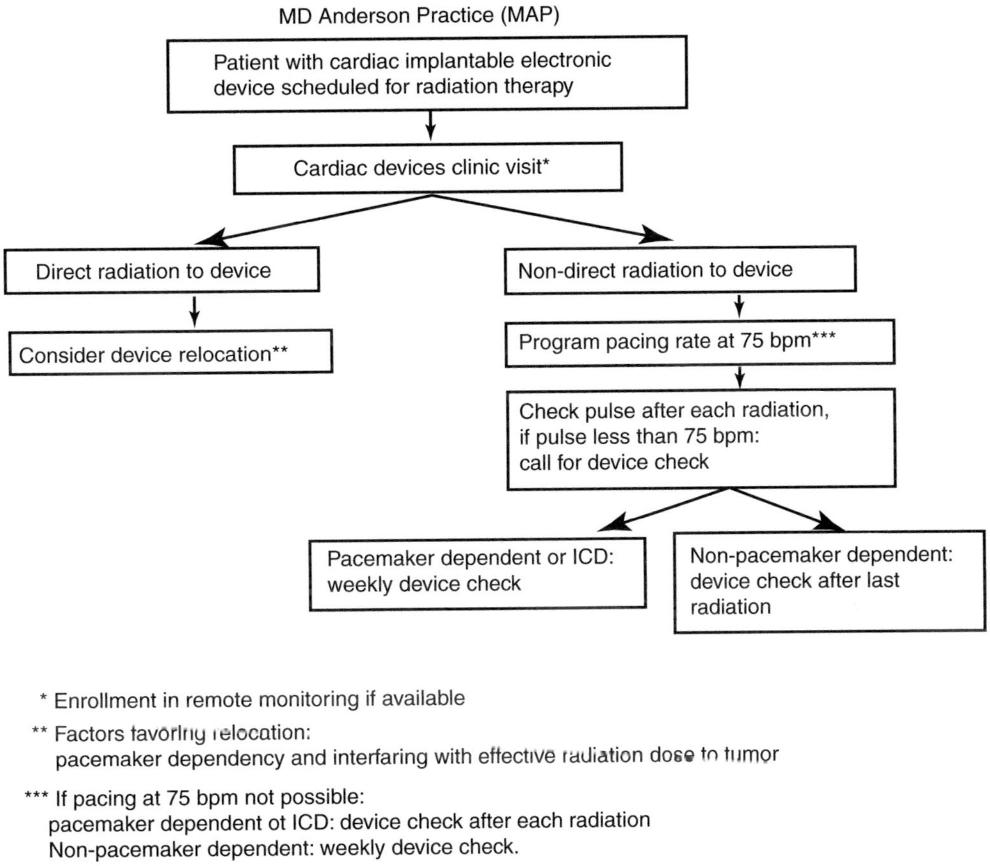

Fig. 14.2 Management of cardiac implantable electronic devices

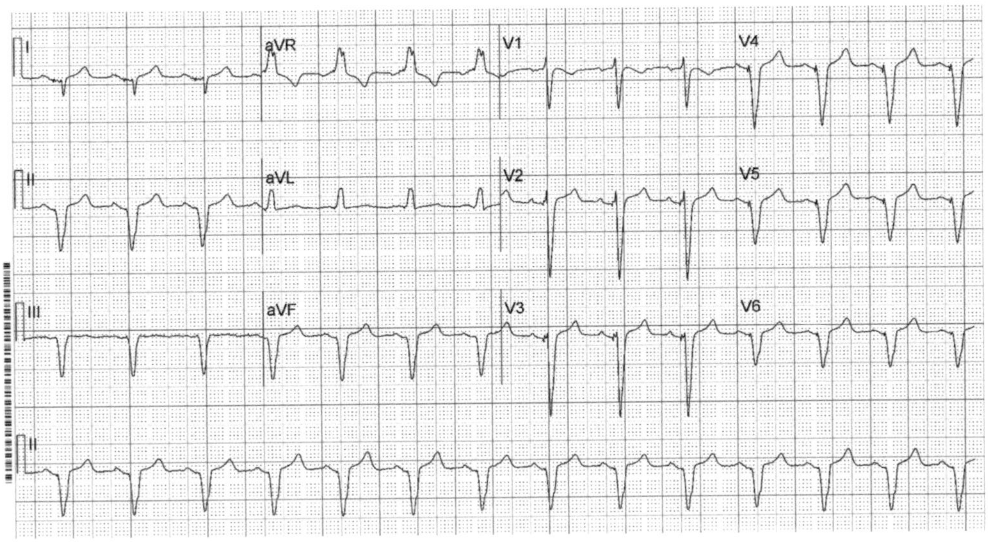

Fig. 14.3 Shows an ECG with biventricular paced rhythm

Case Presentation

A 47 year old woman with metastatic breast cancer who was scheduled to undergo left mastectomy and radiation therapy. She had prior history of non-ischemic cardiomyopathy with severe left ventricular systolic dysfunction, ejection fraction of 20–25% with NYHA class 3 symptoms and left bundle branch block. She underwent biventricular defibrillator implantation 2 years prior to cancer diagnosis and had echocardiographic response with improvement of LVEF to 40–45% and symptomatic improvement to NYHA class 2 symptoms.

She was referred to the cardiac device clinic for repositioning of the defibrillator generator as it was interfering with effective radiation to the tumor and lymph nodes.

Figure 14.3 shows an ECG with biventricular paced rhythm.

Figure 14.4 shows the biventricular-implantable cardioverter defibrillator (BiV-ICD).

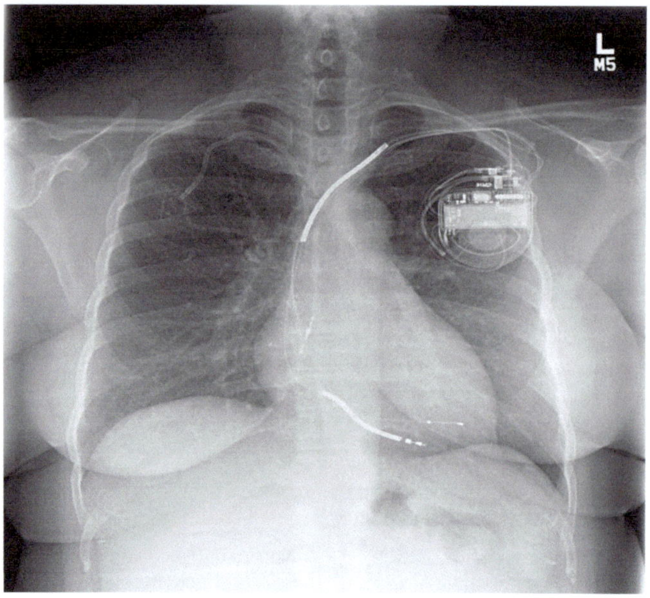

Fig. 14.4 Chest-x-ray showing the BiV-ICD with RA, RV and LV leads

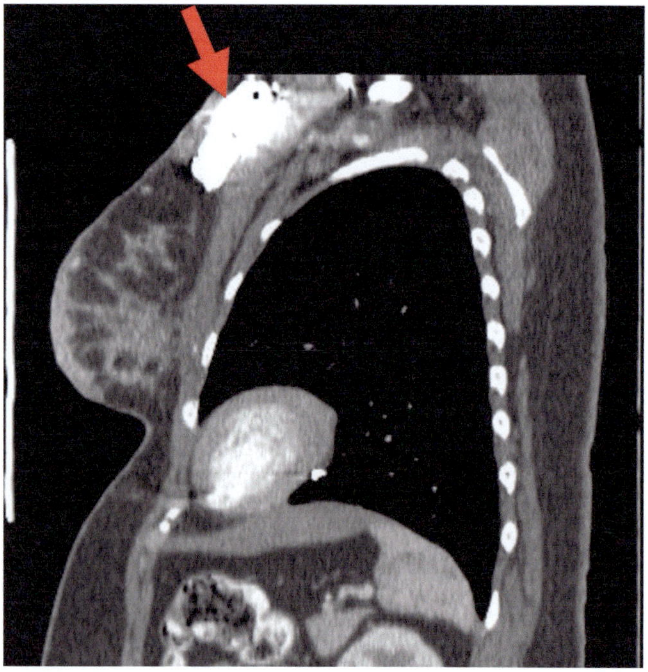

Fig. 14.5 A CT chest showing the device in the left pectoral site, interfering with effective radiation to tumor and lymph nodes. The *red arrow* points to the device

Figure 14.5 shows the device in the left pectoral site, interfering with effective radiation to tumor and lymph nodes.

There are four different options to handle this situation:

1. Implantation of new BiV-ICD in right pectoral site and abandonment of old ICD system in the left side. This option will leave the patient with six leads in the heart and SVC and potential risk for infection and SVC syndrome.
2. Implantation of new BiV-ICD in the right pectoral site after extraction of Old ICD leads in the left side. This option will expose the patient to a high risk procedure of lead extraction with potential mortality and morbidity.
3. Explant the BiV-ICD generator and re-implantation after completion of radiation. In this scenario, patient will lose benefit of biventricular pacing and there is risk for deterioration of LV systolic function.
4. Repositioning BiV-ICD generator to the right pectoral site using lead extenders.

We felt that that the repositioning of the BiV-ICD generator to the right pectoral site using lead extenders was the safest and least invasive option for the patient. Repositioning of the device to the right pectoral site was performed in the operation room after mastectomy, using five lead extenders: right atrial lead, left ventricular lead and right ventricular high voltage lead with three pins (RV sense/pace, RV coil, SVC coil) (Fig. 14.6).

Device repositioning to the right pectoral site was uneventful. Patient was able to undergo radiation therapy after mastectomy and device repositioning.

Polymorphic Ventricular Tachycardia/ Torsade de Pointes

A 73 year old man with hypertension, hyperlipidemia, coronary artery disease and carotid artery disease. He was diagnosed with chordoma of the clivus and suprasellar region and hydrocephalus. He was admitted for surgical resection of his tumor. His hospital course was complicated by multiple bilateral subsegmental pulmonary emboli (PE) (s/p IVC filter placement, started on Lovenox therapy) and multiple small subacute ischemic cerebrovascular accidents (CVAs) leading to discovery of a patent foramen ovale (PFO) causing paradoxical emboli. He underwent trans-nasal resection, his post-operative course was complicated by recurrent respiratory failure due to aspiration and failure to clear secretions, with an episode of post-operative atrial fibrillation with rapid ventricular response (RVR) (likely due to ongoing respiratory failure and fluid shifts). He was treated with amiodarone drip which was discontinued due to QTc prolongation. He continued to have recurrent episodes of respiratory failure requiring reintubation and extubation. Below is his ECG after he was chemically cardioverted with amiodarone which showed prolonged QTc interval of 493 ms (Fig. 14.7).

He continued to have prolonged QTc interval despite discontinuation of amiodarone drip. He was not receiving any QTc prolonging drug. He had signs and symptoms of increased intracranial pressure. Unfortunately he arrested due to polymorphic ventricular tachycardia in the setting of extremely prolonged QTc interval (Torsades de pointes). Below is his ECG prior to VT arrest with significant QTc prolongation: QTc of 533 ms (Fig. 14.8). Also the tracings shows PVCs and

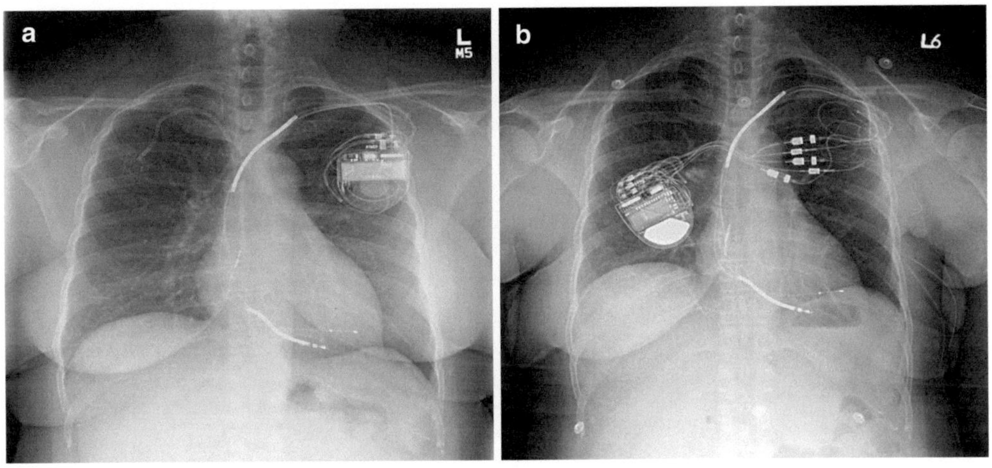

Fig. 14.6 (**a**) Chest-x-ray before repositioning of the BiV-ICD. (**b**) Chest-x-ray, after repositioning of the device to the right pectoral site, using five lead extenders: right atrial lead, left ventricular lead and right ventricular high voltage lead with three pins (RV sense/pace, RV coil, SVC coil)

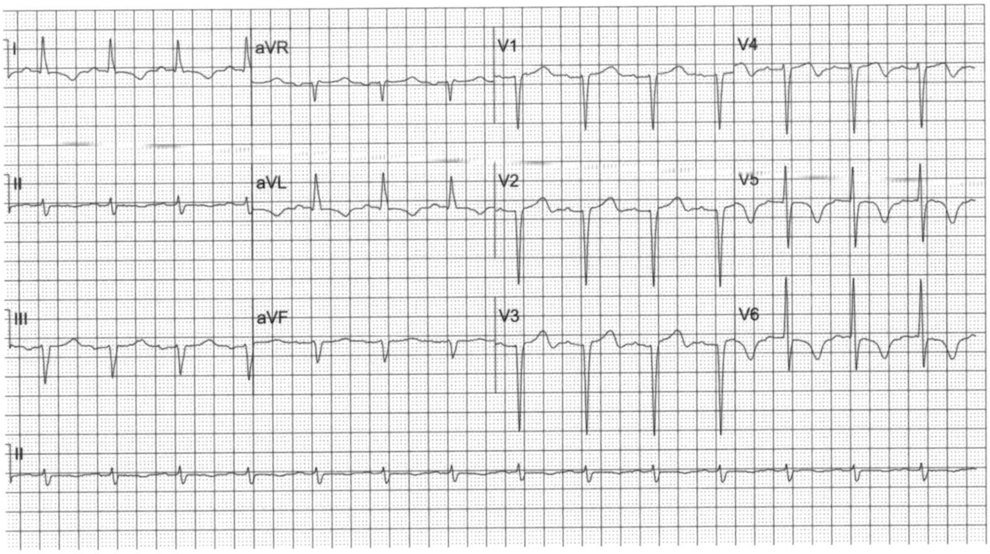

Fig. 14.7 A 12 lead ECG showing a prolong QTc interval of 493 ms

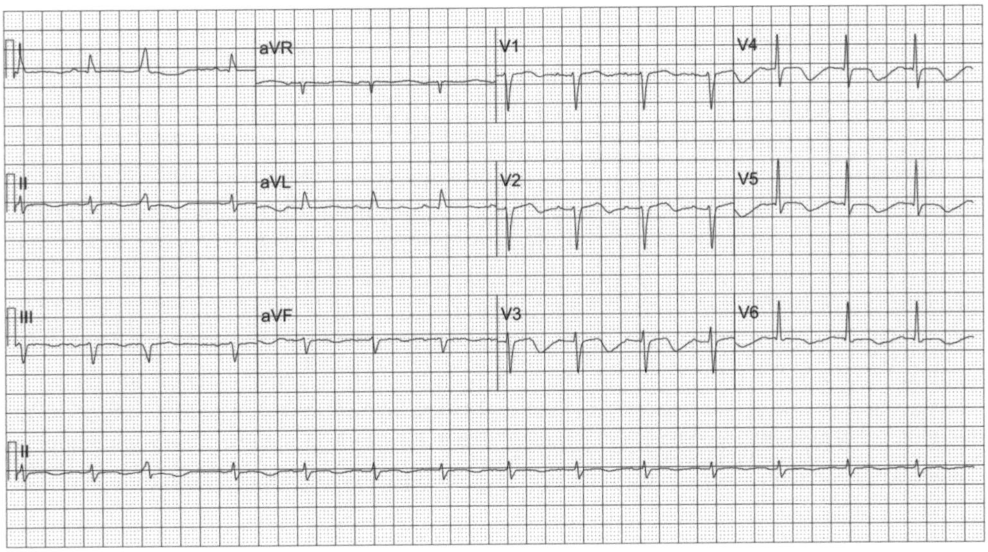

Fig. 14.8 A 12 lead ECG showing a prolong QTc interval of 533 ms

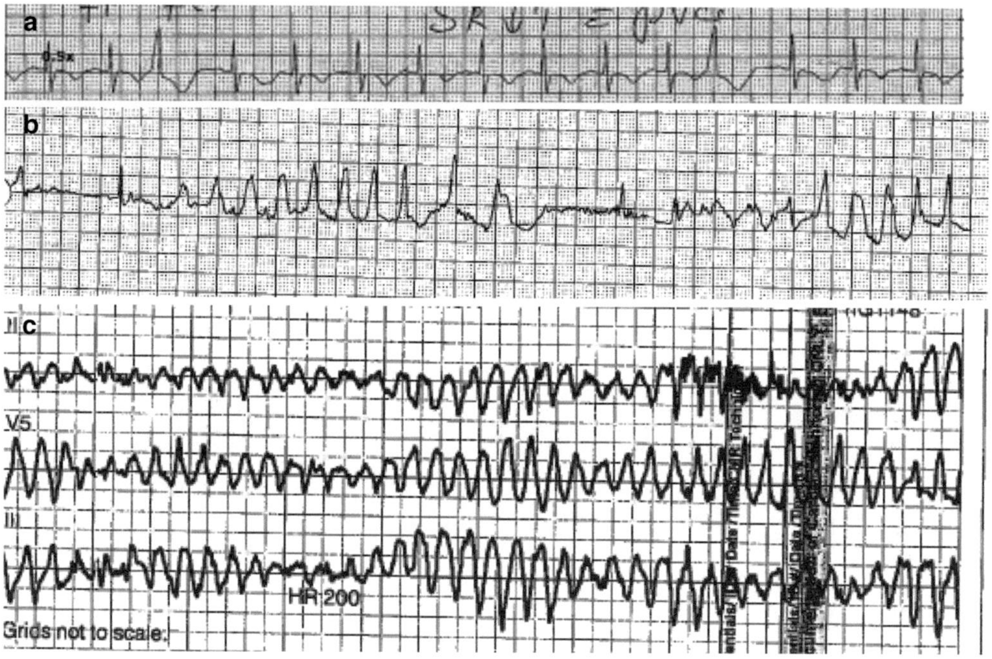

Fig. 14.9 Tracings shows PVCs (**a**), and runs of non-sustained ventricular tachycardia (**b**), few minutes prior to episode of cardiac arrest with R on T phenomenon (**c**)

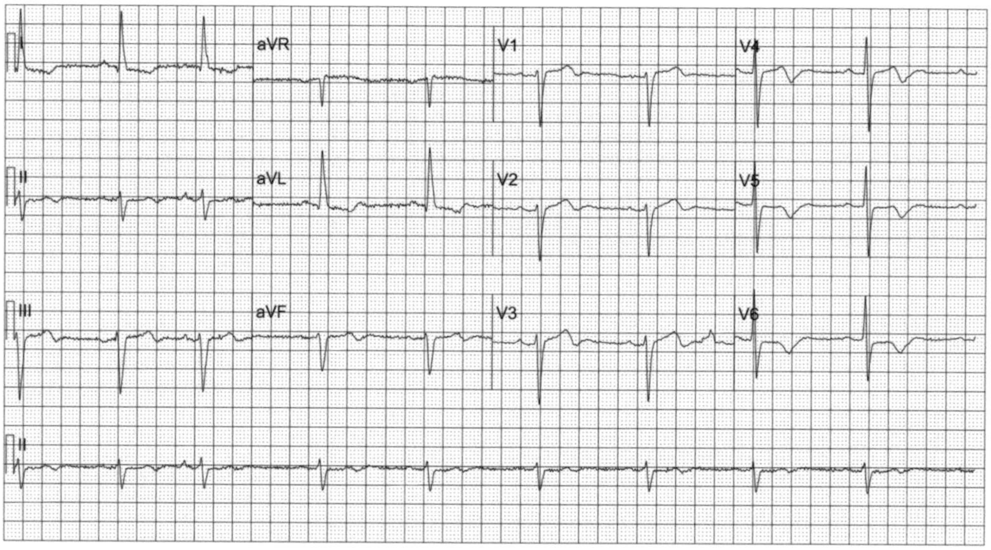

Fig. 14.10 A 12 lead ECG showing a QTc interval of 447 ms

runs of non-sustained ventricular tachycardia few minutes prior to episode of cardiac arrest with R on T phenomenon (Fig. 14.9). He was resuscitated and received external shock which resulted in termination of polymorphic VT.

Ischemic work up was negative for significant coronary artery disease. Echocardiogram revealed mildly depressed LV systolic function with ejection fraction of 45%. He was subsequently treated with lidocaine drip and his electrolytes were replaced but continued to have QTc prolongation in 500 ms range. He underwent VP shunt placement for CSF leak. He had second episode of cardiac arrest due to polymorphic VT in the setting of long QTc interval a week after first episode. His QT interval gradually shortened over the following few weeks in the hospital. He was discharged home with a regimen of Mexiletine. An external defibrillator (Lifevest) was placed prior to discharge for secondary prevention of sudden cardiac death. During subsequent follow up visits in cardiology clinic his QTc interval remained in upper limit of normal (440–460 ms). He did not receive shock from his external defibrillator. Fig.14.10 shows his ECG during follow up visit with QTc 447 ms (Fig. 14.10).

During follow up visits in cardiology clinic, we discovered that his QTc interval was at upper limit of normal even prior to diagnosis of cancer. He denied any family history of sudden cardiac death or any prior history of syncope, presyncope, dizziness and lightheadedness. We performed genetic testing for long QTc syndromes which did not reveal any mutation in LQTS genes. After long conversation with the patient and his wife, implantation of defibrillator was recommended in light of borderline QTc prolongation at baseline and two episodes of polymorphic VT arrest in the setting of significant QTc prolongation. A defibrillator was implanted by his local electrophysiologist.

Discussion: Torsades de pointes is a specific form of polymorphic VT in patients with a long QTc interval. It is characterized by rapid, irregular QRS complexes, which appear to be twisting around the ECG baseline. This arrhythmia may cease spontaneously or degenerate into ventricular fibrillation. It causes significant hemodynamic compromise and often death. Diagnosis is by ECG. Treatment is with IV magnesium, measures to shorten the QTc interval, and direct-current defibrillation when ventricular fibrillation is precipitated.

Episodes of drug-induced TdP usually start with a short-long-short pattern of R-R cycles consisting of a short-coupled premature ventricular complex (PVC) followed by a compensatory pause and then another PVC that typically falls close to the peak of the T wave [6]. However, because of the underlying long-QTc interval, this R-on-T PVC does not have the short coupling interval that is characteristic of idiopathic ventricular fibrillation. This short-long-short sequence is thought to promote TdP by increasing heterogeneity of repolarization across the myocardial wall. In contrast to ventricular fibrillation that does not terminate without defibrillation, TdP frequently terminates spontaneously, with the last 2–3 beats showing slowing of the arrhythmia. However, in some cases, TdP degenerates into ventricular fibrillation and causes sudden cardiac death.

There is a gradual increase in risk for TdP as the heart rate-corrected QTc interval (QT_c) increases. Each 10-ms increase in QT_c contributes approximately a 5–7% exponential increase in risk for TdP in these patients [7, 8]. Chronic administration of amiodarone markedly prolongs the QTc interval, yet it is very rarely associated with TdP [9]. It has been postulated (although as yet unproven) that unlike high-risk drugs that selectively prolong repolarization in myocytes located in the mid myocardium (M cells), amiodarone uniformly delays repolarization in all layers of the myocardial wall. As a result, there is only QTc prolongation and no transmural heterogeneity of repolarization, which is the necessary substrate for the development of a reentrant arrhythmia.

In hospitalized patients, TdP is commonly associated with acquired prolongation of the uncorrected or rate-corrected QTc interval, with or without underlying genetic predisposition, often in the presence of a noncardiac drug that is known (or not known) to prolong the QTc interval. Of note, the risk for TdP increases significantly with concurrent use of more than 1 QTc prolonging drug. Bradycardia is an additional important risk factor for TdP in patients when other predisposing findings are present [10]. Prolonged ventricular cycle length can take the form of simple sinus bradycardia, complete atrioventricular block, or any rhythm in which sudden long cycles may lead to arrhythmogenic early after depolarizations [11].

Brain injury-related ECG abnormalities have been recognized for more than five decades and are particularly common after SAH where they are reported in 49–100% of cases. The most common findings are ST segment changes, flat or inverted T waves, prominent U waves, and prolongation of the QTc interval [12]. Excessive prolongation of the QTc interval may be a cause of sudden cardiac death after brain injury. It is of note that QTc interval prolongation persists in patients with an unfavourable outcome after SAH but improves in those who have a good outcome. The true incidence of malignant arrhythmias is uncertain because they may be the cause of pre-hospital mortality in some patients. The exact mechanism of sudden cardiac death after brain injury is unclear, but severe QTc prolongation, driven by abnormalities in the insula, is thought to be responsible. Drugs that prolong the QTc interval should therefore be avoided after brain injury, even into the rehabilitation phase.

Similar ECG changes have been described in nonvascular intracranial lesions like meningitis and intracranial tumors and increased CSF pressure [13]. The mechanism by which these changes are produced is not clear. The various mechanisms which have been suggested by different workers including actual damage to the myocardium in the form of sub-endocardial haemorrhage, electrolyte imbalance, and raised intracranial tension and vagotonicity.

In our patient, extremely long QTc interval was thought to be secondary to increased intracranial pressure and confirmed by increased in measured CSF pressure in the setting of mild electrolyte abnormalities. He was not receiving any QTc prolonging agents except intravenous amiodarone which he received only for less than 24 h. His second episode of cardiac arrest due to polymorphic VT in the setting of long QTc was about 10 days after discontinuation of amiodarone and aggressive correction of electrolyte abnormalities. His QTc interval remained prolonged most likely due to increased intracranial pressure: elevated CSF pressure.

References

1. Calfee RV. Therapeutic radiation and pacemakers. Pacing Clin Electrophysiol. 1982;5(2):160–1.
2. Crossley GH, Poole JE, Rozner MA, Asirvatham SJ, Cheng A, Chung MK, Ferguson TB Jr, Gallagher JD, Gold MR, Hoyt RH, Irefin S, Kusumoto FM, Moorman LP, Thompson A. The Heart Rhythm Society (HRS)/American Society of Anesthesiologists (ASA) Expert Consensus Statement on the perioperative management of patients with implantable defibrillators, pacemakers and arrhythmia monitors: facilities and patient management. Heart Rhythm. 2011;8(7):1114–54.

3. Hurkmans CW, Knegjens JL, Oei BS, Maas AJ, Uiterwaal GJ, van der Borden AJ, Ploegmakers MM, van Erven L, Dutch Society of Radiotherapy and Oncology (NVRO). Management of radiation oncology patients with a pacemaker or ICD: a new comprehensive practical guideline in The Netherlands. Radiat Oncol. 2012;7:198.
4. Kapa S, Fong L, Blackwell CR, Herman MG, Schomberg PJ, Hayes DL. Effects of scatter radiation on ICD and CRT function. Pacing Clin Electrophysiol. 2008;31(6):727–32.
5. Hurkmans CW, Scheepers E, Springorum BG, Uiterwaal H. Influence of radiotherapy on the latest generation of implantable cardioverter-defibrillators. Int J Radiat Oncol Biol Phys. 2005;63(1): 282–9.
6. Kay GN, Plumb VJ, Arciniegas JG, Henthorn RW, Waldo AL. Torsade de pointes: the long-short initiating sequence and other clinical features: observations in 32 patients. J Am Coll Cardiol. 1983;2:806–17.
7. Moss AJ, Schwartz PJ, Crampton RS, Tzivoni D, Locati EH, MacCluer J, Hall WJ, Weitkamp L, Vincent GM, Garson A Jr, Robinson JL, Benhorin J, Choi S. The long QT syndrome: prospective longitudinal study of 328 families. Circulation. 1991;84:1136–44.
8. Zareba W, Moss AJ, Schwartz PJ, Vincent GM, Robinson JL, Priori SG, Benhorin J, Locati EH, Towbin JA, Keating MT, Lehmann MH, Hall WJ. Influence of genotype on the clinical course of the long-QT syndrome: International Long-QT Syndrome Registry Research Group. N Engl J Med. 1998;339:960–5.
9. Lazzara R. Amiodarone and torsade de pointes. Ann Intern Med. 1989;111:549–51.
10. Roden DM. Drug-induced prolongation of the QT interval. N Engl J Med. 2004;350:1013–22.
11. Dı́iaz-Castro O, Puchol A, Almendral J, Torrecilla EG, Arenal A, Martínez-Selles M. Predictors of in-hospital ventricular fibrillation or torsades de pointes in patients with acute symptomatic bradycardia. J Electrocardiol. 2004;37(1):55–60.
12. Grunsfeld A, Fletcher JJ, Nathan BR. Cardiopulmonary complications of brain injury. Curr Neurol Neurosci Rep. 2005;5:488–93.
13. Hersch C. Electrocardiographic changes in subarachnoid haemorrhage, meningitis and intracranial space occupying lesions. Br Heart J. 1964;26:785–93.

Endocarditis

15

Syed Wamique Yusuf, Steven C. Napierkowki,
Jose Banchs, Javier A. Adachi, and Saamir A. Hassan

Abstract

Endocarditis, defined as infection of the native or prosthetic heart valve, endocardial surface or an intracardiac device, occurs worldwide and though uncommon, can be associated with considerable morbidity and mortality.

In this chapter we present some common clinical cases and discuss the treatment options.

Keywords

Endocarditis • Valve • Prosthetic valve • Cardiac devices

Introduction

Endocarditis

The exact prevalence of endocarditis in large population afflicted with cancer in not known, but in a small study of 200 patients with solid tumor, the prevalence of cardiac valvular vegetation was 19% [1].

In another study of 645 patients with cancer, in whom echocardiogram was obtained for a suspected diagnosis of endocarditis, the prevalence of endocarditis, as diagnosed by Modified Duke Criteria was 7% [2].

It has also been suggested that infective endocarditis may be a potential marker of occult cancer, as in one study of 8445 patients with endocarditis, 997 (12%) cancers were identified after a median follow up of 3.5 years [3]. In particular, there appears to be a relationship between streptococcus bovis endocarditis and/or bacteremia and the presence of colorectal cancer [4].

S.W. Yusuf (✉) • S.C. Napierkowki • J. Banchs • S.A. Hassan
Department of Cardiology, University of Texas MD Anderson Cancer Center, Houston, TX 77030, USA
e-mail: syusuf@mdanderson.org; jbanchs@mdanderson.org

J.A. Adachi
Department of Infectious Diseases, Infection Control and Employee Health, University of Texas MD Anderson Cancer Center, Houston, TX 77030, USA

Infective Endocarditis

Infective endocarditis (IE) is a microbial infection of the endocardial surface of the heart. It most commonly involves heart valves but may also occur at other sites e.g. on the chordae tendineae, site of a septal defect, or on the mural endocardium, prosthetic cardiac valves and indwelling cardiac devices.

The cardinal features of endocarditis is a vegetation, which consists of a dense aggregate of microorganisms, fibrin, platelet-rich thrombus, and inflammatory leucocytes [5, 6].

Rheumatic heart disease remains the commonest key risk factor for IE in low-income countries and underlies up to two-thirds of cases [7, 8].

In developed high income countries, rheumatic fever is uncommon, however, degenerative valve disease, diabetes, cancer, intravenous drug use, and congenital heart disease have replaced rheumatic heart disease as the major risk factors for infective endocarditis [5].

The age at which IE used to afflict patients has also changed over the last 40 years. Compared to the average age of mid-40s during the early 1980s, it has now shifted to older than 70 years in 2001–2006 [5].

S.W. Yusuf, J. Banchs (eds.), *Cancer and Cardiovascular Disease*, https://doi.org/10.1007/978-3-319-62088-6_15

Non-bacterial Thrombotic Endocarditis

Microscopically, the lesions of NBTE are described as agglutinated blood and platelet thrombi with an absence of inflammatory reaction [9, 10].

It is classically associated with malignancy and has been reported in almost all types of cancer [10]. It is also found in other conditions like connective tissue disorder e.g. systemic lupus erythematosus (SLE), hypercoagulable state, septicemia, severe burn or chronic illness like tuberculosis, AIDS and uremia. The prevalence of NBTE is autopsy series ranges from 0.3 to 9.3% [10].

Mitral and aortic valve is most commonly involved [10].

NBTE typically causes embolization. The prevalence of emboli in different autopsy studies of NBTE, has been reported to be between 14 and 91% [10].

Treatment of NBTE is directed towards the underlying condition and in cases with no contraindication, anticoagulation, with either intravenous unfractionated heparin (UFH) or subcutaneous low molecular weight heparin (LMWH) is recommended [11].

The First Case Is an Example of Catheter-Related Endocarditis

Case 1: Catheter-Related Endocarditis

A 32 year old man with past medical history of multiple myeloma, diabetes mellitus and end-stage renal disease, who was on scheduled hemodialysis via a right internal jugular vein tunneled dialysis catheter, presented to an outside hospital with fevers and chills and was diagnosed with MRSA bacteremia and endocarditis of the mitral valve. He was started on intravenous (IV) vancomycin with adequate therapeutic levels and his tunneled dialysis catheter removed and later replaced. About 10 days later, he was referred to our hospital for a second opinion. On examination he had subungual embolic lesion.

A transesophageal echocardiogram (TEE) was done which showed a persistent mitral valve vegetation and moderate mitral regurgitation (Fig. 15.1). His vancomycin therapy was changed to IV daptomycin 800 mg IV q48 h for a total of 6 weeks of therapy. He responded to therapy and was discharged home.

Discussion

Patients with indwelling catheters are at increased risk for infective endocarditis as defined by the modified Duke's criteria. A significant proportion of patients with indwelling central venous catheters are those who are undergoing dialysis with the use of a hemodialysis (HD) catheter. In one study, HD catheter patients made up 20% of all cases of infective endocarditis [12]. *Staphylococcus aureus* is the most common pathogen. Infective endocarditis in hemodialysis patients carries a poor prognosis, with a 1 year mortality of about 50% even amongst patients who underwent valve replacement for endocarditis [13].

According to the 2009 Infectious Diseases Society of America (IDSA) guidelines, diagnosis of a catheter related blood stream infection is based on either a roll plate culture of the catheter tip if the catheter is removed, or from paired blood samples drawn from a peripheral vein and catheter. In patients for whom the diagnosis is made while the catheter is still in place, a decision will need to be made regarding catheter removal. The decision for catheter removal is based on clinical grounds, but the current recommendation is to remove the catheter and to treat with 4–6 weeks of antibiotics after catheter removal [14].

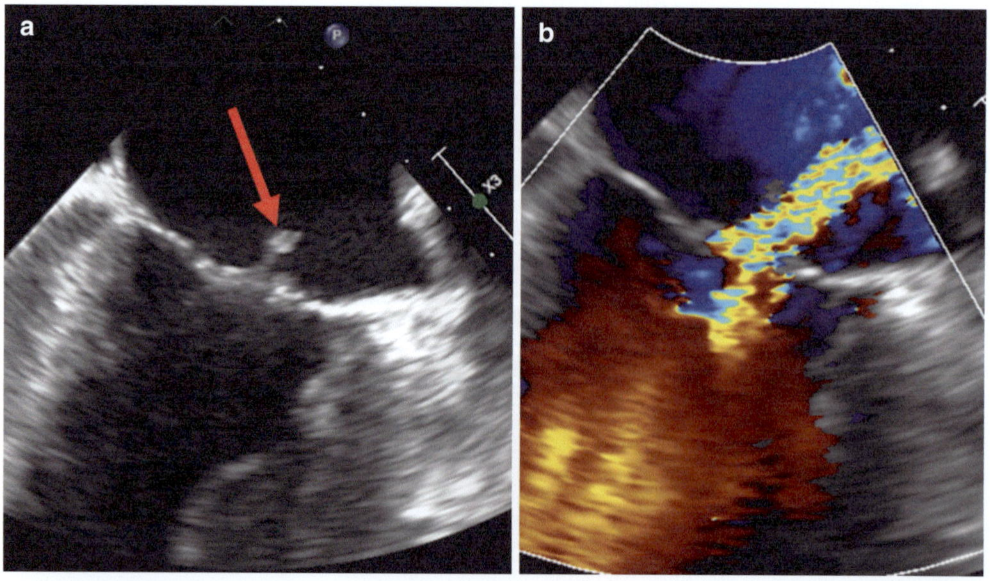

Fig. 15.1 (**a**) TEE showing mitral valve vegetation. The *red arrow* points to the vegetation. (**b**) TEE showing moderate mitral valve regurgitation

Infective Endocarditis in a Patient with a Cardiac Implantable Electronic Device Is Exhibited in the Next Case

Case 2: Intracardiac Device Infection/ Vegetation

The case presented is of a 72 year old man with history of non-small cell lung cancer, atrial fibrillation, sick sinus syndrome for which he had undergone a dual-chamber pacemaker placement in the past. He presented with dyspnea and cough for 2 weeks and was diagnosed with pneumonia by his primary care physician.

For his pneumonia, he was treated with levofloxacin for 2 days prior to blood cultures being drawn, which did not reveal any organism.

An echocardiogram revealed a mobile echogenicity attached to his right atrial pacing lead (Fig. 15.2).

He underwent lead/device extraction and a course of treatment with IV daptomycin, IV ceftriaxone and oral doxycycline. He made a full recovery.

Discussion

Pacemaker and other implantable cardiac electronic devices (ICED) may also become infected, and is associated with considerable morbidity and mortality [15]. A distinction should be made between a cardiac device related infective endocarditis (CDRIE) and a local device infection. CDRIE is defined as infection extending into the electrode leads, cardiac valve leaflets or endocardial surface [16]. Another definition of implantable cardiac electronic devices associated native or prosthetic valve endocarditis is when the Duke criteria for definite endocarditis is satisfied with echocardiographic evidence of valve involvement in a patient with an implantable cardiac electronic device in situ [15].

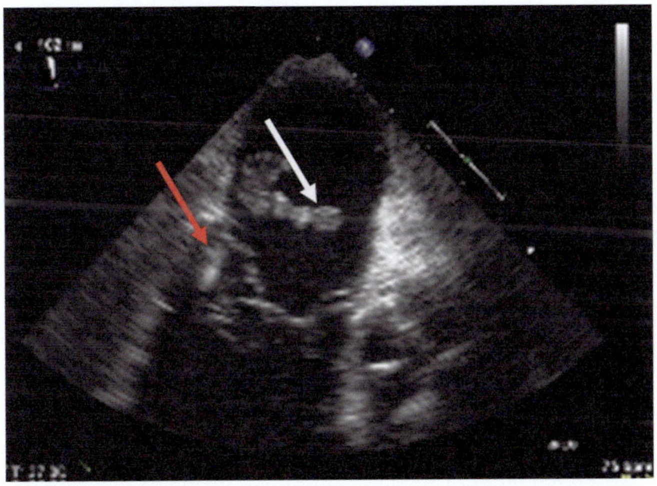

Fig. 15.2 TEE showing a pacemaker wire and a vegetation attached to the right atrial pacing lead. The *red arrow* points to the pacing lead and the *white arrow* points to the vegetation

Staphylococci, in particular coagulase negative *Staphylococcus* accounts for the majority of cases [15].

The diagnosis of CDRIE can be challenging. Due to complimentary role of both TTE and TEE, it is recommended that both TTE and TEE should be performed in suspected cases of CDRIE [16]. A TEE should be performed independent of the result of TTE. Additional tests that may be employed and are helpful includes; intracardiac echocardiogram, radiolabelled scintigraphy and ^{18}F-FDG PET/CT scanning [16].

For diagnosis purposes at least three or more sets of blood cultures are recommended before prompt initiation of antimicrobial therapy and in cases where the device is explanted the lead tip culture should be obtained [16].

The treatment of cardiac device related infective endocarditis relies on both total removal of all cardiac hardware (device and leads) and a prolonged course of antimicrobial therapy [15, 16].

Antibiotic therapy is generally done for 4–6 weeks and hard ware removal can often be performed percutaneously, even in the setting of sizeable vegetations (vegetations > 10 mm) [16].

The Following Case Illustrates Infective Endocarditis with an Indication for Valve Replacement

Case 3

The case presented is of a 59 year old man with past medical history of acute lymphoblastic leukemia who was admitted with altered mental status. His blood and urine cultures grew *Enterococcus faecium*.

This echocardiogram (Fig. 15.3) showed aortic valve vegetation, severe aortic regurgitation and aortic root abscess.

He was treated with IV streptomycin and IV vancomycin, with adequate therapeutic levels, for a total of 6 weeks of therapy and underwent aortic valve replacement.

Discussion

Both the ESC and AHA guidelines [16, 17] have specific indications for cardiac surgery in the setting of infective endocarditis as listed in the table below. The guidelines are very similar although some differences exist as highlighted. The ESC divides their indications based on three categories: resultant heart failure, uncontrolled infection, and prevention of embolism [16]. The ESC [16] and AHA guidelines [17] can both fall within this system and are adapted as such in the Table 15.1 While surgery may be indicated, it is

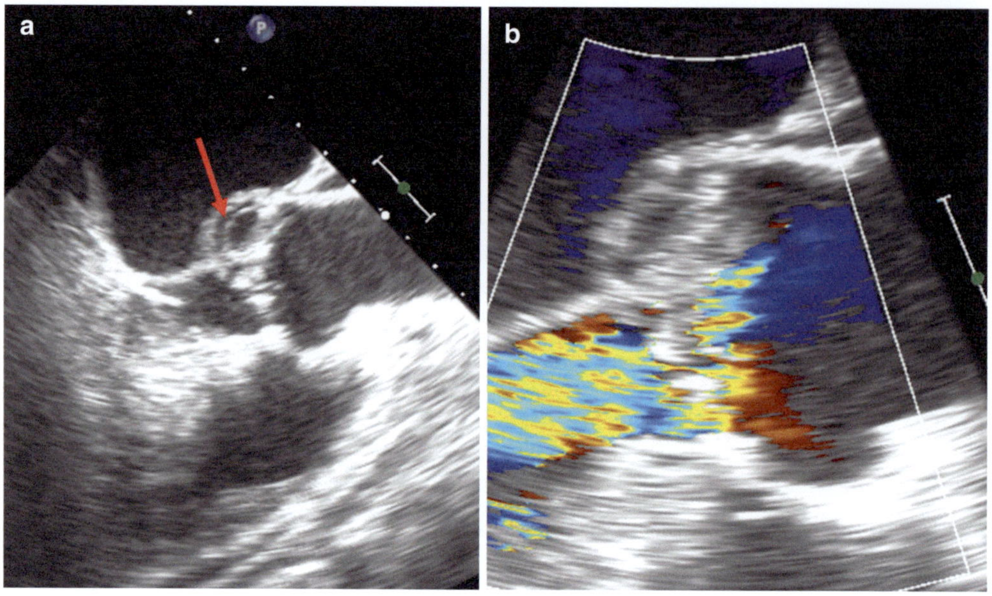

Fig. 15.3 (**a**) TEE showing perivalvular abscess in a patient with aortic valve vegetations. The *red arrow* points to the abscess. (**b**) TEE (same patient as in **a**) showing severe aortic regurgitation

Table 15.1 Indications for surgery in left-sided infective endocarditis

Surgical indication	AHA	ESC
Heart failure		
Valvular damage resulting in symptoms or signs of heart failure	**IB**	**IB**
Uncontrolled infection		
Resulting in abscess, fistula or local destruction	**IB**	**IB**
Resulting in heart block	**IB**	
Persistent positive blood cultures in spite of adequate antibiotic therapy and infectious source control	**IB**	**IIaB**
Persistence of infection, manifested by persistent bacteremia or fever for more than 5–7 days in spite of adequate antibiotic therapy and infectious source control in native valve infectious endocarditis	**IB**	
Infection secondary to fungi or resistant organisms	**IB**	**IC**
Infection secondary to *Staphylococcus aureus* or non-HACEK gram-negative bacteria involving a prosthetic valve		**IIaC**
Relapsing prosthetic valve endocarditis	**IIaC**	
Embolic risk		
Vegetation >10 mm when surgery is otherwise indicated	**IIbC**	**IIaB**
Vegetation >10 mm and severe valve regurgitation	**IIaB**	**IIaB**
Recurrent embolization in spite of antibiotic therapy (prosthetic valve) and persistent or growing vegetation (native valve)	**IIaB**	
Native or prosthetic valve with persistent vegetations >10 mm after one or more embolic episode despite being on appropriate antibiotic therapy		**IB**
Vegetation >30 mm		**IIaB**
Vegetation >15 mm and no other indication		**IIbC**

Indications are for both prosthetic and native valves unless otherwise indicated. Adapted from Habib et al. [16] and Baddour et al. [17]

Table 15.2 Indications for surgery in right-sided infective endocarditis

Surgical indication	AHA and ESC
Heart failure	
Right heart failure secondary to severe tricuspid regurgitation that does not respond to diuretic therapy	**IIaC**
Infection	
Resistant organisms or bacteremia >7 days in spite of appropriate antimicrobial therapy	**IIaC**
Embolic risk	
Persistent tricuspid valve vegetation >20 mm after recurrent pulmonary emboli	**IIaC**

Adapted from Habib et al. [16] and Baddour et al. [17]

ultimately a clinical decision and is individualized based on each patient's factors (Tables 15.1 and 15.2).

The Next Case Is an Example of Infective Endocarditis Complicated by Stroke

Case 4

A 58 year old man with history of oral squamous cell carcinoma which was in remission, was admitted with 4 months of weakness, involuntary weight loss, dyspnea, and fevers. A magnetic resonance imaging (MRI) of the brain revealed a ring enhancing lesion in his temporal lobe (Fig. 15.4). He also complained of floaters and blurry vision in his right eye and, and an ophthalmological examination showed findings consistent with endophthalmitis.

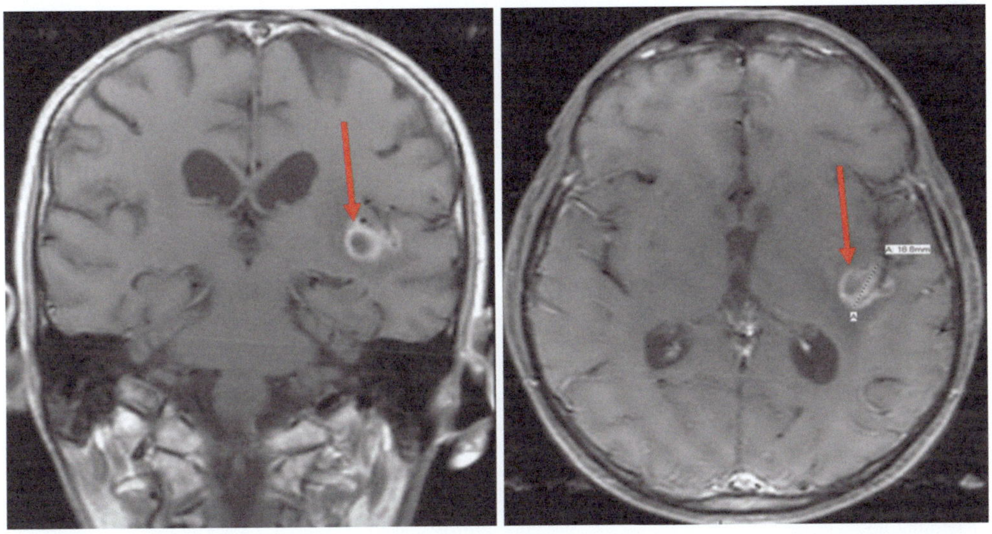

Fig. 15.4 MRI showing a ring enhancing lesion in the temporal lobe. The *red arrow* points to the lesion

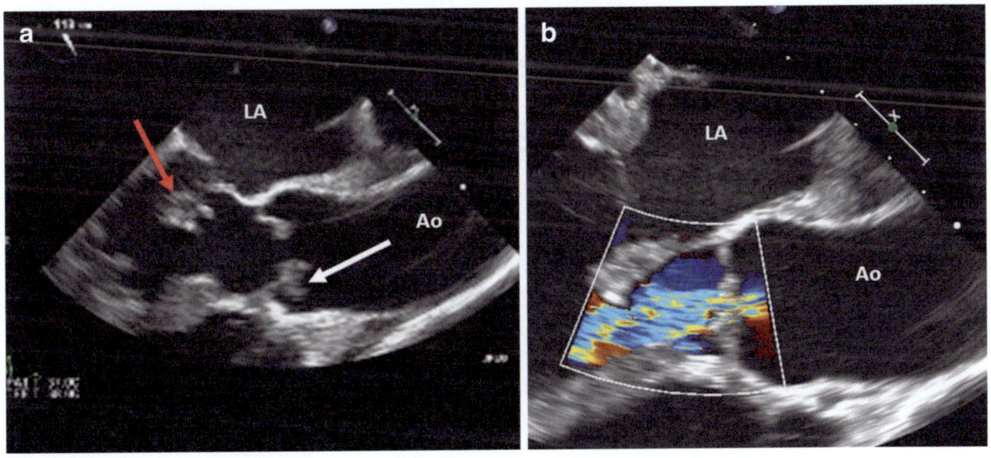

Fig. 15.5 (**a**) TEE showing mitral and aortic valve vegetations. The *red arrow* points to the mitral valve and the *white arrow* points to the aortic valve. (**b**) TEE showing moderate aortic regurgitation. *LA* Left atrium, *Ao* Aorta

Blood cultures were positive for *Streptococcus mutans*. A TEE (Fig. 15.5) showed mitral and aortic valve vegetation, with moderate aortic regurgitation.

The patient underwent therapy with 8 weeks of IV ceftriaxone, followed by four additional therapy with amoxicillin and minocycline. He had repeat echocardiogram 5 months later that showed larger mass and he was referred for surgical evaluation. However due his general condition, surgery was not performed at that time and it was decided to manage him medically. He later had an unexplained neurological event, with no residual deficits while on a vacation. Finally, repeat echocardiogram on 10/22/14 confirmed resolution of the vegetation.

Discussion

Endocarditis, by its nature is a systemic disease. Multiple organ systems can become involved either by direct intravascular bacterial seeding or through rheumatological phenomena, as outlined in Table 15.3.

According to both the ESC and AHA guidelines, a stroke due to endocarditis/vegetation, is an indication for surgery (See Table 15.1) and should be performed without delay [16, 17]. However, if an intracranial hemorrhage is found, then surgery should be delayed for at least 1 month [16, 17]. The AHA guidelines also state that surgery may be considered in the presence of a stroke and residual vegetation [17].

A Case of Infective Endocarditis Involving a Prosthetic Valve Is Demonstrated Below

Case 5: Prosthetic Valve Endocarditis

The case presented is of a 50 year old woman with past medical history of Hodgkin's lymphoma, treated with chemo radiation therapy. Her treatment was complicated by radiation-induced coronary artery disease, heart block and valvular disease. In the past she had undergone a coronary artery bypass grafting (CABG) in 2001 and a re-do CABG in 2005,

Table 15.3 Systemic manifestations of Endocarditis

Organ system	Lesions	Diagnosis
Neurologic [18]	Embolic brain infarction, TIA, cerebral hemorrhage, meningitis, brain abscess, toxic encephalopathy, headache	Full neurological exam, brain CT scan, lumbar puncture
Ophthalmologic [19]	Roth (or Litten) spots (retinal hemorrhages with white centers), conjunctival hemorrhage, endophthalmitis	Ophthalmologic exam
Dermatologic [20]	Osler's nodes (tender palpable nodules on finger tips), Janeway's lesions (non-tender erythematous lesions on palms and soles), purpura, conjunctival hemorrhages	Full skin exam. Biopsy and culture of Osler's nodes or Janeway's lesions may yield the causative organism
Splenic [21]	Splenic infarcts	Abdominal CT scan
Pulmonary [21]	Septic infarct, abscess	Chest x-ray, CT scan
Renal [21]	Renal infarcts, abscess, glomerulonephritis, or antibiotic treatment-induced complications including acute interstitial nephritis	Abdominal CT, urinalysis, complement levels, rheumatoid factor
Rheumatologic [22]	Septic arthritis, aseptic synovitis, back pain, vertebral osteomyelitis, myalgia	X-ray, CT scan, arthrocentesis, serum cryoglobulins, complement levels

permanent pacemaker insertion for complete heart block, and an mechanical aortic valve replacement 12 years prior to current admission. She also had renal failure for which she was on hemodialysis via a tunneled dialysis catheter.

She presented with septic shock requiring pressors. A chest x ray showed infiltrates and serum troponin was elevated with a peak level of 1.78 ng/mL. Tracheal aspirates grew *Pseudomonas aeruginosa* and she was treated with IV ceftazidime and IV ciprofloxacin. A TTE showed an aortic valve vegetation, attached to the prosthetic valve (Fig. 15.6).

The patient continued to deteriorate and died of multiorgan failure 13 days after the echocardiogram.

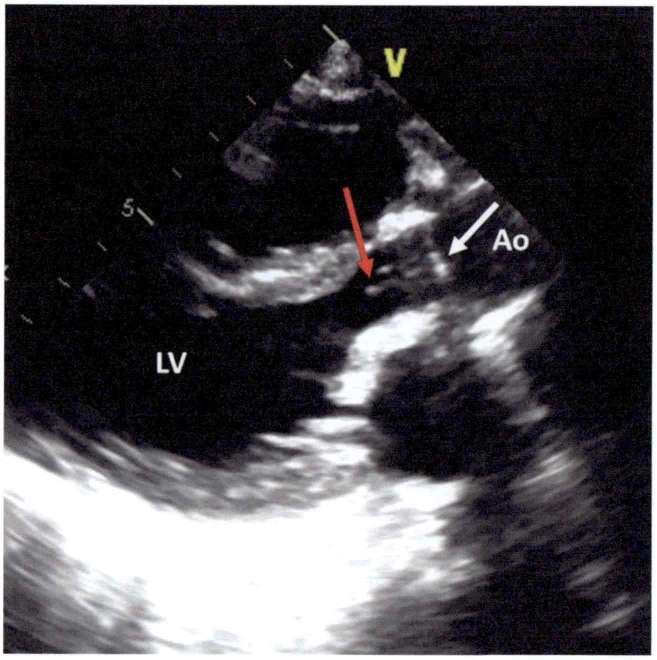

Fig. 15.6 TTE showing an aortic valve vegetation, attached to the prosthetic valve. The *red arrow* points to the vegetation and the *white arrow* shows the prosthetic valve. *Ao* Aorta, *LV* Left ventricle

Discussion

Prosthetic valve endocarditis (PVE) accounts for about 20% of all cases of infective endocarditis [16]. It is classified as either early, those cases diagnosed within 1 year of implantation, or late, occurring >1 year after surgery. Early PVE is associated with more virulent organisms including *S. aureus*, gram negative bacteria and fungi, while late PVE is associated with more typical endocarditis species including oral streptococci, besides staphylococci and enterococci. The risk thromboembolic events in PVE is higher than in native valve endocarditis. If endocarditis is suspected in a patient with a prosthetic valve, then transesophageal echocardiography (TEE) should also be obtained and is mandatory [16, 23]. Other investigations that are helpful includes 18 FDG PET/CT or leucocyte labelled SPECT/CT and cardiac CT [16]. Finally, the Duke criteria is not as sensitive in PVE as in native valve endocarditis. Hence patients with a clinical suspicion should be investigated by imaging techniques outlined above.

Treatment of PVE is based on patient risk stratification. According to the 2015 ESC guidelines [16], patients with high-risk features such as persistent fever, abscess, severe prosthetic dysfunction or heart failure, should be considered for an early surgical strategy (see Table 15.1). Otherwise a course of antimicrobial therapy is given similar for patients with NVE. Patients should be frequently reassessed during antibiotic treatment for complications [16].

Fungal Endocarditis Is Demonstrated in the Next Case

Case 6: Fungal Endocarditis

A 34 year old woman with refractory acute myelocytic leukemia, who was being treated for presumed fungal pneumonia. Figure 15.7 shows the CT scan of the chest. TTE showed a tricuspid valve (TV) vegetation with features suggestive of a fungal vegetation as shown (Fig. 15.8).

She was treated with IV voriconazole and IV caspofungin. Due to profound neutropenia and thrombocytopenia, she was not a candidate for surgery. She later had two consecutive admissions related to invasive fungal infection. The first was for fungal sinusitis and the second for severe sepsis. She died 22 days after this echocardiogram was performed due to sepsis.

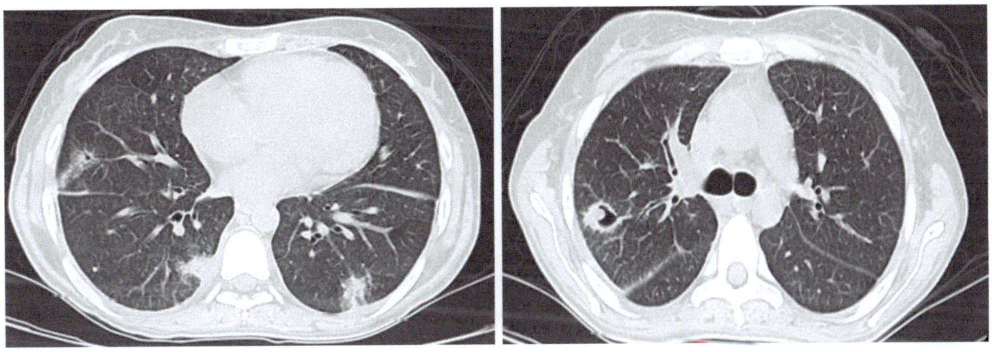

Fig. 15.7 CT scan of the chest shows opacities consistent with fungal infection

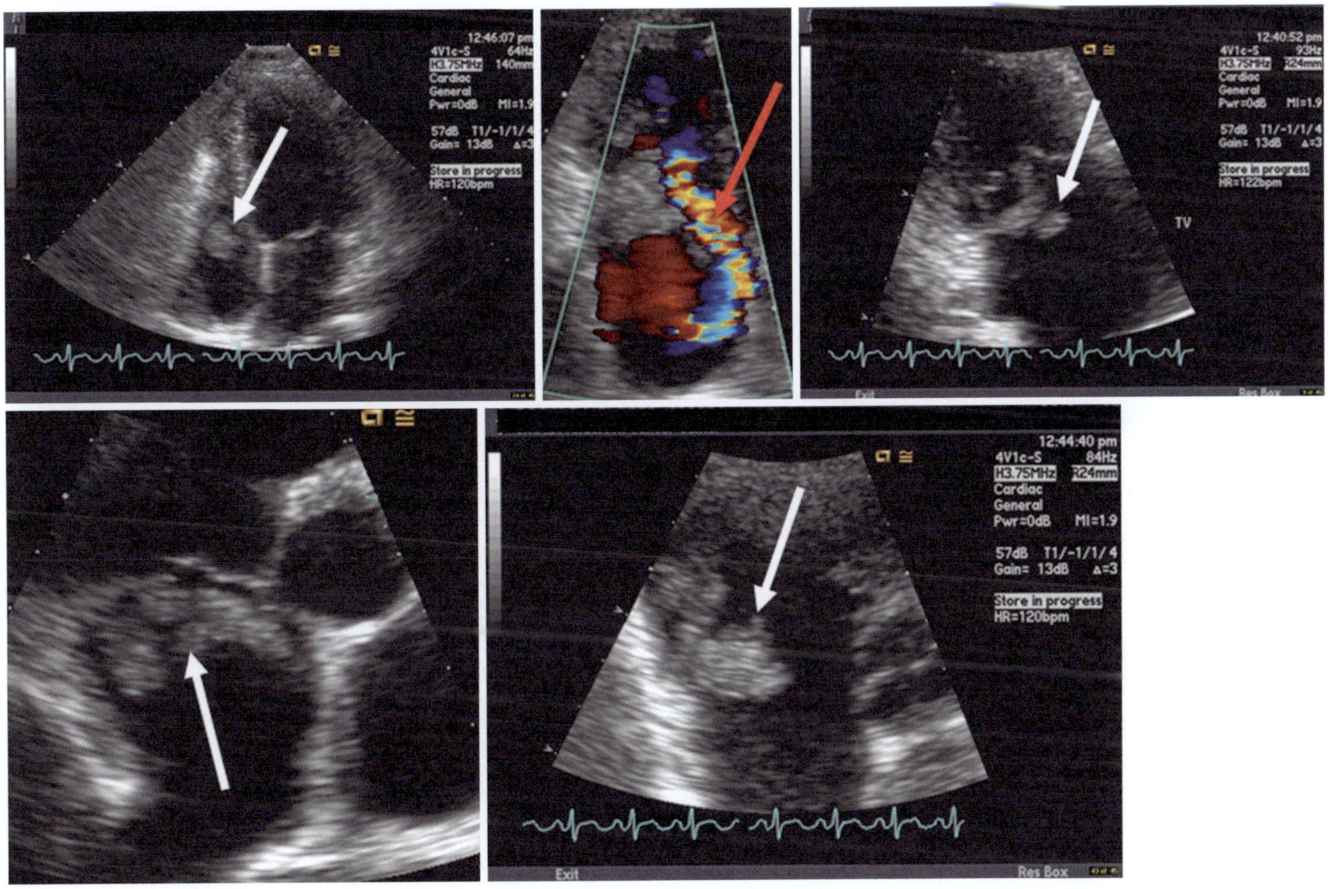

Fig. 15.8 TTE (multiple views) showing tricuspid valve vegetation. The *white arrow* in each image points to the vegetation. The *red arrow* points to the tricuspid regurgitation

Discussion

Less than 2% of endocarditis cases are due to a fungal pathogen. Fungal infection is more frequently observed in patients with PVE, central venous catheter, IV drug abusers and immunocompromised patients [24]. Half of reported cases of fungal endocarditis from 1995 to 2000 were of patients who had central venous catheters and broad-spectrum antibiotic use, prosthetic valves made up the other half with less than 5% being due to recreational IV drug use. The majority of cases are secondary to *Candida* (50–80%) and *Aspergillus* species [24].

Diagnosis of fungal endocarditis, like bacterial endocarditis, is based on the Modified Duke criteria. However, fungal endocarditis is classically a more difficult diagnosis and symptoms have been known to persist for over a month before the diagnosis is made. Therefore, a high index of suspicion is necessary in at risk patients. It should also be noted that while *Candida* will grow in over 90% of blood cultures, blood cultures in a patient with *Aspergillus* endocarditis is rarely positive. Antigenic detection is being developed for the diagnosis of *Candida* (Mannan and anti-mannan antibodies, B-1, 3 D-Glucan) and *Aspergillus* (Galactomannan) [25, 26], with inconclusive results.

Surgical valvular replacement is the mainstay of fungal endocarditis treatment in patients who are candidates and valve replacement in fungal endocarditis is a class I level of evidence C and class I level of evidence B recommendation in the ESC and AHA guidelines respectively [16, 17]. This is done in conjunction with long-term antifungal therapy.

The Following Two Cases Illustrate Tricuspid Valve Endocarditis

Case 7: Tricuspid Valve Vegetation

A 55 year female with history of relapsed diffuse large B-cell lymphoma status post stem cell transplant 1 month, was admitted to the ICU for respiratory distress and pneumonia.

An echocardiogram was done as part of evaluation which showed a tricuspid valve vegetation and also revealed cardiomyopathy with ejection fraction of 30–35%.(Fig. 15.9).

She had already been treated with vancomycin and meropenem for persistent neutropenic fever. The patient's blood cultures were negative. Suspicion of viral causes, *Stenotrophomonas*, or atypical infections such as *Legionella* were raised. She was treated with broad spectrum antibiotic coverage with IV acyclovir, IV caspofungin, IV daptomycin, IV meropenem and IV Bactrim. However, her condition continued to deteriorate and her blood pressure continued to drop in spite of pressor support. She died 9 days after the echocardiogram.

Case 8: Tricuspid Valve Vegetation

The case presented is of a 46 year old man with history of sigmoid adenocarcinoma, for which he had undergone surgery and was on chronic total parenteral nutrition via a right sided port-a-cath. He was admitted with fever and rigors in Nov 2010.

Blood cultures, catheter tip culture, and urine culture were positive for *Enterococcus faecalis*. A transesophageal echocardiogram (TEE) was done which showed a large TV valve vegetation (Fig. 15.10).

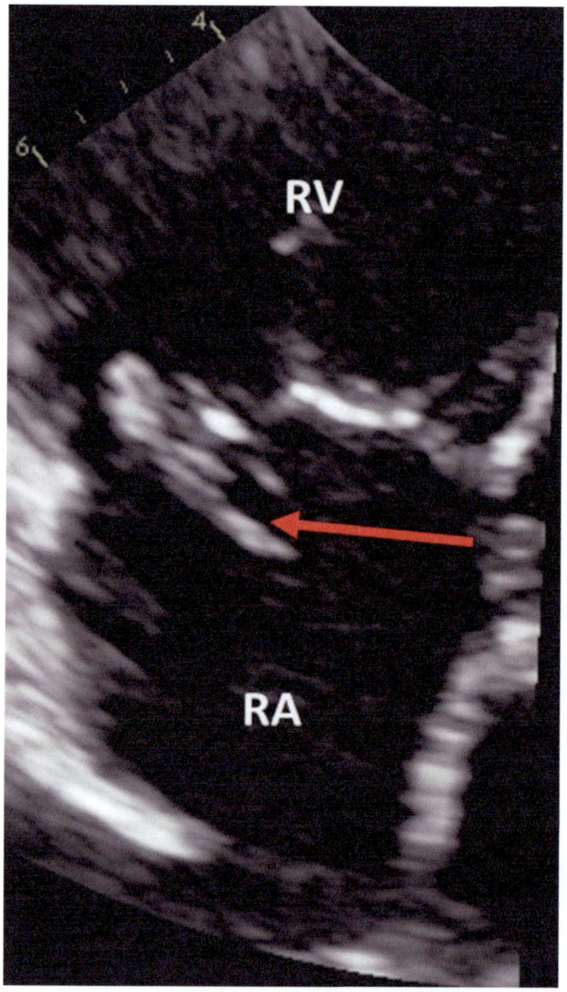

Fig. 15.9 TTE showing the tricuspid valve vegetation. The *red arrow* points to the vegetation. *RV* right ventricle, *RA* right atrium

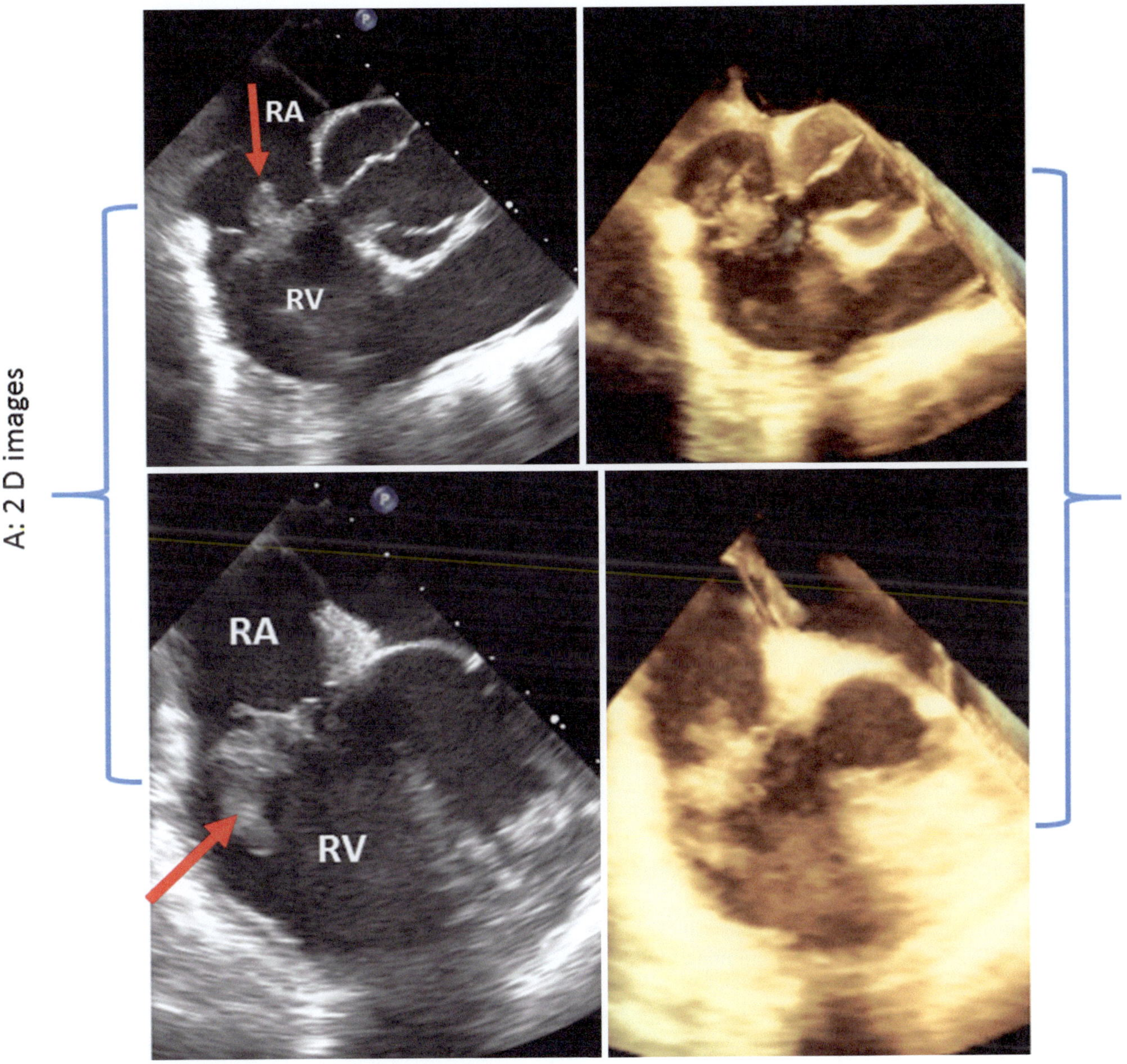

Fig. 15.10 TEE (**a**: 2 D images. **b**: 3 D images) showing the tricuspid valve vegetation

He was transferred to an outside hospital for surgical valve replacement, but was not considered a surgical candidate and ultimately was treated medically with ampicillin for a total of 8 weeks.

He responded well to medical therapy. An echocardiogram in Jan 2012 showed complete resolution of the vegetation. From a cardiovascular point of view he was doing well, when last seen in Feb 2017.

Discussion

Tricuspid valve endocarditis is a disease that most commonly affects intravenous drug abusers and patients with indwelling lines, including central venous catheters and pacemakers. Organisms are typically more virulent than those causing left-sided endocarditis. *Staphylococcus aureus* is the most common microorganism found, followed by *Pseudomonas aeruginosa* and *Alpha Streptococcus* [27]. Signs and symptoms are generally related to septic pulmonary emboli; however, if a patent foramen ovale is present, paradoxical systemic embolization may also occur. The "tricuspid syndrome" is the constellation of recurrent pulmonary illness, anemia, and microscopic hematuria and these findings should alert one to the possibility of tricuspid valve endocarditis [28].

Current ESC guidelines give a IIa recommendation for surgical treatment/valve replacement only if an organism is difficult to treat, the bacteremia lasts for more than 7 days in spite of appropriate antibiotic therapy, there is a tricuspid valve vegetation >20 mm after recurrent pulmonary embolism, or if there is severe tricuspid regurgitation leading to right heart failure that does not respond well to diuretic therapy. Patients should otherwise be treated medically [16].

One of our patient had *Enterococcus faecalis* which is an uncommon cause of tricuspid valve endocarditis. In one study about 13% of IE cases were due to enterococcal strain, of which 52% were due to *E. faecium* and 48% were due to *E. faecalis* [29]. In this study the tricuspid valve was affected in only 20% of all cases. These cases are often nosocomial and are most commonly associated with hemodialysis and indwelling central venous catheters [29].

The Subsequent Three Cases Illustrate Non-bacterial Thrombotic Endocarditis

Case 9: Non-bacterial Thrombotic Endocarditis

A 46 year old man with history of pancreatic cancer with metastases to the liver, presented with a pulmonary embolism and cerebrovascular accident (CVA). The blood cultures were normal and troponin I was elevated with a peak of 0.74 ng/mL. A TTE showed typical findings of marantic endocarditis affecting the mitral valve (Fig. 15.11). Given the patient's clinical presentation, typical findings on echocardiogram and the negative blood cultures, he was diagnosed with non-bacterial thrombotic endocarditis (marantic).

Resumption of anticoagulation was recommended.

During investigations a CT abdomen showed renal infarct (Fig. 15.12).

The patient went into hepatorenal syndrome on this same admission, his condition deteriorated, and he died 11 days after this echocardiogram.

Case 10: Non-bacterial Thrombotic Endocarditis

The case presented is of a 60 year old man with metastatic gastric adenocarcinoma, who was diagnosed with a deep vein thrombosis and a pulmonary embolism 6 weeks prior to presentation. He was as admitted with confusion and an

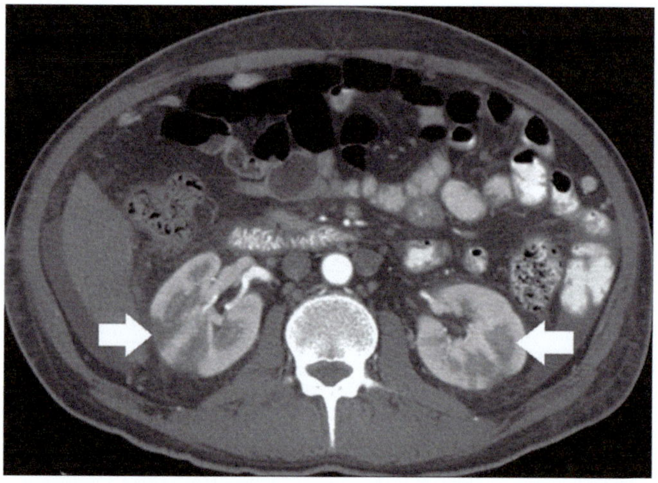

Fig. 15.12 CT scan abdomen showing bilateral wedge-shaped renal infarcts. The *white arrows* points to the infarct

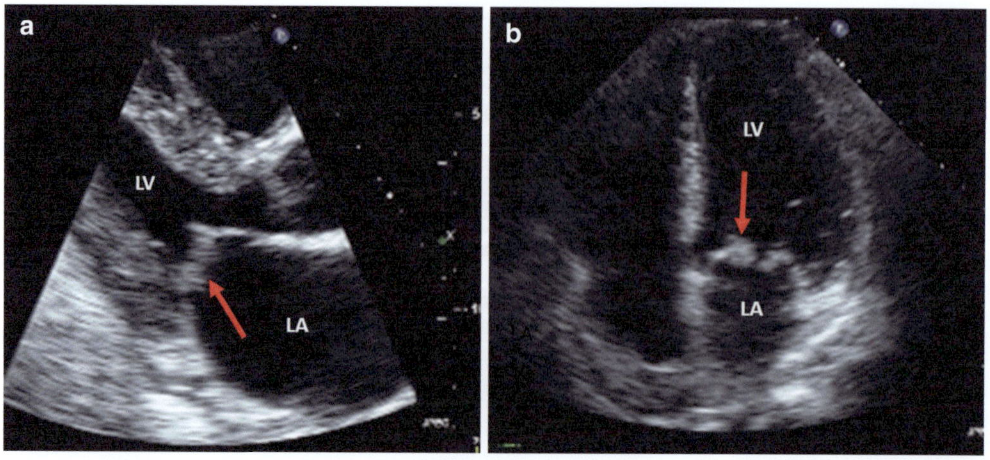

Fig. 15.11 (**a**) TTE (parasternal view) showing mitral valve vegetation. (**b**) TTE (apical 4 chamber view) showing mitral valve vegetation. The *red arrow* points to the vegetations. *LA* Left atrium, *LV* left ventricle

MRI of the brain showed multiple embolic infarcts (Fig. 15.13). As a part of the investigation a TEE echocardiogram was obtained which showed findings suggestive of marantic endocarditis affecting the aortic valve (Fig. 15.14). Besides suffering an acute stroke he also had a gastrointestinal tract bleed.

Blood cultures were negative.

The patient underwent embolization by interventional radiology for his bleeding ulcer, followed by radiation for his malignancy and also received anticoagulation. He was discharged home on low molecular weight heparin (LMWH).

Case 11: Non-bacterial Thrombotic Endocarditis

A 71 year old man with stage IV lung cancer, myocardial infarction, diabetes mellitus and paroxysmal atrial fibrillation underwent a routine MRI brain as a part of staging. The MRI revealed embolic infarcts (Fig. 15.15). Subsequently a TEE was obtained which showed findings suggestive of maranatic endocarditis (Fig. 15.16). Prior to his TEE, empiric antibiotics were started. However, cultures were negative and the lesion appeared to be consistent with marantic endocarditis, so these were stopped. Since he

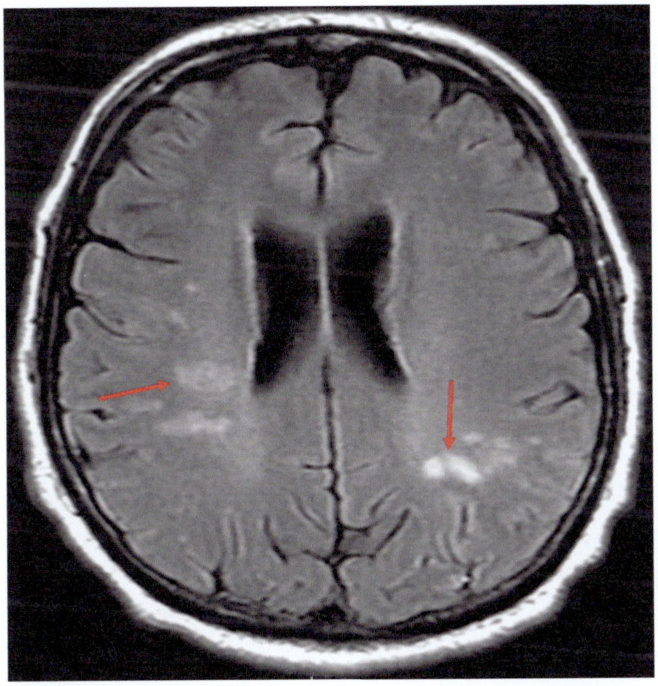

Fig. 15.13 MRI of the brain showing multiple infarcts. The *red arrow* points to the infarcts

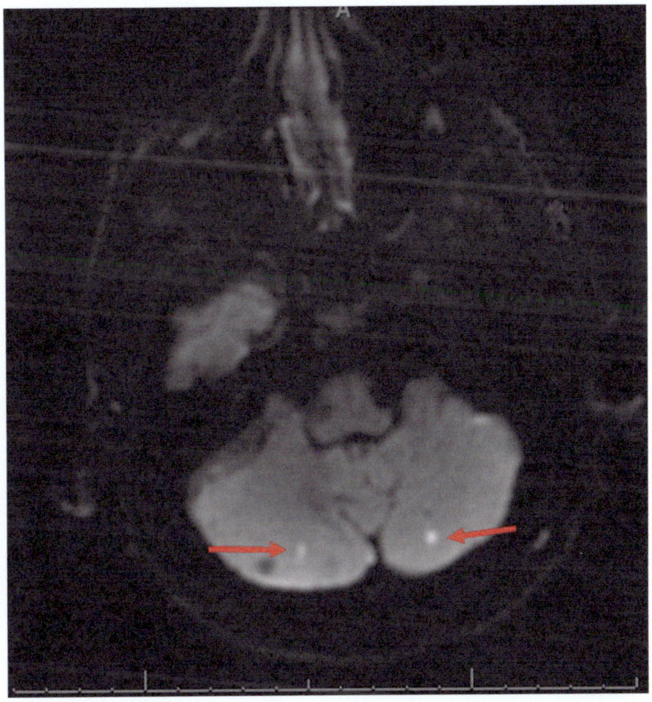

Fig. 15.15 MRI of the brain showing embolic infarcts. *Red arrow* points the infarct

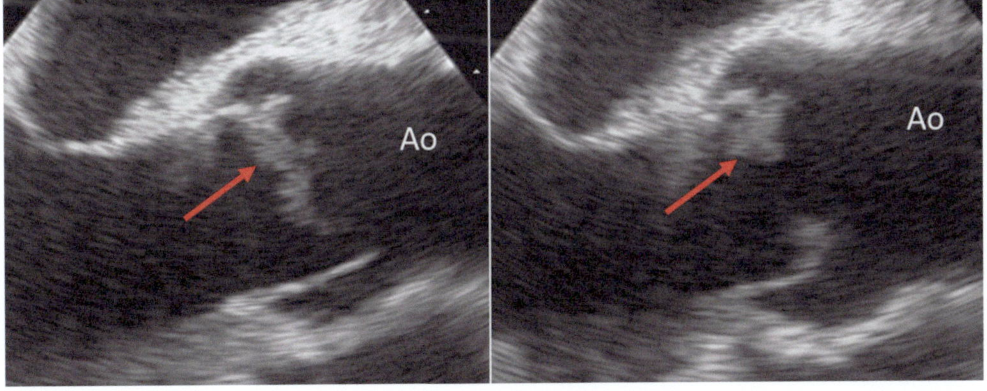

Fig. 15.14 TEE showing aortic valve vegetation. The *red arrow* points to the vegetation. *Ao* aorta

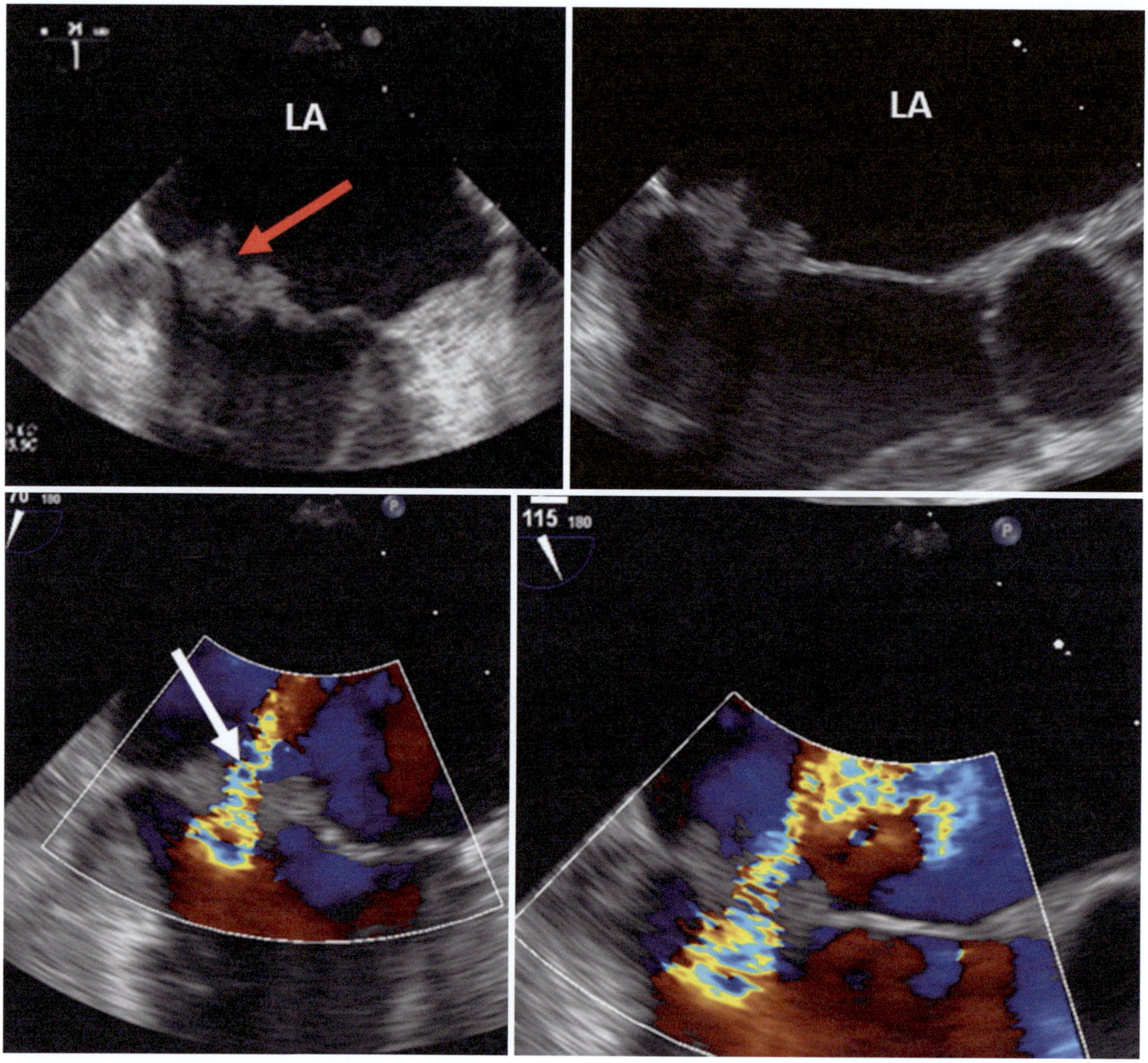

Fig. 15.16 TEE (multiple views) showing mitral valve vegetations and mitral regurgitation. The *red arrow* points to the vegetation and the *white arrow* points to the regurgitation. *LA* Left atrium

also had brain metastases, only aspirin was given for anticoagulation. He was discharged home with outpatient palliative radiation therapy for his brain metastases. He passed away 26 days after the echocardiogram was performed.

Discussion

Nonbacterial thrombotic endocarditis (NBTE), also called marantic endocarditis, is a non-infectious phenomenon that occurs in patients with a hypercoagulable state. Common predisposing conditions are cancer, lupus, or the antiphospholipid syndrome. It can also occur in patients with sepsis, burns or indwelling catheters [10]. They can occur in up to 4% end-stage cancer patients [30] and 11% of lupus patients [31]. The form seen in SLE is also known as Libman-Sacks endocarditis.

NBTE carries a high risk of embolization, in multiple territories [32].

The diagnosis of NBTE can be challenging and begins with a thorough understanding of the patient's underlying history. Clues suggesting malignancy, lupus, or the

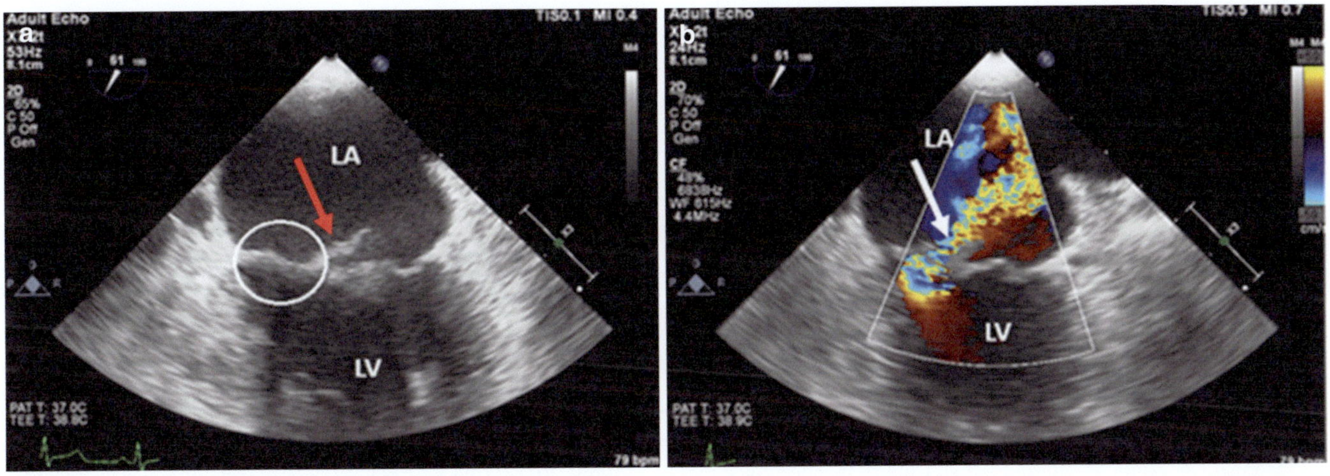

Fig. 15.17 (**a**) TEE view with the *red arrow* on a large vegetation, circle on area of suspected perforation, confirmed perforation on panel (**b**) with jet clearly to left of vegetation. (**b**) Same image now with over imposed color Doppler. Please note that the jet comes to the left of the vegetation in area that looked intact without color. The *white arrow* points to the mitral regurgitation jet

antiphospholipid syndrome should raise the possibility of NBTE. The characteristic lesion of NBTE is a sterile bland thrombus [33]. Lesions typically affect the aortic or mitral valves but it can also affect other valves [11]. Adherence to the Duke criteria for classification of infective endocarditis can help rule out an infectious cause for the lesion as well. Definitive diagnosis is often made on autopsy study.

Therapy of NBTE includes treatment of the underlying disease and unfractionated heparin. Warfarin has not been proven to prevent embolic disease. The use of anticoagulation with heparin in NBTE is a Grade 2C recommendation by the American College of Chest Physicians [11]. This differs from guidelines on infective endocarditis in that routine anticoagulation in native valve infective endocarditis is contraindicated [34] since it increases the risk of cerebral hemorrhage [35].

Case 12: Recurrent Embolic Phenomenon

The case presented is of a 42 year old gentleman with a history of stage III mantle cell lymphoma. He presented with transient loss of vision and dyspnea on exertion. Patient had three episodes of transient visual defect affecting his left eye, with recovery within an hour. Investigations included a CT angiogram of the carotids which was normal and a TTE which showed a vegetation on the mitral valve. A TEE confirmed the vegetation on the posterior mitral leaflet measuring approximately 1.0 × −0.5 cm, with perforation of the posterior mitral leaflet (Fig. 15.17).

He was treated with intravenous ceftriaxone and vancomycin, with adequate therapeutic levels and underwent an urgent successful mitral valve replacement with a bioprosthetic valve. Pathology of the mitral valve showed myxoid degeneration and valve cultures did not reveal any organism.

Discussion

The patient presented with recurrent transient visual symptoms, likely due to do micro embolism, from the mitral valve vegetation. The clinical presentation and the mitral valve findings on TEE, are indications for valve replacement [16, 17].

References

1. Edoute Y, Haim N, Rinkevich D, et al. Cardiac valvular vegetations in cancer patients: a prospective echocardiographic study of 200 patients. Am J Med. 1997;102:252–8.
2. Yusuf SW, Ali SS, Swafford J, et al. Culture-positive and culture-negative endocarditis in patients with cancer: a retrospective observational study, 1994-2004. Medicine. 2006;85:86–94.
3. RW T, Parkas DK, Friis S, et al. Endocarditis and risk of cancer: a Danish nationwide cohort study. Am J Med. 2013;126:58–67.
4. Gupta A, Madani R, Mukhtar H. Streptococcus bovis endocarditis, a silent sign for colonic tumor. Colorectal Dis. 2010;12:164–71.
5. Cahill TJ, Prendergast BD. Infective endocarditis. Lancet. 2016;387:882–93.
6. Vanassche T, Peetermans WE, Herregods MC, Herijgers P, Verhamme P. Antithrombotic therapy in infective endocarditis. Expert Rev Cardiovasc Ther. 2011;9(9):1203–19.
7. Carapetis JR, Steer AC, Mulholland EK, Weber M. The global burden of group A streptococcal diseases. Lancet Infect Dis. 2005;5:6855.
8. Marijon E, Ou P, Celermajer DS, et al. Prevalence of rheumatic heart disease detected by echocardiographic screening. N Engl J Med. 2007;357:470.

9. Gross L, Friedberg CK. Nonbacterial thrombotic endocarditis. Classification and general description. Arch Intern Med. 1936;58:620–40.
10. Lopez JA, Ross RS, Fishbein MC, Siegel RJ. Nonbacterial thrombotic endocarditis: a review. Am Heart J. 1987;113:774–84.
11. Whitlock RP, Sun JC, Fremes SE, Rubens FD, Teoh KH. Antithrombotic and thrombolytic therapy for valvular heart disease: antithrombotic therapy and prevention of thrombosis, 9th ed: American College of Chest Physicians Evidence-Based Clinical Practice Guidelines. Chest. 2012;141(2 Suppl):e576S–600S.
12. Cabell CH, Jollis JG, Gail EP, Corey R, et al. Changing patient characteristics and the effect on mortality in endocarditis. Arch Intern Med. 2002;162:90–4.
13. Leither MD, Shroff GR, Ding S, et al. Long term survival of dialysis patients with bacterial endocarditis undergoing valvular replacement surgery in the United States. Circulation. 2013;128: 344–51.
14. Mermel LA, Allon M, Bouza E, et al. Clinical practice guidelines for the diagnosis and management of intravascular catheter-related infection: 2009 Update by the Infectious Diseases Society of America. Clin Infect Dis. 2009;49(1):1–4.
15. Sandoe JA, Barlow G, Chambers JB, et al. Guidelines for the diagnosis, prevention and management of implantable cardiac electronic device infection. Report of a joint Working Party project on behalf of the British Society for Antimicrobial Chemotherapy (BSAC, host organization), British Heart Rhythm Society (BHRS), British Cardiovascular Society (BCS), British Heart Valve Society (BHVS) and British Society for Echocardiography (BSE). J Antimicrob Chemother. 2015;70: 325–59.
16. Habib G, Lancellotti P, Antunes MJ, et al. 2015 ESC Guidelines for the management of infective endocarditis: the Task Force for the Management of Infective Endocarditis of the European Society of Cardiology (ESC). Eur Heart J. 2015;36(44):3075–128.
17. Baddour LM, Wilson WR, Bayer AS, et al. Infective endocarditis in adults: diagnosis, antimicrobial therapy, and management of complications. A scientific statement for healthcare professionals from the American Heart Association. Circulation. 2015;132: 1435–86.
18. Heiro M, Nikoskelainen J, Engblom E, et al. Neurologic manifestations of infective endocarditis: a 17-year experience in a teaching hospital in Finland. Arch Intern Med. 2000;160(18):2781–7. doi:10.1001/archinte.160.18.2781.
19. Loughrey PB, Armstrong D, Lockhart CJ. Classical eye signs in bacterial endocarditis. QJM. 2015;108(11):909–10.
20. Servy A, Valeyrie-Allanore L, Alla F, et al. Prognostic value of skin manifestations of infective endocarditis. JAMA Dermatol. 2014;150(5):494–500.
21. Cunha BA, Gill MV, Lazar JM. Acute infective endocarditis. Diagnostic and therapeutic approach. Infect Dis Clin North Am. 1996;10:811–34.
22. Thomas P, Allal J, Bontoux D, et al. Rheumatologic manifestations of infective endocarditis. Ann Rheum Dis. 1984;43:716–20.
23. Yusuf SW, Sharma J, Durand JB, Banchs J. Endocarditis and myocarditis: a brief review. Expert Rev Cardiovasc Ther. 2012;10(9): 1153–64.
24. Tattevin P, Revest M, Lefort A, Michelet C, Lortholary O. Fungal endocarditis: current challenges. Int J Antimicrob Agents. 2014;44(4):290–4. doi:10.1016/j.ijantimicag.2014.07.003. (//www.sciencedirect.com/science/article/pii/S0924857914002349). ISSN: 0924-8579.
25. Lefort A, Chartier L, Sendid B, Wolff M, Mainardi J-L, Podglajen I, Desnos-Ollivier M, Fontanet A, Bretagne S, Lortholary O. Diagnosis, management and outcome of Candida endocarditis. Clin Microbiol Infect. 2012;18(4):E99–109. doi:10.1111/j.1469-0691.2012.03764.x. (//www.sciencedirect.com/science/article/pii/S1198743X1461466X). ISSN: 1198-743X.
26. Tacke D, Koehler P, Cornely OA. Fungal endocarditis. Curr Opin Infect Dis. 2013;26:501–7.
27. Chan P, Ogilby JD, Segal B. Tricuspid valve endocarditis. Am Heart J. 1989;117(5):1140–6.
28. Heydari AA, Safari H, Sarvhad MR. Isolated tricuspid valve endocarditis. Int J Infect Dis. 2009;13:e109–11.
29. Forrest GN, et al. Single center experience of a vancomycin resistant enterococcal endocarditis cohort. J Infect. 2011;63:420–8.
30. Chomette G, Auriol M, Baubion D, de Frejacques C. Non-bacterial thrombotic endocarditis. Autopsy study, clinico-pathological correlations. Ann Med Interne (Paris). 1980;131(7):443–7.
31. Moyssakis I, Tektonidou MG, Vasilliou VA, Samarkos M, Votteas V, Moutsopoulos HM. Libman-Sacks endocarditis in systemic lupus erythematosus: prevalence, associations, and evolution. Am J Med. 2007;120(7):636–42.
32. Bathina JD, Daher IN, Plana JC, Durand J-B, Yusuf SW. Acute myocardial infarction associated with nonbacterial thrombotic endocarditis. Tex Heart Inst J. 2010;37(2):208–12.
33. Kim HS, Suzuki M, Lie JT, Titus JL. Nonbacterial thrombotic endocarditis (NBTE) and disseminated intravascular coagulation (DIC): autopsy study of 36 patients. Arch Pathol Lab Med. 1977;101(2):65–8.
34. Delahaye JP, Poncet P, Malquarti V, Beaune J, Gare JP, Mann JM. Cerebrovascular accidents in infective endocarditis: role of anticoagulation. Eur Heart J. 1990;11(12):1074–8.
35. Tornos P, Almirante B, Mirabet S, Permanyer G, Pahissa A, Soler-Soler J. Infective endocarditis due to Staphylococcus aureus: deleterious effect of anticoagulant therapy. Arch Intern Med. 1999;159(5): 473–5.

Pericardial Disease, Constrictive Pericarditis and Restrictive Cardiomyopathy in Patients with Cancer

16

Saamir A. Hassan, Poojita Shivamurthy, and Syed Wamique Yusuf

Abstract

Pericardial disease, specifically acute pericarditis, constrictive pericarditis, and pericardial tamponade, are seen in cancer patients due to the malignant process or from radiation therapy. In this chapter we present an overview of acute pericarditis, constrictive pericarditis and pericardial tamponade. We also discuss restrictive cardiomyopathy and its differences from constrictive pericarditis.

Keywords

Pericardial disease • Cardiac tamponade • Constrictive heart disease • Restrictive heart disease

Acute Pericarditis

Acute pericarditis presents as chest pain, electrocardiogram (ECG) changes, and pericardial friction rub in patients with an acute inflammation of their pericardium. Acute pericarditis can occur in up to 4% of patients with chest pain [1]. There are many cause of acute pericarditis as shown in Table 16.1 and they include infectious, autoimmune, metabolic, malignant, drug-induced, and idiopathic etiologies [2]. To make the diagnosis of acute pericarditis patients need to have two of the following four criteria: typical chest pain, audible pericardial friction rub, diffuse ST-segment elevation, and new or worsening pericardial effusion [3].

Figure 16.1 shows an ECG of a patient who presented with sudden, sharp chest pain which was worse with inspiration and improved with sitting. On physical exam the patient had a pericardial rub. The ECG in patients with acute pericarditis generally shows wide spread ST-segment elevation and diffuse PR depression, except in lead AVR where there is ST depression and PR segment elevation. The ECG changes in pericarditis evolve over four stages. Stage 1 ECG changes last for hours to days and are comprised of ST segment elevation and PR depression. Stage 2 has normalization of the PR and ST segment to baseline. Stage 3 shows diffuse T-wave inversions. Stage 4 shows normalization of the T-wave inversions to baseline.

Echocardiograms in patients with acute pericarditis may show a pericardial effusion which is typically small in 60% of cases [4]. CT and MRI show inflammation-related pericardial enhancement.

Table 16.1 Etiology of pericarditis

Type	Causes
Infectious	Viral, bacterial, mycobacterial, fungal, Q fever
Noninfectious	Metastatic cancer, idiopathic, uremia, hypothyroidism, thoracic radiation
Autoimmune	Lupus, rheumatoid arthritis, arteritis, inflammatory bowel syndrome, post-myocardial infarction
Drug-Induced	Phenytoin, procainamide, hydralazine, cyclosporine
Trauma	Thoracic surgery, thoracic duct injury, chest trauma causing hemopericardium

S.A. Hassan (✉) • P. Shivamurthy • S.W. Yusuf
Department of Cardiology, University of Texas MD Anderson, Houston, TX, USA
e-mail: sahassanl@mdanderson.org

S.W. Yusuf, J. Banchs (eds.), *Cancer and Cardiovascular Disease*, https://doi.org/10.1007/978-3-319-62088-6_16

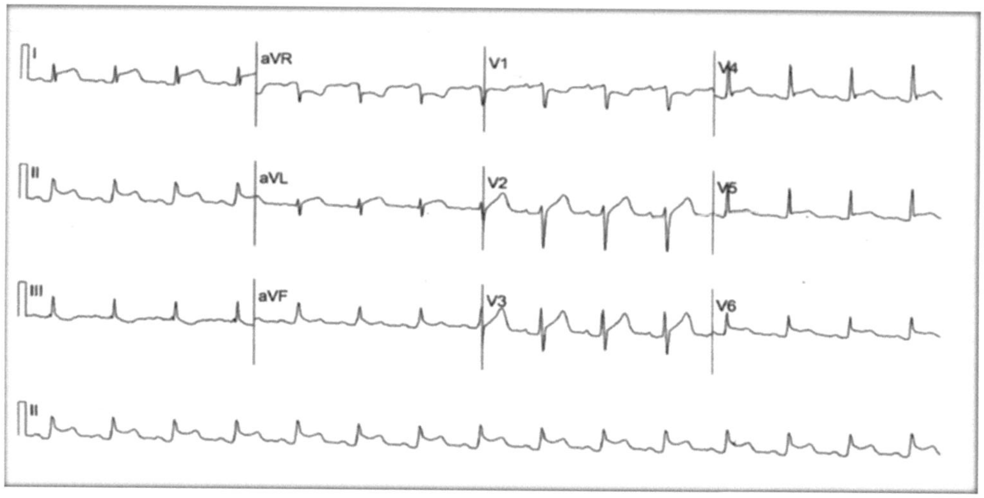

Fig. 16.1 ECG of a patient with positional chest pain and pericardial rub. ECG shows diffuse ST elevation and PR depression in all leads except AVR which shows ST depression with PR segment elevation

Table 16.2 Treatment of acute pericarditis

	Dose	Initial attack
(First line)		
Aspirin	750–1000 mg TID	1–2 weeks
NSAIDs (e.g. Ibuprofen)	600–800 mg TID	1–2 weeks
Colchicine	0.5 mg BID	3 months
	0.5 mg/day (<70 kg or intolerant to high dose)	
(Second line)		
Steroids (prednisone)	0.25–05 mg/kg/day	1–2 weeks

Treatment of acute pericarditis is directed toward symptom relief and decreasing the chance of recurrence. Aspirin, non steroidal anti-inflammatory drugs (NSAIDs), and colchicine are first-line choice for therapy. Colchicine should be added to aspirin/NSAIDS in the initial management of acute pericarditis, as studies have shown significantly reduced recurrence rate with addition of colchicine. Steroids should not be used as first line treatment due to high rates of relapse when stopped. Steroids should only be used when first line treatment choices are contraindicated or in refractory cases [3]. For post myocardial infarction (MI) pericarditis, Aspirin is the drug of choice and colchicine added if high-dose aspirin is ineffective [5]. In post-MI pericarditis steroids and NSAID are not recommended and can be harmful [5]. Table 16.2 summarizes the different medication used in the treatment of acute pericarditis.

Constrictive Pericarditis

Constriction is caused by pericardial scarring, calcification and thickening, although, up-to 18% have normal pericardial thickness [6]. Mediastinal irradiation accounts for 13% cases of constrictive pericarditis [6], other causes are pervious surgery, tuberculosis, and malignant pericardial disease. In constriction, there is dissociation of intra-thoracic and intra-cardiac pressures leading to enhanced inter-ventricular dependence with significant respiratory variation in ventricular diastolic filling. Decrease in left ventricular filling occurs during inspiration with simultaneous increase in right ventricular preload and the opposite changes occur in expiration.

Presenting symptoms are dyspnea and edema in patients with a remote history of radiation. Clinical features include jugular venous distension, Kussmaul's sign, pleural effusions, ascites and a pericardial knock. Diagnosis requires clinical suspicion with imaging evidence of constriction.

Figure 16.2 shows the case of a patient with Hodgkin's lymphoma who received prior radiation and presented with congestion and dyspnea due to constrictive pericarditis. Echocardiographic findings that are highly suggestive of constriction are ventricular septal bounce, medial mitral annulus e′ velocity $\geq$ 9 cm/s, hepatic vein expiratory diastolic reversal ratio $\geq$ 0.79, plethoric inferior vena cava [7, 8]. Reduction in mitral inflow velocity during inspiration and increase during expiration is an important finding [7] (Fig. 16.2). There is decreased longitudinal strain in anterolateral and RV free walls due to restricted motion of the myocardium adjacent to constricted pericardium. Pericardial calcification can be seen on echocardiogram, chest X-ray and CT imaging.

Cardiac magnetic resonance (CMR) is a validated test to detect pericardial thickening, pericardial-myocardial adherence (myocardial tagging), respiratory variation in septal excursion and real time cine-imaging with greater than 25% respiratory variation in mitral inflow velocities [9].

Definitive diagnosis is possible by simultaneous left and right ventricular pressure tracings [10]. Early rapid

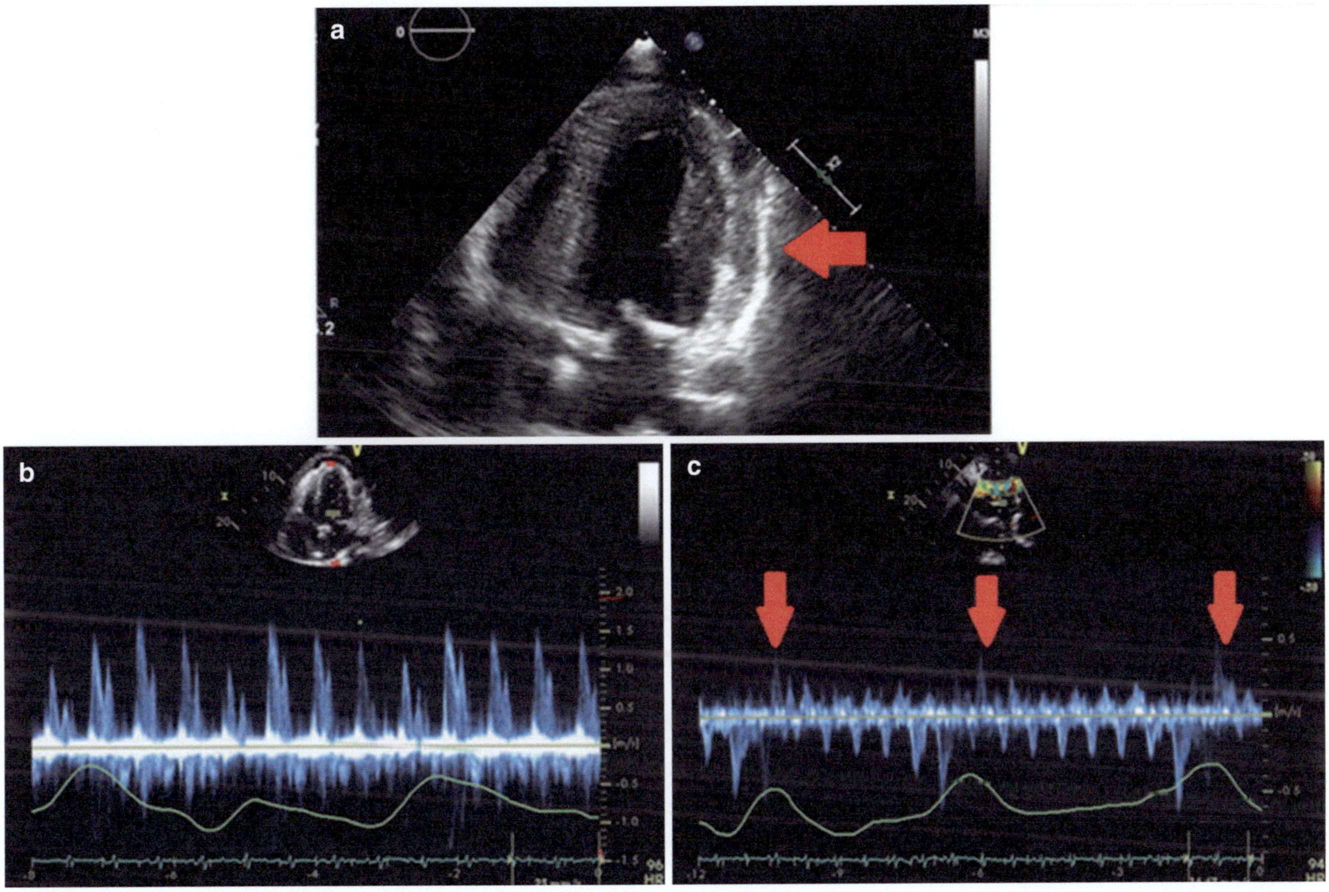

Fig. 16.2 Patient with Hodgkin's lymphoma who underwent radiation therapy in 1984. In 2007, he presented with congestion and dyspnea due to constrictive pericarditis. (**a**) The *red arrow* shows portion of markedly thickened pericardium longitudinally along the lateral wall. (**b**) Mitral inflow variation in constriction, with the typical decreased flow velocities with inspiration, which recover with expiration. (**c**) Hepatic vein diastolic flow reversal at the onset of expiration (see *red arrows*) (With the permission from Yusuf SW et al. 2016 [2])

filling with characteristic dip and plateau of ventricular diastolic pressures and equalization of end diastolic pressures is seen in all four chambers. This is sensitive but not specific to constriction [10]. There is inspiratory decrease in left ventricular (LV) volume with increase in right ventricle (RV) volume and vice-versa, implying ventricular discordance (Fig. 16.3). Systolic area index i.e. ratio of RV area to LV area in inspiration versus expiration greater than 1.1 is the most specific (100%) and sensitive (97%) diagnostic test [11].

Pericardiectomy is the definitive treatment with mortality rate of 6–12%. Complete normalization of hemodynamics is seen in only 60% of the patients [12].

Restrictive Cardiomyopathy

Restrictive cardiomyopathy in cancer patients can occurs as a consequence of cardiac amyloidosis in multiple myeloma, tumor infiltration of myocardium or transfusion induced hemosiderosis. It can also result from mediastinal radiation induced (>30-Gy dose) myocardial damage and fibrosis [9]. It manifests as heart failure from a stiff myocardium causing diastolic dysfunction.

Figure 16.4 shows an echocardiogram in a patient with a history of multiple myeloma who presented with signs and symptoms of congestive heart failure and had biopsy proven cardiac amyloid. 2D Echocardiographic features in patients with amyloid heart disease, include increased thickness of the LV myocardium, a small LV cavity, and increased atrial size (Fig. 16.4a). As a result, early rapid rise in LV pressure is seen during diastolic filling. Transmitral flow pattern will show short mitral E deceleration time and a low A wave velocity resulting in a high E/A ratio consistent with restrictive filling. E′ velocity by tissue Doppler imaging is usually decreased (Fig. 16.4b). Longitudinal strain in patients with cardiac amyloidosis classically shows a relative apical sparing (Fig. 16.5). A 12 lead ECG in patients with amyloid heart disease may show a pseudo-infarct pattern and low voltage complexes (Fig. 16.6).

Simultaneous LV and RV pressure tracings will show dip-plateau pattern of early diastolic filling. There is no

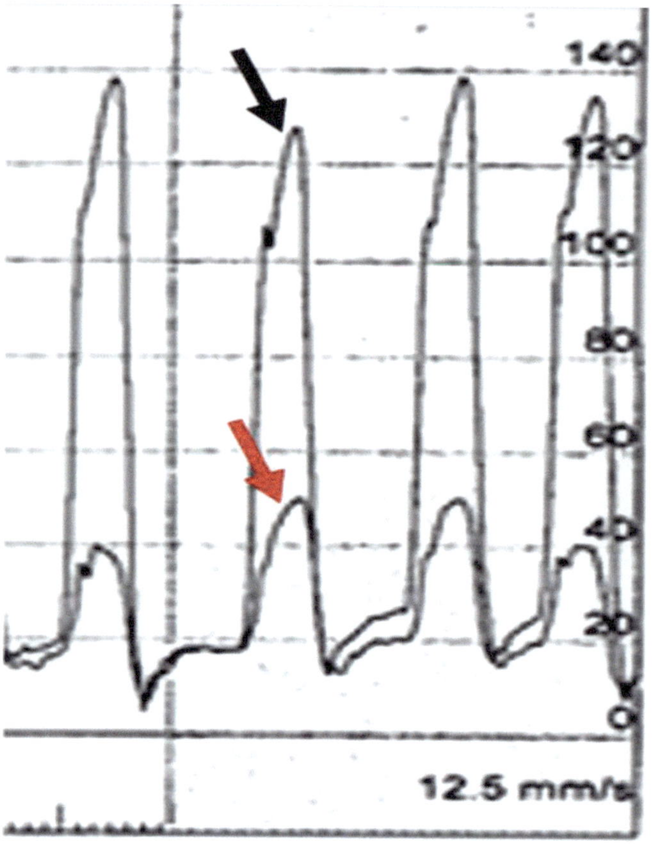

Fig. 16.3 Constrictive Pericarditis: Hemodynamics showing ventricular discordance (Interdependence) with an increase in right ventricular (RV) pressure and a simultaneous decrease in left ventricular (LV) pressure during inspiration in a patient with constrictive pericarditis due to previous thoracic surgery. (The *red arrow* points to the RV and the black arrow points to the LV)

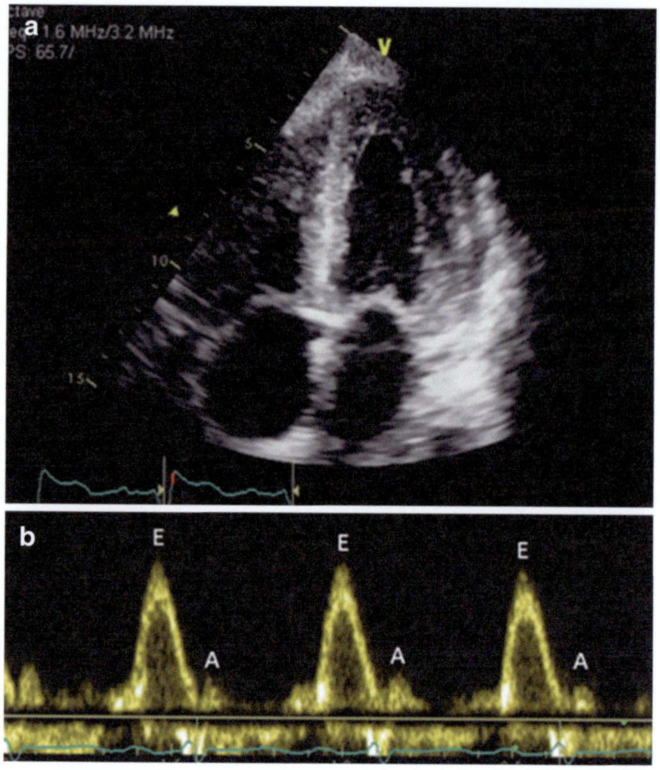

Fig. 16.4 (**a**) Four chamber echocardiographic view in a patient with restrictive cardiomyopathy from cardiac amyloidosis. A thickened left ventricle with small LV cavity and enlarged atria are seen. (**b**) Transmitral flow showing a short mitral E deceleration time and low A velocity resulting in high E/A ratio, consistent with restrictive filling

dissociation of intra-thoracic and intra-cavitary pressures and hence, there is equal lowering of pulmonary wedge and LV diastolic pressures [13]. LV and RV pressures are in concordance during respiration unlike constrictive pericarditis (Fig. 16.7), showing no enhanced inter-ventricular dependence. Other features of restriction pattern that are not specific include LV end-diastolic pressure exceeding RV end diastolic pressure by 5 mmHg or more, pulmonary artery systolic pressure greater than 50 mmHg and RV end-diastolic pressure less than 1/3rd of systolic pressure [13]. Differentiating constriction from restrictive cardiomyopathy can be clinically challenging and the two entities often co-exist. Table 16.3 describes the distinguishing features of both.

Cardiac MRI as a tool to detect myocardial fibrosis is promising but its role remains unclear. T1 mapping can be used to quantify the concentration of gadolinium-based extracellular contrast agents in the myocardium, which is related to collagen content/fibrosis [13]. In patients with cardiac amyloidosis which can lead to restrictive cardiomyopathy, the cardiac MRI shows thickening of the myocardium, atrial enlargement, and global transmural or subendocardial

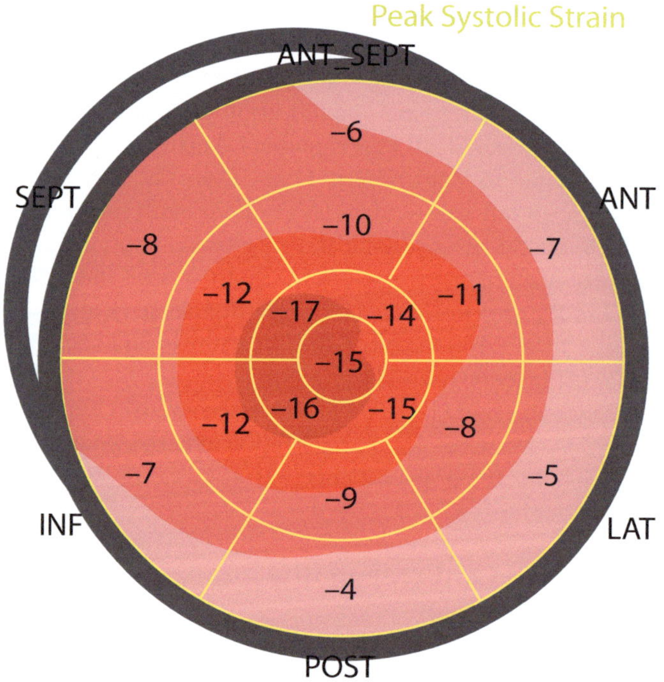

Fig. 16.5 Longitudinal strain in a patient with cardiac amylodosis showing relative apical sparing

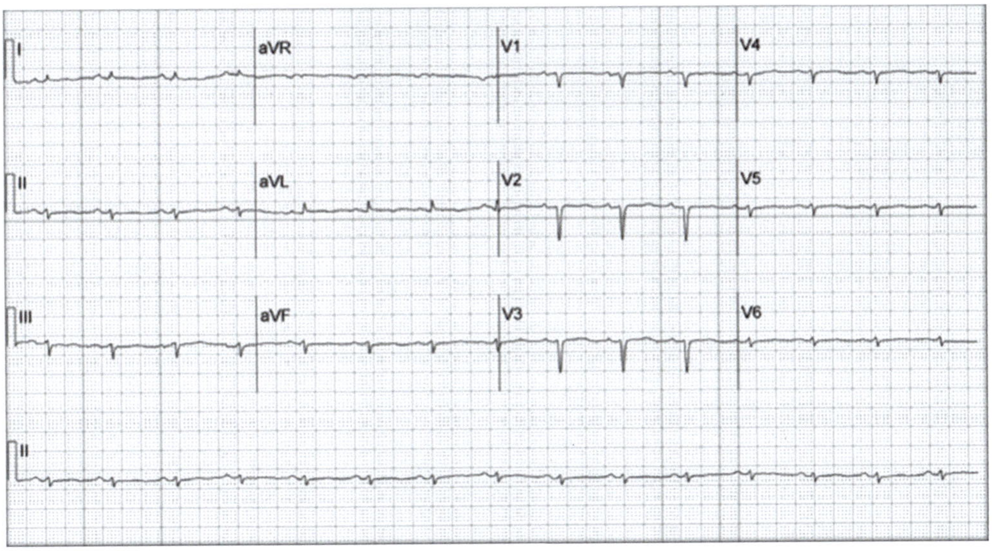

Fig. 16.6 A 12 lead ECG from a patient with cardiac amyloidosis, showing pseudo-infarct pattern and low voltage complexes

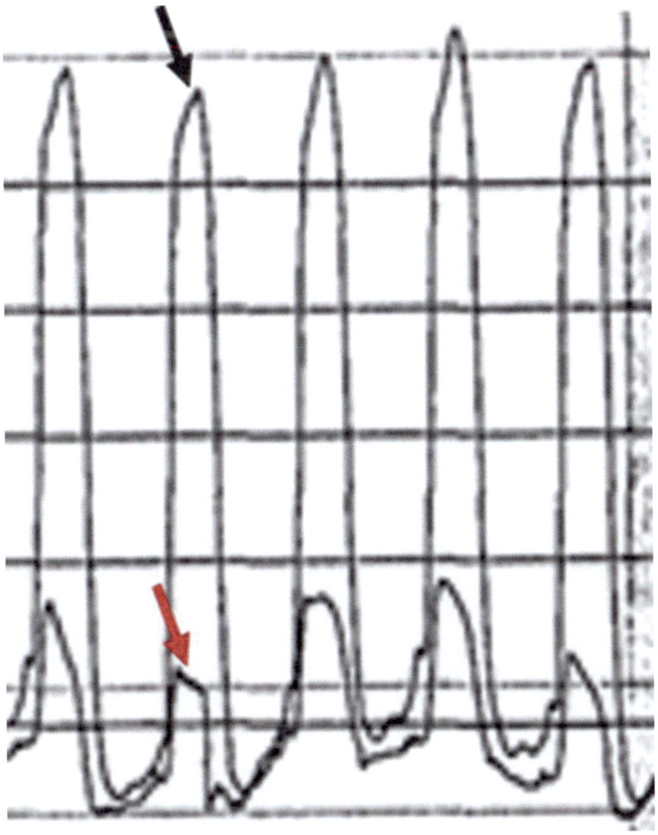

Fig. 16.7 Restrictive cardiomyopathy: Hemodynamics showing ventricular concordance with a concomitant decrease in LV pressure and a RV pressure during inspiration in a patient with restrictive cardiomyopathy due to cardiac amyloidosis. (The *red arrow* points to the RV and the black arrow points to the LV)

late enhancement of the myocardium as in Fig. 16.8 [14]. Treatment of restrictive cardiomyopathy is challenging and includes management of heart failure and in appropriate cases, cardiac transplantation.

Table 16.3 Differentiating features of constrictive and restrictive cardiomyopathy

Features	Constriction	Restriction
Pericardial thickening	Present	Absent
Pericardial knock	Present	Absent
Rapid 'y' descent in JVP	Present	Absent
Inter-ventricular septal bounce	Present	Absent
Respiratory variation >25% in mitral Inflow	Present	Absent
Mitral annulus medial e' velocity	Normal/increased	Decreased
Hepatic vein flow diastolic reversal in expiration	Present	Absent
Simultaneous LV/RV tracings	Discordant pattern	Concordant pattern
Systolic area index	>1.1	<1.1
Pulmonary artery systolic pressure >50 mmHg	Uncommon	Often present
RVEDP/RVSP	>1/3	<1/3
LVEDP—RVEDP	<5 mmHg	>5 mmHg

Pericardial Tamponade

Pericardial tamponade is the accumulation of fluid into the pericardial space that can lead to reduction in ventricular filling and hemodynamic compromise. Patients may present with symptoms of shortness of breath, tachycardia, hypotension, pulsus paradoxus, and eventually cardiogenic shock due to a drop in cardiac output.

12 Lead ECG

The ECG in cardiac tamponade classically shows electrical alternans, but while it has a high positive predictive value in detecting cardiac tamponade, its negative predictive value is

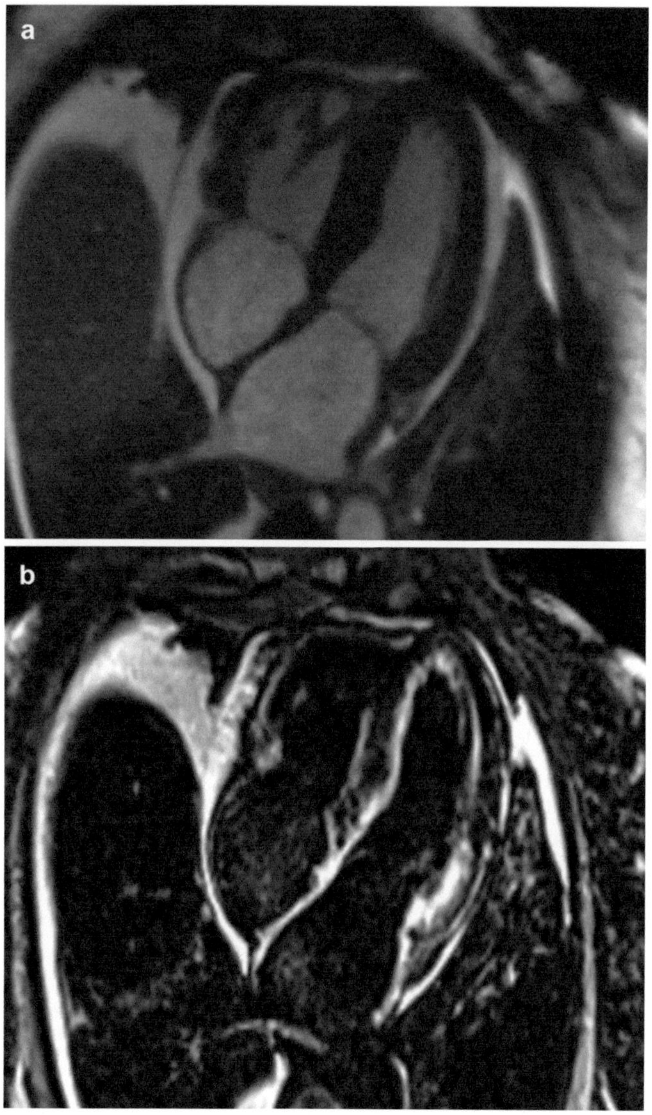

Fig. 16.8 Cardiac MRI of a patient with cardiac amyloidosis. Image (**a**) shows thickening of the myocardium along with dilated atria. The T1 image (**b**) shows global subendocardial hyperenhancement which is characteristic of cardiac amyloid

low. Hence due to a low negative predictive value, a 12-lead ECG cannot be used as a screening tool to exclude cardiac tamponade [15] (Fig. 16.9).

2D Echocardiographic and Doppler Evaluation

Echocardiography is the diagnostic test of choice for diagnosis of pericardial tamponade. Echocardiography can help determine the size and location of the pericardial fluid. Furthermore, it allows the determination of whether cardiac tamponade physiology is present.

With increased in pericardial pressure due to the accumulation of fluid in the pericardial space, there is a reduction in RV chamber size, collapse of the RV during early diastole, and RA inversion during atrial diastole [16, 17]. In particular, with RV collapse there is an associated 21% decrease in cardiac output [18]. RA inversion or collapse can also be seen with cardiac tamponade. In particular, a RA inversion time index ≥0.34 has the highest sensitivity and specificity in detecting cardiac tamponade in patient with a large pericardial effusion [19].

Table 16.4 list the sensitivity and specificity of echocardiographic signs for cardiac tamponade.

Figure 16.10 shows a subcostal view of an echocardiogram of a patient with evidence of RV chamber collapse who presented with shortness of breath, tachycardia and hypotension. Figure 16.11 shows RA collapse of a different patient who presented with similar symptoms.

Doppler echocardiographic measurements are also altered in cardiac tamponade. E-velocity changes with respiration have been demonstrated across the mitral and tricuspid valves in patients with cardiac tamponade. The percentage change in E-velocity was determined as (INSP-EXP)/EXP where INSP was defined as the first beat of inspiration and EXP was defined as the first beat of expiration. In one early study, with cardiac tamponade the

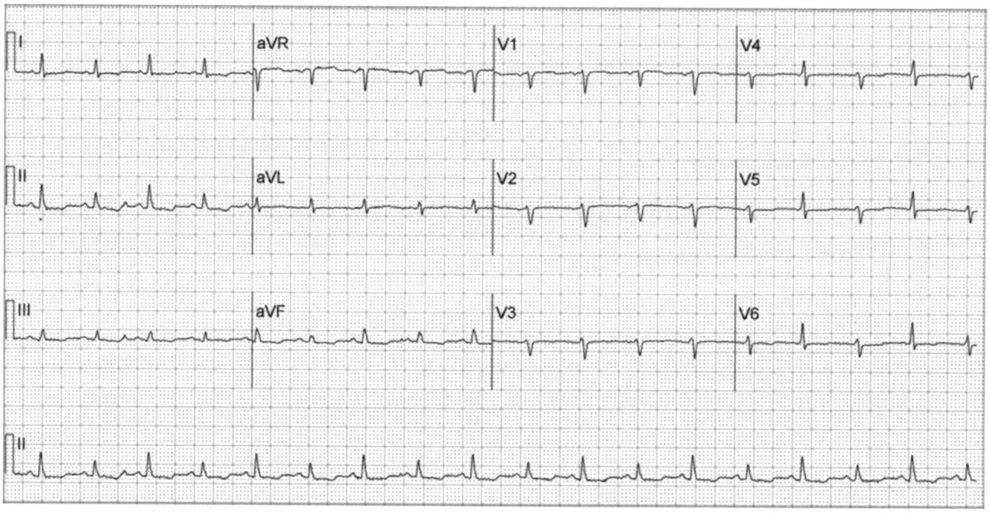

Fig. 16.9 A 12 lead ECG showing low voltage complexes and electrical alternans, in a patient with large pericardial effusion and tamponade

Table 16.4 Sensitivity and specificity of signs of pericardial tamponade in patient with large pericardial effusions (modified from *Shrairer et al. Cardiology in Review. 2011; 19; 233-238*)

	Sensitivity (%)	Specificity (%)	PPV (%)	NPV (%)
RA collapse	55	88	10	99
RA collapse-1/3 cardiac cycle	94	100	–	–
RV collapse	48	95	38	99
IVC plethora	97	66	7	99
Large PEF	73	97	45	99

RA right atrium, *RV* right ventricle, *IVC* inferior vena cava, *PEF* pericardial effusion, *PPV* positive predictive value, *NPV* negative predictive value

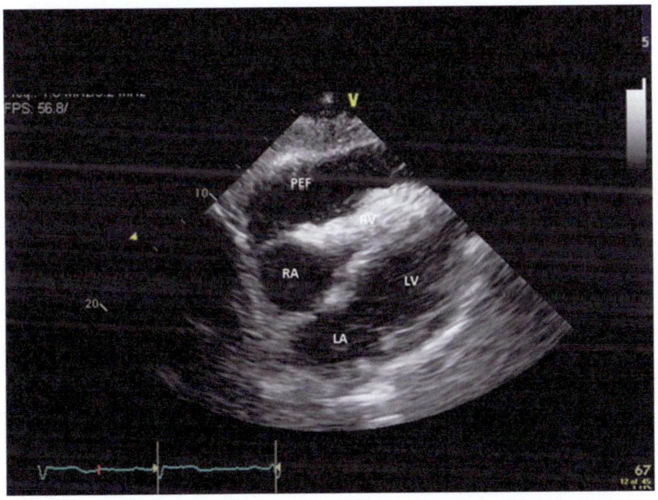

Fig. 16.10 Echocardiogram showing RV chamber collapse. *RA* right atrium, *RV* right ventricle, *LA* left atrium, *LV* left ventricle, *PEF* pericardial effusion

mitral E-velocity decreased by 43% during inspiration. The tricuspid E-velocity increased by 85% with inspiration [20].

Figures 16.12 and 16.13 show the mitral and tricuspid valve velocity in a patient with cardiac tamponade who presented with dyspnea and tachycardia. In general, variations in E-wave velocities during respiration across the mitral valve and tricuspid valve greater than 25% and 50%, respectively, may indicate cardiac tamponade. However, when evaluating for changes across the valves, other disease states such as COPD, pericardial constriction, and severe tricuspid regurgitation should be accounted for. One way to distinguish between cardiac tamponade and COPD, is that the maximal change in e-velocity during inspiration will occur in the very first beat after inspiration as opposed to the more gradual drop seen in e-wave velocity with pulmonary conditions such as asthma [21].

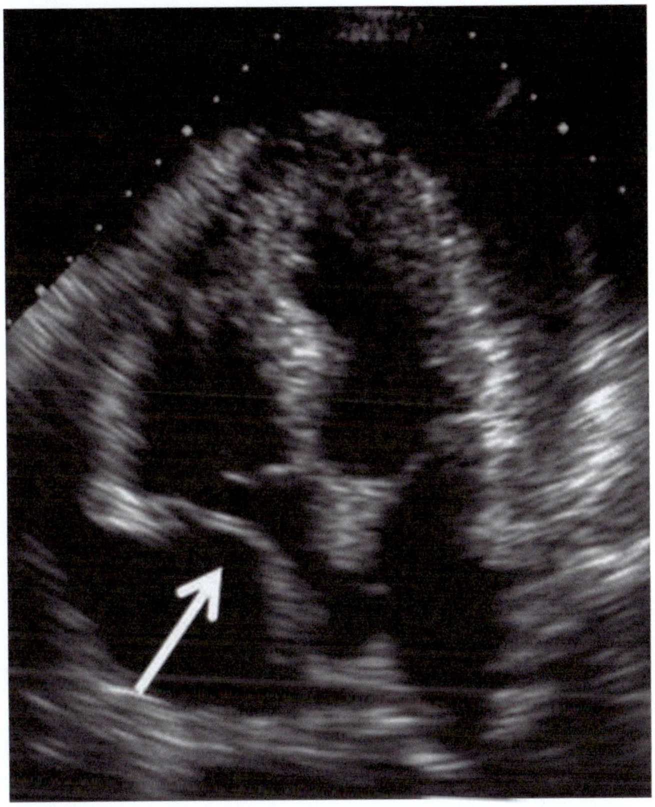

Fig. 16.11 Echocardiogram showing RA chamber inversion/collapse (*arrow*)

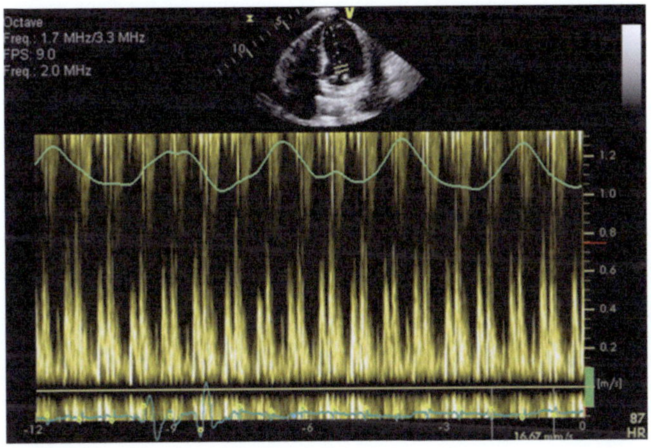

Fig. 16.12 E-wave velocity across the MV valve showing >25% respiratory variation

With hemodynamically significant pericardial effusions and cardiac tamponade, RA pressure will invariably be increased which leads to dilation of the inferior vena cava that can be easily studied by echocardiography. An estimated RA pressure can be calculated form these findings [22].

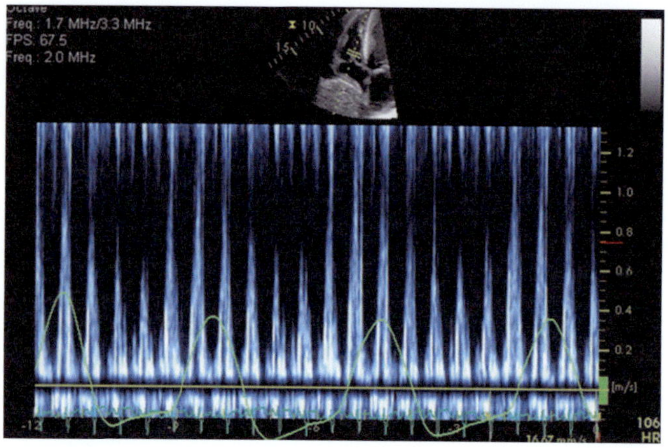

Fig. 16.13 E-wave velocity across the TV valve showing >50% respiratory variation

Large pericardial effusion or effusion with tamponade can be drained via percutaneous approach. For recurrent pericardial effusion a pericardial window is indicated.

References

1. Fruergaard P, Launbjerg J, Hesse B, et al. The diagnoses of patients admitted with acute chest pain but without myocardial infarction. Eur Heart J. 1996;17(7):1028–34.
2. Yusuf SW, Hassan SA, Mouhayar E, et al. Pericardial disease: a clinical review. Expert Rev Cardiovasc Ther. 2016;14(4):525–39.
3. Adler Y, Charron P, et al. 2015 ESC guidelines for the diagnosis and management of pericardial diseases: the task force for the diagnosis and management of pericardial diseases of the European Society of Cardiology (ESC) endorsed by: the European Association for Cardio-Thoracic Surgery (EACTS). Eur Heart J. 2015;36(42):2921–64.
4. Imazio M, Demichelis B, Cecchi E, et al. Cardiac troponin I in acute pericarditis. J Am Coll Cardiol. 2003;42(12):2144–8.
5. O'Gara PT, Kushner FG, Ascheim DD, et al. 2013 ACC/AHA guideline for the management of ST-elevation myocardial infarction. Circulation. 2013;127(4):e362–425.
6. Ling LH, Jae KO, et al. Constrictive pericarditis in the modern era: evolving clinical spectrum and impact on outcome after pericardiectomy. Circulation. 1999;100:1380–6.
7. Welch TD, Ling LH, Espinosa RE, Anavekar NS, Wiste HJ, Lahr BD, Schaff HV, Oh JK. Echocardiographic diagnosis of constrictive pericarditis: mayo clinic criteria. Circ Cardiovasc Imaging. 2014;7(3):526–34.
8. Syed FF, Schaff HV, Oh JK. Constrictive pericarditis-a curable diastolic HF. Nat Rev Cardiol. 2014;11(9):530–44.
9. Lancellotti P, et al. Expert consensus for multi-modality imaging evaluation of cardiovascular complications of radiotherapy in adults: a report from the European Association of Cardiovascular Imaging and the American Society of Echocardiography. J Am Soc Echocardiogr. 2013;14:721–40.
10. Little WC, Freeman GL. Pericardial disease. Circulation. 2006;113:1622–32.
11. Talreja DR, et al. Constrictive pericarditis in the modern era. Novel criteria for diagnosis in the cardiac catheterization laboratory. J Am Coll Cardiol. 2008;51(3):315–9.
12. Alder Y, et al. 2015 ESC guidelines on the diagnosis and management of pericardial diseases. Eur Heart J. 2015;36:2921–64.
13. Paul Sorajja MD. Invasive hemodynamics of constrictive pericarditis, restrictive cardiomyopathy, and cardiac tamponade. Cardiol Clin. 2011;29:191–9.
14. Syed IS, Glockner JF, Feng D, Araoz PA, Martinez MW, Edwards WD, Gertz MA, Dispenzieri A, Oh JK, Bellavia D, Tajik AJ, Grogan M. Role of cardiac magnetic resonance imaging in the detection of cardiac amyloidosis. JACC Cardiovasc Imaging. 2010;3(2):155–64.
15. Argula RG, Negi SI, Banchs J, et al. Role of a 12-lead electrocardiogram in the diagnosis of cardiac tamponade as diagnosed by transthoracic echocardiography in patients with malignant pericardial effusion. Clin Cardiol. 2015;38:139–44.
16. Singh S, Wann L, Klopfenstein H, et al. Usefulness of right ventricular collapse in diagnosing cardiac tamponade and comparison to pulsus paradoxus. Am J Cardiol. 1986;57:652–7.
17. Armstrong WF, Schilt BF, Helper DJ, et al. Diastolic collapse of the right ventricle with cardiac tamponade: an echocardiographic study. Circulation. 1982;65:1491–6.
18. Leimgruber PP, Klopfenstein HS, Wann LS, et al. The hemodynamic derangements associated with right ventricular diastolic collapse in cardiac tamponade: an experimental echocardiographic study. Circulation. 1983;68:612–20.
19. Gillam LD, Guyer DE, Gibson TC, et al. Hydrodynamic compression of the right atrium: a new echocardiographic sign of cardiac tamponade. Circulation. 1983;68:294–301.
20. Appleton CP, Hatle LK, Popp RL. Cardiac tamponade and pericardial effusion: respiratory variation in transvalvular flow velocities studied by Doppler echocardiography. J Am Coll Cardiol. 1988;11:1020–30.
21. Hoit B, Sahn DJ, Shabetai R. Doppler-detected paradoxus of mitral and tricuspid valve flows in chronic lung disease. J Am Coll Cardiol. 1986;8:706–9.
22. Rudski L, Wai W, Aifalo J, et al. Guidelines for the echocardiographic assessment of the right heart in the adult: a report from the American Society of Echocardiography endorsed by the European Association of Echocardiography, a registered branch of the European Society of Cardiology, and the Canadian Society of Echocardiography. J Am Soc Echocardiogr. 2010;23:685–713.

Exercise Therapy and Cardiovascular Benefits in Patients with Cancer

17

Amy M. Berkman and Susan C. Gilchrist

Abstract
Exercise therapy improves vascular function and survival. In this chapter we briefly review the benefits of exercise therapy in patients with cancer.

Keywords
Exercise therapy • Cardiovascular • Cancer

Introduction

Common treatments for cancer, such as molecular targeted therapies, radiation, and particular chemotherapeutic agents are known to directly contribute to structural heart disease, vascular compromise, and systolic heart failure [1]. In addition, cardiovascular disease (CVD) risk factors, such as body weight, blood pressure, and cardiorespiratory fitness (CRF) worsen in cancer patients post-treatment, compared to pre-diagnosis risk factor burden [2, 3]. Medical therapies, such as aspirin or anticoagulants to prevent or treat thrombotic risk [4] statins, angiotensin-converting enzyme (ACE) inhibitors, or beta-blockers to treat cancer patients who have left ventricular (LV) dysfunction [5, 6]; and protective therapies, such as dexrazoxane, specifically aimed at preventing anthracycline induced cardiotoxicity [7], are currently used to offset cancer related insults to the cardiovascular system. However, the timing of CVD events in cancer patients is unpredictable and can occur years after a cancer diagnosis and treatment, making the timing and choice of medical therapies challenging.

The potential of non-medical therapy, particularly exercise training, is receiving increasing attention as a safe and effective way to mitigate the cardiovascular effects of cancer treatment, as well as promote future all-around health. In non-cancer populations, exercise training has already been shown to reduce recurrent myocardial infarction, improve survival among patients with coronary artery disease, improve LV function, and reduce the risk of stroke [8–12]. In addition, aerobic exercise training has proven to be an effective means of inducing weight loss, decreasing the risk of hypertension, and improving CRF [13–15]. While exercise training has not been studied as extensively in the cancer population, data are promising, with exercise training shown to significantly improve vascular function [16, 17], skeletal muscle function [18, 19], and maintain or improve CRF in cancer patients [19–23], a key predictor of survival [24–28].

Assessment of CRF Prior to Exercise Training in Cancer Patients

Given the role for exercise training to improve the cardiovascular health of cancer patients, it is important to implement standardized clinical measurements and practices across the cancer care spectrum. A good starting point is the measurement of CRF. CRF is an objective measurement of response to aerobic exercise training, as well as a marker of accelerated cardiac aging experienced during cancer treatment, and, importantly, prognostic of survival before and after a cancer

A.M. Berkman
University of Vermont School of Medicine, University of Vermont, Burlington, VT, USA

S.C. Gilchrist (✉)
Department of Clinical Cancer Prevention and Cardiology, The University of Texas M.D. Anderson Cancer Center, 1155 Pressler, Houston, TX 77006, USA
e-mail: sgilchrist@mdanderson.org

S.W. Yusuf, J. Banchs (eds.), *Cancer and Cardiovascular Disease*, https://doi.org/10.1007/978-3-319-62088-6_17

diagnosis [20, 29]. Measurement of CRF (VO_{2peak}), via cardiopulmonary exercise testing (CPET), is clinically feasible and established in the cancer setting [30]. CPET is a non-invasive test performed on a treadmill or stationary bike that measures both gas exchange (requiring a mouthpiece or facemask) and cardiac (ECG) monitoring. Uniquely, it can simultaneously assess multiple organ systems (cardiac, skeletal muscle, pulmonary) impacted by cancer treatment. Additionally, CPET can help clinicians make decisions regarding cardiopulmonary readiness for an exercise training regimen, as well as inform individually tailored exercise prescriptions for cancer patients. A CPET should be performed to make sure that cancer patients participate in aerobic exercise from a cardiopulmonary standpoint and in order to assess current CRF level and heart rate response to exercise. Importantly, exercise intensity recommendations are based on a percent of VO_{2peak} attained during CPET. After cardiopulmonary readiness has been assessed, opportunities to incorporate exercise training in the cancer setting to improve CRF and mitigate decline of cardiac health can be initiated. Below are several case examples of exercise training across different points in the cancer continuum.

Case Examples of Exercise Training in the Cancer Setting

Post Diagnosis/Prior to Surgery

Exercise training prior to surgery (prehabilitation) provides an opportunity to mitigate loss of CRF and enhance functional capacity prior to surgery [31]. A recent systematic review of 18 exercise training trials among 966 cancer patients provides supportive evidence of its effectiveness. A typical patient and exercise prescription are as follows: a 65 year old man presents with stage T2 nonsmall-cell lung cancer. He is a former smoker and is currently overweight with a BMI of 27 kg/m^2 and CRF (VO_{2peak}) of 15.7 mL/kg/min, which is lower than expected for his age. A 5-week exercise prescription, either on cycle ergometer or treadmill, is recommended prior to surgery. The patient is told to exercise 5 days for 20 min each day at an intensity of 60% of VO_{2peak} during the first week of exercise training (Of note, intensity is determined by the patient's peak heart rate (PHR) during CPET, given heart rate is linearly related to VO_2 (40%–85% of VO_{2peak} is equivalent to 50%–90% of PHR)). On weeks 2 and 3 he should continue to exercise 5 days out of the week for 20–25 min sessions and at 60–65% VO_{2peak} On weeks 4 and 5 the patients will perform 3–4 sessions/week at 60–65% VO_{2peak} for 25–30 min as well as 1–2 session/week of interval training (30 s at peak VO_2 followed by active recovery for 60 s with a total of 10–15 intervals). Under this exercise training regimen, the patient can be expected to increase his CRF by 3.3 mL/kg/min, which is a clinically significant change in CRF [32].

During Active Treatment

Based on a systematic review and meta-analysis by Schmitz et al., there is weak evidence for exercise interventions to improve CRF during active treatment in breast cancer [33]. However, the weight of the evidence does suggest that exercise mitigates loss of CRF during active treatment. For example, a 50 year old female breast cancer patient with a BMI of 26.5 kg/m^2 and a VO_{2peak} of 29 mL/kg/min, assessed by CPET, who exercises at the Physical Activity Guidelines for Americans recommended 75 min/week of vigorous aerobic exercise or 150 min/week of moderate aerobic exercise can expect to lose 12% of her CRF over 16 weeks of breast cancer treatment. For this patient, an exercise regimen that can successfully mitigate this fitness loss is as follows: 50–60 min sessions 3 times/week on either a cycle or rowing ergometer, treadmill, or elliptical; weeks 1 and 2 sessions should be performed at an intensity of 55–60% VO_{2peak}, weeks 3 and 4 sessions should be performed at 60–65% VO_{2peak}, weeks 5 and 6 sessions should be performed at 65–70% VO_{2peak}, and remaining weeks 7–16 sessions should be performed at 70–75% VO_{2peak} Following this exercise training prescription, the patient can expect to only lose 9% of her CRF, which is an improvement over the expected loss [21]. This is important given the loss of CRF experienced during active treatment can be substantial (~30%) [29]; as such, maintaining CRF during treatment has the potential to promote quicker recovery and improvement in CRF in the post-treatment setting.

Post Treatment

The benefits of exercise training in the post-treatment setting on CRF have been demonstrated in multiple cancer types. Based on a meta-analysis of randomized controlled trials, a pooled increased in VO_{2peak} of 2.2 mL/kg/min ($p < 0.01$) has been demonstrated among cancer survivors including breast, colorectal, prostate, lung, and lymphoma malignancies [34]. Exercise training post treatment is performed with the goal of getting a patient back to their pre-diagnosis CRF level. This is important regardless of age or cancer diagnosis, but may be particularly important among survivors of childhood cancer who are eager to get back to the pre-diagnosis school and community activities. For example, a 16 year old male survivor of childhood acute lymphoblastic leukemia presents with a BMI of 25.1 kg/m^2 and a VO_{2peak} of 35.2 mL/kg/min. For this patient, a 16 week, home-based exercise training regimen is prescribed, which consists of both strength training and aerobic activity. The strength training prescription includes resistance exercises that target all major muscle groups and should be completed 3–4 times/week. Aerobic exercise, consisting of brisk walking, jogging, or sports, should be undertaken at least three times a week for at least 30 min/session. After completing 16 weeks of training, the patient on average will significantly increase his CRF by 5.4 mL/kg/min [35].

Conclusion

Exercise is a non-pharmacologic strategy to mitigate cardiac insult and promote improvement in CRF across the cancer continuum. We recommend use of CPET prior to exercise training to (1) provide an objective assessment of cardiopulmonary health, (2) determine feasibility to perform exercise training, and (3) provide objective data and exercise goals for patients, oncologists, primary care physicians and others in health care field invested in a cancer patient's recovery. CPET also offers a level platform to begin cancer rehabilitation, specifically aerobic exercise, independent of the cancer rehabilitation model chosen to be cost-effective and feasible across institutions and communities. Integrating this message and delivering personalized exercise prescriptions to patients in the cancer setting should be a priority in cancer care, especially given the impact of exercise training on CRF, as illustrated in the cases above. Ultimately, exercise should be promoted and maintained across all facets of the cancer continuum, including the preventative setting.

References

1. Lenihan DJ, Cardinale DM. Late cardiac effects of cancer treatment. J Clin Oncol. 2012;30:3657–64.
2. Mason C, Alfano CM, Smith AW, Wang CY, Neuhouser ML, Duggan C, Bernstein L, Baumgartner KB, Baumgartner RN, Ballard-Barbash R, McTiernan A. Long-term physical activity trends in breast cancer survivors. Cancer Epidemiol Biomark Prev. 2013;22:1153–61.
3. Jack S, West MA, Raw D, Marwood S, Ambler G, Cope TM, Shrotri M, Sturgess RP, Calverley PM, Ottensmeier CH, Grocott MP. The effect of neoadjuvant chemotherapy on physical fitness and survival in patients undergoing oesophagogastric cancer surgery. Eur J Surg Oncol. 2014;40:1313–20.
4. Lyman GH, Bohlke K, Falanga A, American Society of Clinical Oncology. Venous thromboembolism prophylaxis and treatment in patients with cancer: American Society of Clinical Oncology clinical practice guideline update. J Oncol Pract. 2015;11:e442–4.
5. Seicean S, Seicean A, Plana JC, Budd GT, Marwick TH. Effect of statin therapy on the risk for incident heart failure in patients with breast cancer receiving anthracycline chemotherapy: an observational clinical cohort study. J Am Coll Cardiol. 2012;60:2384–90.
6. Vejpongsa P, Yeh ET. Prevention of anthracycline-induced cardiotoxicity: challenges and opportunities. J Am Coll Cardiol. 2014;64:938–45.
7. Liu H, Wang H, Xiang D, Guo W. Pharmaceutical measures to prevent doxorubicin-induced cardiotoxicity. Mini Rev Med Chem. 2017;17:44–50.
8. Clark AM, Hartling L, Vandermeer B, McAlister FA. Meta-analysis: secondary prevention programs for patients with coronary artery disease. Ann Intern Med. 2005;143:659–72.
9. Adamopoulos S, Schmid JP, Dendale P, Poerschke D, Hansen D, Dritsas A, Kouloubinis A, Alders T, Gkouziouta A, Reyckers I, Vartela V, Plessas N, Doulaptsis C, Saner H, Laoutaris ID. Combined aerobic/inspiratory muscle training vs. aerobic training in patients with chronic heart failure: the Vent-HeFT trial: a European prospective multicentre randomized trial. Eur J Heart Fail. 2014;16:574–82.
10. Goldstein LB. Physical activity and the risk of stroke. Expert Rev Neurother. 2010;10:1263–5.
11. Faulkner J, Lambrick D, Woolley B, Stoner L, Wong LK, McGonigal G. Effects of early exercise engagement on vascular risk in patients with transient ischemic attack and nondisabling stroke. J Stroke Cerebrovasc Dis. 2013;22:e388–96.
12. Lockard MM, Gopinathannair R, Paton CM, Phares DA, Hagberg JM. Exercise training-induced changes in coagulation factors in older adults. Med Sci Sports Exerc. 2007;39:587–92.
13. Slentz CA, Duscha BD, Johnson JL, Ketchum K, Aiken LB, Samsa GP, Houmard JA, Bales CW, Kraus WE. Effects of the amount of exercise on body weight, body composition, and measures of central obesity: STRRIDE–a randomized controlled study. Arch Intern Med. 2004;164:31–9.
14. Giannaki CD, Aphamis G, Sakkis P, Hadjicharalambous M. Eight weeks of a combination of high intensity interval training and conventional training reduce visceral adiposity and improve physical fitness: a group-based intervention. J Sports Med Phys Fitness. 2016;56:483–90.
15. Baster T, Baster-Brooks C. Exercise and hypertension. Aust Fam Physician. 2005;34:419–24.
16. Giallauria F, Vitelli A, Maresca L, Santucci De Magistris M, Chiodini P, Mattiello A, Gentile M, Mancini M, Grieco A, Russo A, Lucci R, Torella G, Berrino F, Panico S, Vigorito C. Exercise training improves cardiopulmonary and endothelial function in women with breast cancer: findings from the Diana-5 dietary intervention study. Intern Emerg Med. 2016;11:183–9.
17. Gilbert SE, Tew GA, Fairhurst C, Bourke L, Saxton JM, Winter EM, Rosario DJ. Effects of a lifestyle intervention on endothelial function in men on long-term androgen deprivation therapy for prostate cancer. Br J Cancer. 2016;114:401–8.
18. Demark-Wahnefried W, Case LD, Blackwell K, Marcom PK, Kraus W, Aziz N, Snyder DC, Giguere JK, Shaw E. Results of a diet/exercise feasibility trial to prevent adverse body composition change in breast cancer patients on adjuvant chemotherapy. Clin Breast Cancer. 2008;8:70–9.
19. Devin JL, Sax AT, Hughes GI, Jenkins DG, Aitken JF, Chambers SK, Dunn JC, Bolam KA, Skinner TL. The influence of high-intensity compared with moderate-intensity exercise training on cardiorespiratory fitness and body composition in colorectal cancer survivors: a randomised controlled trial. J Cancer Surviv. 2016;10:467–79.
20. Dunne DF, Jack S, Jones RP, Jones L, Lythgoe DT, Malik HZ, Poston GJ, Palmer DH, Fenwick SW. Randomized clinical trial of prehabilitation before planned liver resection. Br J Surg. 2016;103:504–12.
21. Courneya KS, McKenzie DC, Mackey JR, Gelmon K, Friedenreich CM, Yasui Y, Reid RD, Cook D, Jespersen D, Proulx C, Dolan LB, Forbes CC, Wooding E, Trinh L, Segal RJ. Effects of exercise dose and type during breast cancer chemotherapy: multicenter randomized trial. J Natl Cancer Inst. 2013;105:1821–32.
22. Wood WA, Phillips B, Smith-Ryan AE, Wilson D, Deal AM, Bailey C, Meeneghan M, Reeve BB, Basch EM, Bennett AV, Shea TC, Battaglini CL. Personalized home-based interval exercise training may improve cardiorespiratory fitness in cancer patients preparing to undergo hematopoietic cell transplantation. Bone Marrow Transplant. 2016;51:967–72.

23. Schmitt J, Lindner N, Reuss-Borst M, Holmberg HC and Sperlich B. A 3-week multimodal intervention involving high-intensity interval training in female cancer survivors: a randomized controlled trial. Physiol Rep. 2016;4. pii: e12693.
24. Robsahm TE, Falk RS, Heir T, Sandvik L, Vos L, Erikssen JE, Tretli S. Measured cardiorespiratory fitness and self-reported physical activity: associations with cancer risk and death in a long-term prospective cohort study. Cancer Med. 2016;5:2136–44.
25. Lakoski SG, Willis BL, Barlow CE, Leonard D, Gao A, Radford NB, Farrell SW, Douglas PS, Berry JD, DeFina LF, Jones LW. Midlife cardiorespiratory fitness, incident cancer, and survival after cancer in men: the Cooper Center Longitudinal Study. JAMA Oncol. 2015;1:231–7.
26. Sawada SS, Lee IM, Naito H, Kakigi R, Goto S, Kanazawa M, Okamoto T, Tsukamoto K, Muto T, Tanaka H, Blair SN. Cardiorespiratory fitness, body mass index, and cancer mortality: a cohort study of Japanese men. BMC Public Health. 2014;14:1012.
27. Schmid D, Leitzmann MF. Cardiorespiratory fitness as predictor of cancer mortality: a systematic review and meta-analysis. Ann Oncol. 2015;26:272–8.
28. Jones LW, Watson D, Herndon JE II, Eves ND, Haithcock BE, Loewen G, Kohman L. Peak oxygen consumption and long-term all-cause mortality in nonsmall cell lung cancer. Cancer. 2010;116:4825–32.
29. Jones LW, Courneya KS, Mackey JR, Muss HB, Pituskin EN, Scott JM, Hornsby WE, Coan AD, Herndon JE II, Douglas PS, Haykowsky M. Cardiopulmonary function and age-related decline across the breast cancer survivorship continuum. J Clin Oncol. 2012;30:2530–7.
30. Jones LW, Eves ND, Haykowsky M, Joy AA, Douglas PS. Cardiorespiratory exercise testing in clinical oncology research: systematic review and practice recommendations. Lancet Oncol. 2008;9:757–65.
31. Silver JK. Cancer prehabilitation and its role in improving health outcomes and reducing health care costs. Semin Oncol Nurs. 2015;31:13–30.
32. Jones LW, Peddle CJ, Eves ND, Haykowsky MJ, Courneya KS, Mackey JR, Joy AA, Kumar V, Winton TW, Reiman T. Effects of presurgical exercise training on cardiorespiratory fitness among patients undergoing thoracic surgery for malignant lung lesions. Cancer. 2007;110:590–8.
33. Schmitz KH, Holtzman J, Courneya KS, Masse LC, Duval S, Kane R. Controlled physical activity trials in cancer survivors: a systematic review and meta-analysis. Cancer Epidemiol Biomark Prev. 2005;14:1588–95.
34. Fong DY, Ho JW, Hui BP, Lee AM, Macfarlane DJ, Leung SS, Cerin E, Chan WY, Leung IP, Lam SH, Taylor AJ, Cheng KK. Physical activity for cancer survivors: meta-analysis of randomised controlled trials. BMJ. 2012;344:e70.
35. Jarvela LS, Kemppainen J, Niinikoski H, Hannukainen JC, Lahteenmaki PM, Kapanen J, Arola M, Heinonen OJ. Effects of a home-based exercise program on metabolic risk factors and fitness in long-term survivors of childhood acute lymphoblastic leukemia. Pediatr Blood Cancer. 2012;59:155–60.

Index

S.W. Yusuf, J. Banchs (eds.), *Cancer and Cardiovascular Disease*, https://doi.org/10.1007/978-3-319-62088-6

D

E

F

MIX
Papier aus verantwortungsvollen Quellen
Paper from responsible sources
FSC® C105338

If you have any concerns about our products,
you can contact us on
ProductSafety@springernature.com

In case Publisher is established outside the EU,
the EU authorized representative is:
Springer Nature Customer Service Center GmbH
Europaplatz 3, 69115 Heidelberg, Germany

Printed by Libri Plureos GmbH
in Hamburg, Germany